SECOND EDITION
REVIEW MANUAL TO
HENRY'S
CLINICAL DIAGNOSIS AND MANAGEMENT
BY LABORATORY METHODS
TWENTY-FIRST EDITION

Commissioning Editor: Michael Houston
Development Editor: Louise Cook and Russell Gabbedy
Project Manager: Gemma Lawson
Design Manager: Stewart Larking
Illustration Manager: Bruce Hogarth
Illustrator: Anne Erickson and Oxford Illustrators
Marketing Manager(s) (UK/USA): Leontine Trieur and Ethel Cathers

SECOND EDITION

REVIEW MANUAL TO
HENRY'S
CLINICAL DIAGNOSIS
AND MANAGEMENT
BY LABORATORY METHODS

TWENTY-FIRST EDITION

Katherine I. Schexneider, MD

LCDR MC USN
Medical Director
Blood Bank
Naval Medical Center Portsmouth
Portsmouth, VA, USA

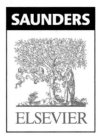

SAUNDERS

ELSEVIER

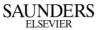

SAUNDERS
ELSEVIER

An imprint of Elsevier Inc

ISBN-13: 978 1 4160 3024 9
ISBN-10: 1 4160 3024 7

British Library Cataloguing in Publication Data
A catalogue record for this book is available from the British Library

Library of Congress Cataloging in Publication Data
A catalog record for this book is available from the Library of Congress

Notice
Medical knowledge is constantly changing. Standard safety precautions must be followed, but as new research and clinical experience broaden our knowledge, changes in treatment and drug therapy may become necessary or appropriate. Readers are advised to check the most current product information provided by the manufacturer of each drug to be administered to verify the recommended dose, the method and duration of administration, and contraindications. It is the responsibility of the practitioner, relying on experience and knowledge of the patient, to determine dosages and the best treatment for each individual patient. Neither the Publisher nor the author assume any liability for any injury and/or damage to persons or property arising from this publication.

The Publisher

 ELSEVIER
your source for books,
journals and multimedia
in the health sciences

www.elsevierhealth.com

The
Publisher's
policy is to use
**paper manufactured
from sustainable forests**

Working together to grow
libraries in developing countries

www.elsevier.com | www.bookaid.org | www.sabre.org

ELSEVIER   BOOK AID International   Sabre Foundation

Printed in China
Last digit is the print number: 9 8 7 6 5 4 3 2

Contents

Contents

PART VIII: Molecular pathology

PART IX: Clinical pathology of cancer

APPENDICES: Examinations

Preface to the Second Edition

My goal in this study guide is to facilitate your reading and review of Henry's Clinical Diagnosis and Management by Laboratory Methods, Twenty First Edition (CDM). In clinical pathology and clinical laboratory science training programs, students often feel daunted by CDM, a work to which they ought to be devoting time, but typically do not. On the surface, the text can appear challenging. It is a comprehensive work frequently used as a reference, but less often studied with the goal in mind of achieving a solid understanding of key principles and themes in clinical pathology. Some have argued that a full grasp of CDM's concepts is sound preparation for the clinical pathology part of the pathology boards. From my experience taking and passing the boards last year, this is absolutely the case. The text is also, of course, a thorough synopsis of the whole of clinical pathology. What this study guide will do, then, is walk you through clinical pathology via CDM, all 76 chapters, reinforcing what are, in my best estimation, the facts and concepts which are likely to be covered on the boards, and those which will help you provide useful, directed consultation to clinicians in the years to come. I have relied for my "best estimation" on board remembrances from pathologists who have recently passed the boards and my own experience as a recently board-certified (AP/CP) pathologist.

What you will need to use this study guide

1. CDM, 21st edition. Questions and discussions come directly from the text. I will always give the page number italicized and in parentheses at the end of the question to which the book should be open as you study. I envision you with this study guide in one hand and CDM in the other.
2. A pencil. This is a workbook as much as it is a question book.
3. A cup of coffee or tea. Rare is the man (or woman) for whom CDM is itself a stimulant.

Format of study guide

1. Chapter review questions. These constitute the bulk of this study guide. They are chiefly in the short answer format, with an occasional true/false or matching type. Answers are provided at the end of each chapter review.

2. Image Simulation Examination. There are several color plates in CDM, and we will make use of these with a 50-question examination using some of these images. They have been incorporated into the workbook.

3. Math Examination. Calculators are allowed on the boards, and this 30-question test will cover topics in hematology, blood banking and chemistry where mathematical formulas are used. The format will be to write in the answer.

4. Comprehensive Examination. This is a 100 multiple choice question test covering all the sections in CDM. There will be a balanced coverage of the sections, with eight questions on laboratory administration, 18 on chemistry, eight on urine and body fluids, 20 on hematology and transfusion medicine, 16 on immunology, 20 on microbiology, and ten on molecular diagnostics.

Good luck in your journey through clinical pathology.

Katherine I. Schexneider, MD
2006

Acknowledgements

I am indebted to Richard McPherson, MD, Matthew Pincus, MD, and Robert Hutchison, MD for their assistance with the early manuscripts of CDM, 21st edition, which I needed to prepare this edition of the Review Manual. Their tireless gathering and e-mailing of chapters is greatly appreciated.

The production team for the 2nd edition was superb. Michael Houston provided the same excellent direction for the work that we have come to expect from him. Rus Gabbedy and Gemma Lawson kept the project on track and answered my many questions quickly and patiently. Finally, Sue Beasley and Sukie Hunter offered solid critiques of the text and certainly improved its content. It has been a pleasure to work with such a professional group.

Dedication

To my late parents, Victor and Margaret; to my husband,
Will; and to Barb, Lin and Marg. Thank you for keeping me
mindful of my roots.

Part I

The clinical laboratory

CHAPTER 1

General concepts and administrative issues

QUESTIONS

● Q 1

In the discussion of leadership and management, leadership is the WHERE WE ARE GOING, and management is the HOW WE WILL GET THERE. What are the four management skills involved in achieving objectives? *(p. 3)*

● Q 2

A popular quality tool in today's business world employs the single mantra of improvement and measures quality by counting the number of defects per million opportunities (DPMO). The name of this tool is _____. *(p. 4)*

● Q 3

The Clinical Laboratory Improvement Act (CLIA '88) has developed suggested guidelines for retention of records, reports, and specimens. These retention guidelines are mandated then by JCAHO, CAP, and HCFA. How long are the following to be retained? *(Table 1–14, p. 9)*

Quality control records: _____

Proficiency testing: _____

Blood bank donor/recipient records: _____

Autopsy reports: _____

Pathology reports: _____

Bone marrow reports: _____

Cytopathology reports: _____

Serum specimens: _____

Routine blood smears: _____

● Q 4

Your laboratory needs to hire a new technician for the evening shift, and your evening shift supervisor writes a job announcement based on the specific tasks the technician will be expected to perform. The Criterion-Based Job Description recommends against this approach. Why? *(p. 6)*

● Q 5

Concerns about the accuracy and regulation of which common screening test was the impetus for the passage of CLIA? *(p. 7)*

● Q 6

Two states and a handful of organizations work outside the CLIA system, being accredited through alternative channels. What are three key organizations that use alternative accreditation? *(Table 1–10, p. 7)*

● Q 7

Differentiate between personal protective equipment (PPE) and work practice controls by defining each. *(p. 8)*

● Q 8

What is an MSDS sheet? *(Table 1–18, p. 10)*

ANSWERS

A1. These skills are planning and prompt decision-making, organizing, leading and controlling.

A2. This is Six Sigma. It can be applied to the clinical laboratory as well as many other business settings.

A3. **20 years:** Many reports *where a diagnosis is made*, including autopsy reports, pathology reports, bone marrow reports, cytopathology reports. (Some recommend keeping paraffin blocks for 20 years to be safe.)
5 years: BB donor/recipient reports, paraffin blocks
2 years: Quality control, proficiency testing, several administrative items
7 days: Routine blood smears.
24 hours: Serum specimens.

A4. This approach to hiring emphasizes roles rather than specific tasks, as the tasks may require changes at some point depending on operations. This is particularly true for evening shift workers who need to be cross-trained to other tasks.

A5. The PAP smear. An investigative article appeared in the Wall Street Journal and stirred congressional interest in regulation of physician-operated laboratories. The key member of Congress responsible for passing CLIA was Senator Barbara Mikulski (D-MD).

A6. The American Association of Blood Banks, the College of American Pathologists and the Joint Commission on Accreditation of Health Care Organizations.

A7. PPE includes clothing, gloves and face shields which physically separate the user from a hazard. Work practice controls are procedures and preventive measures (behaviors) that reduce or eliminate exposure to biological hazards, and include segregation of biological waste and hand washing.

A8. The Material Safety Data Sheet (MSDS) is a summary of the hazardous nature of a chemical used in the workplace. It communicates workplace hazards and preventive/precautionary steps to employees.

CHAPTER 2

Optimizing laboratory workflow and performance

QUESTIONS

• Q 1

Clinical laboratories integrate three phases of the testing process: pre-analysis, analysis and post-analysis. Briefly discuss the activities in each of these phases. *(p. 12)*

• Q 2

Reviewing *Figure 2–2 (pp. 12, 14)*, is another technician or a new analyzer needed to keep up with the workflow on the evening shift?

• Q 3

Refer to *Table 2–2 (pp. 13, 14)* to answer the following question. By relaxing the limits for delta checks and panic values on Analyzer A, the delta checks are reduced from 62 to 15, and the panic values from 23 to 12, per 500 tubes run. What are the total number of reruns and the percentage of reruns, assuming that the other causes for reruns remain the same?

● Q 4

To run a troponin I test for a hospital with a busy emergency department (ED), would the optimal testing system be utilization of a reference laboratory, a batch analyzer, or a random access analyzer? Explain your answer. *(p. 15)*

● Q 5

Reviewing *Figures 2–3 and 2–4 (pp. 15–16)*, how has task mapping improved efficiency in the hematology section of the clinical laboratory depicted?

● Q 6

Distinguish between *breakthrough technology* and *derivative technology*. *(pp. 16–17)*

● Q 7

Consolidation, standardization and integration are three interrelated strategies used to make laboratories and groups of laboratories more efficient and effective. Which strategy is defined by the descriptions below? *(p. 18)*

A. Services, such as laboratory data, at one location are coordinated, shared and connected to those at a separate site: _____

B. Using a single site to perform testing on samples from several facilities to lower per unit costs: _____

C. The adoption of uniform policies, methods and equipment to facilitate the cross-training of staff and simplify operations: _____

Q 8

A house officer admits a 32-year-old male with jaundice to his ward and suspects acute viral hepatitis. As part of his admission laboratory tests, he orders daily hepatitis A (HAV) IgM titers, and one-time hepatitis B surface antigen (HBsAg) and hepatitis C (HCV) viral genotyping. Give three reasons that this ordering strategy will negatively impact on hospital revenue. *(p. 18)*

ANSWERS

A1. Pre-analysis involves the activities which take place prior to testing, such as test ordering and sample collection. Analysis is the actual performance of testing on an automated analyzer. Post-analysis includes reporting of results and interpretation of those results.

A2. Here, where the test density, the number of tests per sample, is high compared with that on the day shift, a new analyzer would solve the problem of keeping up with the workflow. It would still take the same number of technicians to load the samples onto the analyzer, but a system with a higher throughput would complete the testing in a timely fashion.

A3. The total number of reruns is now 67, and the percentage is 67/500 = 13.4%.

A4. Random access analyzers continually process samples and can be interrupted to process an emergency sample at any time. This is what would be needed to support a busy ED. A reference laboratory would clearly take too long to report a result, and batch analyzers cannot be interrupted once a batch has begun its cycle.

A5. By mapping the tasks performed, the laboratory manager was able to determine that some tasks could be combined or deleted. The number of steps to complete a task was reduced, thus improving efficiency.

A6. Breakthrough technology is technology that fundamentally changes workflow, consolidates workstations, saves labor and improves service. However, because this technology is new, it is costly, and often ridden with glitches. Derivative technology, on the other hand, is the same technology some months or years down the road. Here, the cost of the technology is less because several vendors are competing for the same customer, and the glitches have been identified and addressed.

A7. A. This is integration.
     B. This is consolidation.
     C. This is standardization.

A8. First, inpatient laboratory tests are generally not reimbursed. Second, many tests sent to reference laboratories, such as viral genotyping, are very costly. Finally, test repetition, such as repeating the HAV IgM daily (to catch it as soon as the patient seroconverts!), is not cost-effective.

CHAPTER 3

Pre-analysis

QUESTIONS

Q 1

A 43-year-old well-trained female distance runner completes a 12-mile run and immediately provides a blood sample for a creatine phosphokinase (CK) level in a research study. The next day, a rest day with no exercise, she submits a second sample. How will each CK level compare with those of a sex- and age-matched non-athletic control? *(p. 20)*

Q 2

What is the effect of a high-protein diet, such as the Atkins diet, on blood urea nitrogen (BUN)? *(p. 21)*

Q 3

Describe the effect of an upright posture on serum albumin. *(p. 21)*

Q 4

What preservative maintains blood glucose stability and is chosen for glucose testing?
How does this preservative work? *(p. 24)*

Q 5

Name two common blood collection tubes would be inappropriate for serum calcium levels? *(Table 3–5, pp. 23–24)*
_____ (color) top tube contains _____
_____ (color) top tube contains _____

Q 6

A clinician brings a hemolyzed sample to the laboratory and asks if *any* of the following tests can be performed with reasonable accuracy: sodium, potassium, phosphate, AST and LDH. *(p. 22)* You reply:

Q 7

What preservative, if any, is recommended for a 24-hour urine collection for catecholamines and vanillylmandelic acid? *(p. 28)*

Q 8

A clinician is preparing to collect cerebrospinal fluid (CSF) from a patient with a pressure of 125 mmHg, measured in a sterile manometer. How much CSF can be removed for various studies? *(p. 28)*

Q 9

All serum or plasma laboratory measurements should ideally be performed within 1 hour after collection, and certain tests must be performed immediately. If analysis cannot be performed within 4 hours, at what temperature should serum/plasma be stored? *(p. 29)*

Q 10

A centrifuge spins down a sample for 10 minutes at 8200 rpm. The distance from the axis of rotation to the center of the tube is 20 cm. What is the relative centrifugal force (RCF) on the tube? *(p. 29)*

ANSWERS

A1. Immediately after strenuous exercise, the CK will be elevated. The next day, however, the CK will be *lower* than that of the control, as chronic aerobic exercise lowers baseline CK levels.

A2. A high-protein diet will increase the BUN. Excess protein cannot be fully utilized and is metabolized into urea for excretion.

A3. The upright posture increases hydrostatic pressure. As water and small electrolytes leak out of the vascular compartment, the concentration of serum proteins such as albumin increase.

A4. Fluoride, which is added to heparin, inhibits glycolysis to maintain a stable glucose level. Otherwise, RBCs continue to utilize glucose at a rate of 5% per hour.

A5. The lavender top tube contains ethylenediamine tetra-acetic acid, and the blue top tube contains a buffered citrate, both of which bind calcium to inhibit the coagulation cascade.

A6. Only the test for sodium can still be performed. All the other analytes exist in significantly high concentrations inside erythrocytes, and are thus increased in serum/plasma with hemolysis.

A7. 10 mL of 6 N hydrochloric acid should be added to a 3- or 4-liter urine collection container.

A8. This is a normal CSF pressure, so 20 mL may be removed.

A9. The specimen should be stored at 4–6°C.

A10. The formula for RCF is $1.118 \times 10^{-5} \times r \times (\text{rpm})^2$ where 1.118×10^{-5} is a constant, and r is the radius in cm. The duration of centrifugation is not part of the formula. In this case, $1.118 \times 10^{-5} \times 20\,\text{cm} \times (8200)^2 = 1.504 \times 10^4$, or 15 035 times the force of gravity.

CHAPTER 4

Analysis:
principles of instrumentation

QUESTIONS

• Q 1

There is a relationship between the concentration of a substance in solution (such as bilirubin in serum) and the amount of radiant energy absorbed or transmitted through that solution under controlled conditions. This is the principle underlying spectrophotometry. The equation that mathematically describes this relationship is the Beer–Lambert law.

State the law in words. *(p. 33)*

The equation is:

$$A = abc = 2 - \log \%T$$

where A = absorbance, a = absorptivity of compound under standard conditions, b = light path of solution, c = concentration of compound, $\%T$ = percent transmittance.

• Q 2

What is the chief use of atomic absorption spectrophotometry in today's laboratories? *(p. 34)*

Q 3

What is the chief advantage of fluorescence spectroscopy? *(p. 40)*

Q 4

In nephelometry, the Rayleigh–Debye theory describes the scattering of light in relationship to the light wavelength and the size of the particles encountered by the light. If the wavelength and the size of the particles are approximately the same, then some light will scatter at an angle and some will scatter forward. What is the main application of nephelometry in the clinical laboratory? *(Fig. 4–15, p. 40)*

Q 5

Bacterial growth in broth cultures, clot formation in coagulation studies, and protein levels in urine and CSF are often measured by _____, which measures the reduction of light in the forward direction. *(Fig. 4–15, pp. 40–41)*

Q 6

Osmometry is the measurement of the osmolality of a solution. Although Henry does not dwell on this, let's take a moment to recall that osmolality is millimoles of solute per kilogram of solvent. This is the measurement we see for serum and urine concentrations. Serum osmolality is 275–295 mOsm/kg, urine is 300–900 mOsm/kg. The closely related term, osmolarity, is only occasionally used, and refers to milliosmoles of solute per liter of solution.

Osmometry is based on measuring the changes in the colligative properties of a solution. These four properties are: *(p. 41)*

The one most commonly used in the clinical laboratory is _____

Q 7

In flow cytometry, cells are suspended in fluid and pass single file through a sensing point where the quantity and characteristics of the cell can be determined. Scattered light from an argon beam travels both forward, giving an indication of cell _____ , and in the 90 degree, or side scatter direction, showing cell _____ . *(Fig. 4–16, pp. 41–42)*

• Q 8

What is the main use of the electrical impedance method, which measures the change in electrical resistance across an aperture when a particle in a conductive liquid passes through the aperture? *(p. 44)*

• Q 9

What is the glass electrode used to measure? *(p. 43)*

• Q 10

Potentiometry is the measurement of voltage between two electrodes in a solution. If you have an unknown concentration of an ion, such as Na, and a metal of that same sodium ion across a membrane, you can measure the electrical potential across the interface between the ion and the metal. The measured cell potential is related to the molar concentration of Na (or any ion) by what equation? *(p. 42)*

• Q 11

Electrophoresis is the separation of compounds, usually proteins, based on their electrical charge. The proteins with greater net charges move (circle correct choice) *(p. 44)*

faster   slower

• Q 12

What does densitometry add to simple electrophoresis? *(p. 44)*

• Q 13

Gas chromatography is used to measure volatile substances and those that can be converted to a volatile form. We can change the retention time of compounds (how long they stay in the column) by changing what parameter? *(Fig. 4–19, pp. 45–46)*

• Q 14

Liquid chromatography (LC) is more effective than gas chromatography for compounds that are unstable or have poor volatility. Older types of LC include paper, thin-layer, ion exchange, and exclusion. The newer method is called high-performance liquid chromatography (HPLC). How does HPLC compare with the older methods in terms of analysis time? *(p. 46)*

OK, now why?

• Q 15

True/False. A disadvantage to HPLC is the need to regenerate the columns with each new run. This adds to the cost of running each test. *(Fig. 4–20, pp. 46–47)*

• Q 16

Characteristic fragmentation of molecules when bombarded with electrons or fast atoms such as argon describes the technique called *(Fig. 4–21, pp. 46, 48)*

• Q 17

What is a key application of the method of scintillation counting, the measurement of flashes of light that occur when gamma rays interact with matter? *(p. 48)*

• Q 18

Briefly describe the composition and advantages of the most common type of glassware used for volume measurements in the clinical laboratory. *(p. 52)*

ANSWERS

A1. Beer–Lambert law: the concentration of a substance is directly proportional to the amount of light absorbed or inversely proportional to the logarithm of transmitted light.

A2. Measurement of metals such as lead, and others in the field of toxicology (heavy metals, industrial exposures, etc.).

A3. Fluorescence spectroscopy, or luminescence, is characterized by high sensitivity.

A4. Ag–Ab reactions, particularly to measure proteins, such as apolipoproteins and immunoglobulins, and drugs.

A5. This is turbidimetry.

A6. The four colligative properties are osmotic pressure, freezing point, boiling point, and vapor pressure. Freezing point osmometers are in common use.

A7. Forward scatter relates to cell size. Side scatter relates to cell complexity features, such as granularity.

A8. Hematology. This method is used to count WBCs, RBCs, and platelets. This method also makes size-based criteria for these three cell types.

A9. The glass electrode is still used to measure the hydrogen ion concentration. This is the pH electrode.

A10. The Nernst equation.

A11. Faster. The greater the negative charge, the faster the molecule will move toward the positively charged anode.

A12. Densitometry quantifies the protein fractions.

A13. Column temperature can be increased to reduce the retention time and speed up the throughput of gas chromatography.

A14. Shorter analysis time is achieved by the high pressure used to push the liquids through.

A15. False. The columns can be used many times without regeneration.

A16. This is mass spectrometry. This technique is used extensively in toxicology and therapeutic drug monitoring.

A17. Radioimmunoassays for hormones is the key application.

A18. This is borosilicate glass. It is characterized by a high degree of thermal resistance, low alkali content, and does not contain such elements or substances as magnesium, lime, zinc, heavy metals, arsenic or antimony.

CHAPTER 5

Analysis:
clinical laboratory automation

QUESTIONS

• Q 1

What is the disadvantage of a parallel testing configuration, such as that in the SMAC II® analyzer? *(p. 57)*

• Q 2

What is the major task in the pre-analytical stage of testing? *(p. 57)*

• Q 3

What step in specimen handling has been eliminated by the serum separator tube? *(p. 57)*

• Q 4

Define carry-over. *(p. 59)*

● Q 5

Distinguish between an open and a closed reagent system. *(p. 59)*

● Q 6

State the main drawbacks or challenges of total laboratory automation (TLA). *(p. 61)*

ANSWERS

A1. Parallel testing performs a measurement of every analyte on every sample in the batch. If a clinician only wants a glucose measurement on his patient, he would get an entire seven-test panel, for example.

A2. This is sample or specimen processing.

A3. The double spin technique has been eliminated. Prior to the development of the serum separator tube, plain red top tubes had to be spun twice to fully remove the clot and free the serum. This technique required decapping the container and risking exposure to blood either directly or via aerosol.

A4. Carry-over is the contamination of one sample by the previous sample. For example, if sample 33 has a glucose concentration of 500 mg/dL, then carry-over would result in sample 34 testing as perhaps 150 mg/dL instead of a correct 90 mg/dL.

A5. An open reagent system allows the laboratory to use reagents other than those made by the instrument manufacturer. It might be cheaper to use reagents from Company A on Analyzer X, and an open system will permit that. A closed reagent system only allows the use of reagents made by the instrument manufacturer. This system is restrictive, and may be costly to the laboratory. An analogy is when you attend a sporting event at a stadium where you cannot bring food into the venue. You can only buy refreshments from the concession stands. You can eat, all right, but you pay $4.75 for a hot dog.

A6. TLA requires a considerable financial investment and increased floor space. Skilled technical personnel are needed to operate and troubleshoot the system. The laboratory infrastructure must be remodeled and personnel teams developed, and software must be interfaced with other laboratory or hospital systems. Some TLA systems do not allow for the processing of stat samples.

CHAPTER 6

Point-of-care and physician office laboratories

QUESTIONS

Q 1

What does CLIA stand for? *(p. 64)*

Q 2

Using the CLIA definition, describe the function of a laboratory. *(p. 64)*

Q 3

Which government agency issues certificates allowing laboratories to analyze human specimens? *(p. 64)*

Q 4

What are the three tiers of laboratories in the CLIA system? *(pp. 64–65)*

● Q 5

Certain simple laboratory tests are exempt from rigorous quality assurance, personnel, and proficiency testing. Still, the Department of Health and Human Services (HHS) can conduct spot checks to ensure that these smaller laboratories are performing only such tests. A common theme in the exempt tests is that they are usually performed with equipment made for home/individual use. List three of these tests, which are commonly performed by patients at home as well as by waived laboratories. *(p. 65)*

● Q 6

What government agency designates certain laboratory tests as moderately complex? *(p. 65)*

● Q 7

Are screening tests and other measures of wellness generally covered by Medicare? *(p. 67)*

● Q 8

At what level of laboratory complexity is the position of laboratory director required by CLIA? *(Table 6–2, p. 66)*
Does CLIA require that the director be a licensed physician?

Q 9

Point-of-care (POC) tests are those which can be performed near the patient, sometimes even at the bedside. Review the features of POC instrumentation. *(p. 66)*

Size: _____

Durability: _____

Complexity of quality control (QC): _____

Throughput: _____

Unit cost (per test): _____

Q 10

True/False. Competency assessment is not required for personnel performing POC tests. *(p. 66)*

. . . .

ANSWERS

A1. Clinical Laboratories Improvement Act. These amendments were passed in 1988. They greatly expanded federal regulation of physician office laboratories. Prior to CLIA, these laboratories were unregulated.

A2. A laboratory is 'a facility for the … examination of materials derived from the human body for the purpose of providing information for the diagnosis, prevention, or treatment of any disease ….'

A3. The Department of Health and Human Services issues a certificate for each procedure that is to be performed.

A4. These are waived test/waived laboratories, moderate complexity, and high complexity.

A5. Some examples are UA using dipstick, whole blood glucose, and urine pregnancy.

A6. Food and Drug Administration (FDA).

A7. No. However, the screening PSA was recently added under Medicare coverage.

A8. Moderate complexity laboratories must have a director. Although this person may be a physician, he/she need not be so. A person with a bachelor's degree and appropriate experience may also function as the director.

A9. POC instruments are typically small, often hand-held, durable and have simple QC requirements. Throughput is low, and unit cost is high; these are the price to pay for convenience.

A10. False. Personnel must still be trained, the training documented, and competency assessed in the POC arena.

CHAPTER 7

Post-analysis:
medical decision-making

QUESTIONS

• Q 1

True/False. The reference interval is defined as representing the central 95% tendency of measurements from the general population. *(p. 68)*

• Q 2

Refer to *Table 7–1 (p. 69)* for the following question. A husband and wife have fasting total cholesterol measurements performed on Tuesdays of 2 consecutive weeks. The wife's first result is 160 mg/dL, the second is 178 mg/dL. Her husband's results are 192 mg/dL and 187 mg/dL. Does either show increased intra-individual variability? _____ Is the inter-individual variation within what is expected with this analyte? _____

• Q 3

The probability that a patient in a given population with a positive test result has the disease of interest is called *(Table 7–4, pp. 70–71)* _____.

• Q 4

The likelihood of a positive test result when the patient has the disease of interest is the *(p. 70)* _____.

• Q 5

The likelihood of a negative or normal test when the patient does not have the disease of interest is the *(p. 70)* _____.

• Q 6

Bayes theorem calculates the probability that event B will occur when event A has occurred. This theorem is the foundation for determining diagnostic *(p. 71)* _____ , _____ and _____
_____

• Q 7

Review the format for the truth table, also called the 2×2 table as it is set up in *Table 7–3 (p. 70)*. Give the formulae for the following parameters.

		DISEASE	
		+	–
TEST	+	A	B
	–	C	D

A = true-positive   B = false-positive

C = false-negative   D = true-negative

Using this format, let's review:

Sensitivity = _____

Specificity = _____

Positive predictive value = _____

• Q 8

Define diagnostic efficiency. *(p. 73)*

• Q 9

Using the formula for diagnostic efficiency from *Table 7–4 (p. 70)*, calculate the efficiency of the following test. A new test for Strep throat gives positive results in 92 of 100 high-school students with culture-proven disease. It gives negative results in 89 of 100 healthy controls. In an outbreak at a local school of 500 students, 8% of students have Strep throat. The efficiency is:

• Q 10

A receiver operator characteristic (ROC) curve can be used to determine a test's diagnostic efficiency. A curve which closely approximates the upper left-hand corner of the grid has (circle correct choice): *(p. 73)*

high efficiency   low efficiency

• Q 11

The ROC curve can also compare two tests to determine which is more sensitive and which is more specific, or perhaps that one test is superior in both sensitivity and specificity. To determine the more sensitive test, select a particular point of high sensitivity on the *y*-axis, say 97%, as is shown with a dashed line in Figure 7.1. Dropping a vertical line down to the *x*-axis from where 97% intersects each curve, where do tests A and B fall on the *x*-axis? *(Fig. 7–6, pp. 72–73)*

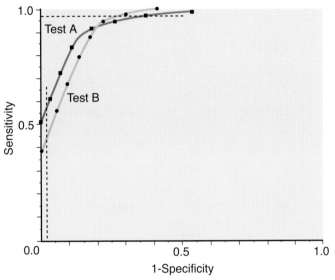

Test A has a value for 1 – specificity (false-positive rate) of _____

Test B has a value for 1 – specificity of _____

At a sensitivity of 97%, test _____ is superior to test _____

_____ and is therefore more specific.

• Q 12

Calculate the likelihood ratio (LR) for the test for Strep throat in Question 9. ____

_____ Does the LR suggest that a positive test

result will accurately predict disease? _____ *(p. 73)*

ANSWERS

A1. False. The reference interval is derived from the 'normal' or 'healthy' individuals in a population, not from the general population, which includes persons with disease.

A2. The wife shows more than the 8.2% variation seen when individuals have this test repeated. The husband's first result is 20% greater than his wife's, and this is within the inter-individual variation typically seen with total cholesterol.

A3. Positive predictive value (PPV). Recall that PPV depends on the prevalence of the disease in a population. The lower the prevalence, the lower the PPV, even with a test with very good specificity.

A4. Sensitivity.

A5. Specificity.

A6. Bayes' 'truth tables' are what we more commonly refer to as 2×2 tables. We use these to calculate diagnostic sensitivity, specificity, and positive predictive value.

A7. Sensitivity = A/A + C
Specificity = D/B + D
PPV = A/A + B

A8. Diagnostic efficiency is the proportion of correct disease classifications made by a test. Mathematically, it is (TP + TN)/TS, where TS is total subjects. Using our scheme here, it would be:
(A + D)/(A + B + C + D)

A9. First, set up the 2×2 table. The total population is 500, and 8%, or 40, have disease, so 460 do not have disease. Out of the 40 with disease, 92% will have a positive test result, or about 37, and 3 will have a false negative result. Of the 460 healthy students, 89% will have a negative result (409), and 460 − 409 = 51 will have false-positive results. The table will look like this:

DISEASE

		+	−
TEST	+	37	51
	−	3	409

The formula for diagnostic efficiency is (TP + TN)/(TP + TN + FP + FN), expressed as a percentage. This is (37 + 409)/(37 + 409 +3 + 51) = 89.2%

A10. A ROC curve that approaches the upper left corner of the grid has high efficiency.

A11. Test A has a false-positive rate of 37%, while test B has a rate of only 30%. Test B is a better test when high sensitivity is most important, as is the case with screening tests.

A12. The formula for the likelihood ratio is simply TP/FP, in this case 37/3 = 12.3. This is fairly high. A positive test is an accurate predictor of disease.

CHAPTER 8

Interpreting laboratory results

QUESTIONS

• Q 1

How does the red cell distribution width (RDW) help one distinguish between iron deficiency anemia, the thalassemias, and anemia of chronic disease (ACD)? *(p. 77)*

• Q 2

How does serum ferritin help one distinguish between iron deficiency and ACD? *(p. 78)*

• Q 3

Total iron binding capacity (TIBC) is usually elevated in iron deficiency, and the ratio of serum iron to TIBC can be helpful in making the diagnosis of iron deficiency. What ratio suggests this diagnosis? *(p. 78)*

Q 4

There are several characteristic laboratory values associated with a hemolytic anemia. Indicate whether the following parameters are elevated, normal or decreased. *(Table 8–1, pp. 77–78)*

Haptoglobin: _____

Indirect bilirubin: _____

Reticulocytes: _____

RDW: _____

Erythroid precursors in marrow: _____

Q 5

What abnormal red cell morphology is seen in renal failure? *(p. 79)*

Q 6

Megaloblastic anemias are typically due to deficiencies of either vitamin B_{12} or folate, although they can also be secondary to alcoholism, liver disease, and myelodysplasia. How is RNA synthesis affected in B_{12} deficiency? *(p. 79)*

How is the RDW affected?

Q 7

Basophilia suggests which type of leukemia? *(p. 80)*

Q 8

Lymphocytosis is seen in which three bacterial infections? *(p. 80)*

Q 9

What laboratory test distinguishes between a leukemoid reaction and CML? *(p. 80)*

• Q 10

Heparin preferentially blocks the _____ coagulation system, resulting in an elevation of _____. *(p. 81)*

• Q 11

An elevated D-dimer is characteristic of disseminated intravascular coagulation (DIC). It is a specific test for activation of the coagulation cascade. It measures (circle correct choice): *(p. 81)*

thrombin   fibrin monomers

cleaved cross-linked fibrin   fibrinogen

• Q 12

Clinical Consultation: A clinician calls you about a patient who has a psychiatric history of compulsive behaviors. Six months ago, he was diagnosed with small cell carcinoma of the lung, and he completed chemotherapy 4 months ago. He is now hyponatremic, with a serum Na of 122, and he seems somewhat confused. It is not clear whether he is drinking excessive amounts of water. Sketch out for the clinician how she can distinguish between hyponatremia due to water intoxication and syndrome of inappropriate ADH (SIADH). *(Table 8–2, pp. 81–82)*

	Water intoxication	SIADH
Serum Na		
Urine Na		
Urine Osm		
Serum K		

• Q 13

Your laboratory has two methods by which it can measure electrolytes, flame photometry and the direct ion-selective electrode. You are called by the laboratory for a serum Na of 125 mEq/L in a patient with type I lipoproteinemia. *(p. 82)* Which method do you suspect the laboratory used to determine his Na?_____

Which method will correct this error? _____

• Q 14

The glomerular filtration rate (GFR) is estimated by the creatinine clearance (C_{cr}). What is the formula for C_{cr}? *(p. 83)*

• Q 15

Acid–base abnormalities will be covered in detail in Chapter 14. Here, we'll review the Henderson–Hasselbalch formula, and a few common causes of acid–base abnormalities.

Recall that at room temperature, we can estimate H_2CO_3 as $0.03 \times P_{CO_2}$. The H–H equation becomes:

$$pH = 6.1 + \log(HCO_3/0.03 \times P_{CO_2})$$

where $6.1 = pKa$ of H_2CO_3.

A type 1 diabetic in ketoacidosis who is vomiting will likely have elements of both (*Table 8–4, p. 84*)

_____ and _____

• Q 16

A 65-year-old smoker with chronic obstructive pulmonary disease will likely have (*Table 8–4, p. 84*)

• Q 17

Give the formula for calculating the anion gap. (*p. 84*)

• Q 18

What malignancy is suggested by a low anion gap of 1–3 mEq/L? (*p. 84*)

• Q 19

In hypercarbic states, where CO_2 is elevated, what is the impetus for respiration? (*p. 85*)

Q 20

Let's review the laboratory definition of diabetes mellitus (DM). There are three possible glucose results that will define DM. List them. *(p. 85)*

_____ fasting serum glucose (on two occasions)

_____ random glucose with classic symptoms of DM (on two occasions)

_____ oral glucose tolerance test (GTT) at 2 hours postload

Q 21

An elevated ammonia level suggests two diagnoses, _____ _____ and _____. These can be readily distinguished because the aminotransferases would likely be extremely elevated in _____ but may well be normal or decreased in _____ _____. *(Table 8–5, p. 86)*

Q 22

There are several biochemical markers used in the diagnosis of acute myocardial infarction (AMI). Some are not specific for cardiac muscle, but rise early after injury, peaking within 12 hours. Others are specific and are considered definitive markers. *(pp. 86–87)*

Identify three useful markers for AMI _____ and _____ and _____ . The one which is now the standard definitive marker and remains elevated for 5–9 days: _____

Q 23

Which coagulation factor is also an acute phase reactant? *(p. 87)*

• •

ANSWERS

A1. In iron deficiency, the RDW is typically elevated. In thalassemia and ACD, it is usually normal.

A2. In iron deficiency, ferritin is low, reflecting decreased iron stores. In ACD, iron stores are abundant, so ferritin is elevated, or at least normal. Recall that ferritin is also an acute phase reactant, so in chronic diseases with an inflammatory component, such as rheumatoid arthritis, ferritin can be elevated due to an acute flare.

A3. 1 : 5.

A4. Haptoglobin is decreased. Indirect bilirubin, reticulocytes, RDW, and erythroid precursors in marrow are all increased.

A5. Burr cells (echinocytes).

A6. RNA synthesis is *not* affected. Recall that B_{12} is part of the thymine pathway, and that RNA uses uracil instead of thymine in nucleic acid synthesis. RDW is elevated.

A7. Chronic myelogenous leukemia (CML).

A8. Tuberculosis, brucellosis, and pertussis/whooping cough.

A9. The neutrophil/leukocyte alkaline phosphatase, which is elevated in the leukemoid reaction and low/absent in CML.

A10. Intrinsic system, with prolonged partial thromboplastin time (PTT).

A11. D-dimer measures cross-linked fibrin which has been cleaved by plasmin.

A12. In water intoxication, urine sodium is low, urine Osm is low, and serum K is low. In SIADH, urine sodium is high, urine Osm is high, and serum K is normal or low.

A13. Pseudohyponatremia is due to excess lipids in serum. Na cannot dissolve in lipids, and the absolute amount of Na estimated by flame photometry includes the lipid-laden serum, giving a falsely low value for Na. The direct ion-selective method does not depend on the volume of serum, and it thus gives an accurate estimate of Na concentration.

A14. $C_{cr} = U_{cr} \times V/P_{cr}$, where U_{cr} is urine creatinine, V is urine flow or volume over time, and P_{cr} is plasma creatinine.

A15. Metabolic acidosis will likely predominate, but metabolic alkalosis may complicate the picture.

A16. Respiratory acidosis due to retained CO_2.

A17. $AG = Na - (Cl + HCO_3)$

A18. Multiple myeloma. Recall that globulins are positively charged proteins. This is why they are down in the gamma region on SPEP, far away from the more negatively charged albumin.

A19. The impetus to breathe is only from hypercarbia-induced hypoxia, which causes chemoreceptors in the aortic arch to signal the brainstem to maintain respiration. If supplemental oxygen is given to patients with hypercarbia, like COPD patients, they may lose their respiratory drive and become apneic.

A20. Fasting $\geq 126\,mg/dL$, or random $\geq 200\,mg/dL$ with classic symptoms, or 2-hour postload $\geq 200\,mg/dL$. Any one of these three is sufficient for the diagnosis of DM. However, this must be confirmed with a repeat test on a subsequent day.

A21. Cirrhosis and acute fulminant liver failure would both show an elevated NH_3. Cirrhotics can often have normal-low AST and ALT because they have few surviving hepatocytes left to release these enzymes. In acute liver failure, the transaminases would be markedly elevated.

A22. Good early markers are creatine kinase, MB fraction (CK-MB), which rises 2–6 hours post-AMI, and myoglobin (MG). Troponin is now the biochemical standard for diagnosing AMI. Tn I is specific for cardiac muscle, becomes elevated fairly early after injury (4–8 hours) and remains elevated for 5–9 days after injury.

A23. Fibrinogen.

CHAPTER 9

Laboratory statistics

QUESTIONS

Q 1

Briefly define and contrast descriptive and comparative statistics. *(p. 91)*

Q 2

The default assumption being tested by a statistical technique is called *(p. 92)*

Q 3

A spread of data in which elements are distributed symmetrically around the mean with most values close to the center is termed _____. *(p. 92)*

Q 4

A mathematical value r describing how well a single straight line fits the relationship observed between two variables measured on the item is termed the _____. *(p. 92)*

Q 5

Which term describes the most common value in a set of data points which exhibit Gaussian distribution? *(p. 92)*

Q 6

The probability that a difference between groups will be detected by a study is the *(p. 92)* _____.

Q 7

A type I error (alpha error) is stating that two groups are statistically _____ _____ when really they are _____. *(p. 92)*

Q 8

What is a type II error? *(p. 92)*

Q 9

When a set of data, such as albumin results from a new lot of QC material, exhibit Gaussian distribution, which three measures of central tendency will be nearly equal? *(p. 93)*

_____ , _____ and _____.

Q 10

If the mean blood glucose in a group of healthy subjects is 72 mg/dL and the standard deviation (SD) is 8 mg/dL, what percentage of the healthy population will have values between 66–80 mg/dL? *(p. 93)*

Q 11

Based on the data in Question 10, what should you establish as your laboratory's reference range? *(p. 93)*

Q 12

A clinical trial studying 50 diabetic subjects, 25 in the treatment group and 25 in the control group, found that subjects in the treatment group showed more improvement in their blood glucose than did the control subjects. However, the *p*-value was only 0.08, so statistical significance could not be demonstrated. What should have been calculated before this trial began? *(p. 95)*

Q 13

You are preparing to incorporate a new method for measuring serum magnesium levels in your laboratory. Your linear regression analysis, in which you compare your new method to your existing one, shows an intercept of 0.4 mEq/L and a slope of 0.67. The correlation coefficient is 0.51. Should you proceed with this new method? *(p. 96)*

Q 14

Define precision. What mathematical measure describes precision? *(p. 98)*

Q 15

The lowest value that an assay can reliably detect is termed _____ _____. *(p. 98)*

ANSWERS

A1. Descriptive statistics analyzes continuous data by calculating or estimating the central tendencies of one group (mean, median, mode) and variations from these central points. Comparative statistics asks the question whether one group differs from another group.

A2. The null hypothesis. If antibiotic A is the standard for treating community-acquired pneumonia, and a pharmaceutical company develops antibiotic B, hoping it will be more effective in clinical trials, then the trials begin with the null hypothesis: A is equally as effective as B, or, said another way, A is no more effective than B.

A3. This is Gaussian distribution. It is also referred to as a parametric distribution of data.

A4. This is the correlation coefficient.

A5. This is called the mode.

A6. Statistical power. It is related to the type II error by the formula 1 – beta.

A7. Type I error is stating that two groups are different when really they are not. I like to think of this as the 'lying pharmaceutical company.' Say that in our previous example, antibiotic B was no more effective than antibiotic A, but the B drug company sponsored a clinical trial, where 'voilà,' B appeared more effective than A. They then publish their 'findings' and start selling antibiotic B. This is a type I error.

A8. Type II error is stating that two groups are not statistically different when they really are. I like to think of this as the 'overly modest pharmaceutical company.'

A9. These are the mean, median and mode.

A10. 68.2% of the healthy population will fall within one SD of the mean.

A11. 56–88 mg/dL would encompass 2 SD on either side of the mean. This is the usual reference range.

A12. The sample size necessary to achieve statistical significance can be calculated. This study was too small to achieve statistical significance.

A13. No. The constant bias of 0.4 mEq/L is far too great, the slope of the regression line is low, demonstrating a proportional bias, and the $r = 0.51$ is unsatisfactory.

A14. Precision is the reproducibility of an assay and is expressed mathematically by the coefficient of variation.

A15. This is analytical sensitivity.

CHAPTER 10

Quality control

QUESTIONS

Q 1

What is the primary purpose of quality control (QC)? *(p. 99)*

Q 2

Are clinical laboratories required to develop written Standard Operating Procedures (SOPs)? *(p. 100)*

Q 3

What is the minimum frequency for performing assay controls, consistent with CLIA regulations? *(p. 101)*

Q 4

The night chemistry technician calls you to report that a QC result has failed an evaluation rule (Westgard rule). A repeat of the control has given the same unacceptable result. The technician believes that the QC material has deteriorated during storage, causing these results. He wants to release the patient results for the shift and resolve the issue on the next a.m. shift. *(p. 104)* What is your response?

• Q 5

When the College of American Pathologists (CAP) sends a control substance to a local hospital, on which it will run an albumin level and report back its findings to CAP for review of the hospital's accuracy, this is an example of *(p. 108)*

• Q 6

After changing method reagent lots, how many patient samples must be analyzed for comparison of performance according to the Clinical and Laboratory Standards Institute? *(p. 105)*

• Q 7

In tracking QC for a given analyte, the control material is analyzed 20 times over at least five different runs at the beginning of a control lot to establish the target mean as well as the standard deviation (SD). From these two values, the laboratory can set acceptable limits on any future result achieved with that control lot. Usually, the acceptable control limits are set at ±2.2–3.2 SD from the target mean. With these parameters set, the daily/periodic controls are plotted on a graph over time to review trends in analyte measurements. Identify the following points on the Levey–Jennings plot (Fig. 10.1). *(Figure 10–4, p. 100)*

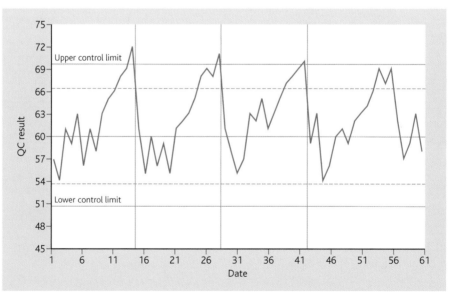

Let's say the analyte is glucose and the units on the *y*-axis are mg/dL.

Lower control limit: _____ mg/dL

Upper control limit: _____ mg/dL

Target mean: _____ mg/dL

On what day did the value first exceed the upper control limit? _____

Does this chart indicate positive, negative, or random bias? _____

Q 8

The Westgard rules help identify trends in running controls and also limit the frequency of false rejections. Review the nomenclature in *Table 10–2* and give the correct Westgard rule for the following: (*p. 102*)
1. The difference between successive control results is 3 SD _____
2. The last three control results (or three results from the same run) are more than 2 SD from the target mean _____
3. The last five consecutive control results are on the same side of the target mean

_____

Q 9

What are delta checks? (*p. 107*)

ANSWERS

A1. The primary purpose of quality control is to statistically sample the measurement process to verify that the method continues to perform within the specifications consistent with acceptable systemic bias and imprecision. In short, QC allows you to trust your patient results.

A2. Yes, this is required by government agencies.

A3. Controls must be performed at least every 24 hours, or more frequently if specified by the manufacturer of the analyzer.

A4. Not so fast. He may be right in his assessment of the cause of the QC results, but you cannot release patient results until the problem is resolved. The measurement should be repeated on a new specimen of QC material first. If this yields an acceptable result, then the patient results can be released.

A5. External proficiency testing.

A6. At least 40 patient samples must be analyzed.

A7. Lower control = 50.5 mg/dL
Upper control = 69.5 mg/dL
Target mean = 60 mg/dL
Day 14 – above upper control
This represents positive bias, as the controls run high.

A8. 1. R_{3S}
2. 3_{2S}
3. 5_m

A9. Delta checks are a patient-based QC technique. Simply, they compare a current laboratory result to previous results for that same patient. For example, if a patient has a glucose value of 572 mg/dL on Tuesday morning of a 10-day hospital stay, but he is not diabetic, and his glucose has consistently been between 73–91 mg/dL, this new value warrants investigation. Is there a problem with the chemistry analyzer? Did a clinician inadvertently give D50 (50% dextrose in water)?

CHAPTER 11

Clinical laboratory informatics

QUESTIONS

• Q 1

Describe clinical laboratory informatics, as defined by the American Board of Pathology. *(p. 112)*

• Q 2

Clinical pathologists are key consultants to clinicians in many areas of laboratory medicine. LIS plays a pivotal role in advising clinicians on which aspects of laboratory testing? *(Table 11–5, p. 117)*

• Q 3

How does electronic order entry empower the client to select the correct test for his patient? *(p. 114)*

11

CHAPTER

• Q 4

Discuss automated mechanisms that make useful interpretive information available to clinicians. *(p. 116)*

• Q 5

What are the established and expected roles of automated surveillance in microbiology LIS? *(p. 117)*

• Q 6

Define HL7. *(p. 119)*

• Q 7

Define DICOM. *(p. 121)*

• Q 8

The government expects healthcare professionals to treat patients' information confidentially, to control access to that information, and to ensure the safety and integrity of electronic patient data. What 1996 Act required this level of security of patient information? *(p. 119)*

Q 9

What two agencies set standards for LIS compliance? *(p. 118)*

Q 10

True/False. Clinical laboratories must prepare, execute and routinely update and test a plan for recovery from a disaster (loss of data). *(p. 118)*

Q 11

Your less than robust LIS system is down, and you must help a clinician read the result of an arterial blood gas from the HLA result transaction. What is the arterial pH, the reference range, and the FiO_2? *(Fig. 11–6, p. 120)*

Q 12

What is the ultimate goal of the LIS? *(p. 117)*

· ·

ANSWERS

A1. Clinical laboratory informatics is that practice of pathology which focuses on the management of information and systems in support of patient care decision-making, education and research.

A2. LIS assists clinicians (as well as laboratories) in pre-analysis, analysis and post-analysis. The management function is utilized by the laboratorians rather than the clinicians.

A3. Electronic order entry details collection requirements, the nature of the test procedure, and expected results. It sometimes discusses the applicability of the test to the diagnostic process.

A4. Interpretive reports and clinical alerts can all be generated from the LIS automatically.

A5. The LIS is already used to detect outbreaks of infectious diseases and to provide disease reporting to various authorities. It may also be used to aid in the detection of bioterrorism events.

A6. Health Level Seven is a widely adopted LIS–HIS interface standard which defines data to be exchanged, the timing of exchanges, and error communication between applications. It standardizes data exchanges and integrates the communication of all information contributions to the comprehensive electronic health record.

A7. Digital Image Communications in Medicine is a technical body of work that formally specifies the encoding and exchange protocol for many digital and nondigital imaging diagnostic modalities. The Visible Light Supplement domain allows pathologists to take and send gross and microscopic images and associated data to others for analysis.

A8. This is the Health Insurance Portability and Accountability Act of 1996 (HIPAA).

A9. These are the Joint Commission on Accreditation of Healthcare Organizations (JCAHO) and the College of American Pathologists (CAP). Additionally, the Clinical Laboratory Improvement Amendments (CLIA) provides regulations for LIS. This answer is not in the text. The author apologizes.

A10. True.

A11. The pH is 7.39, reference range 7.35–7.45, and the neonate is on 100% FiO_2.

A12. The ultimate goal of the LIS is to provide data to clinicians as well as laboratorians, and to incorporate data from multiple computer systems into a single system.

CHAPTER 12

Financial management

QUESTIONS

• Q 1

Business expenses are classified in several ways, one of which is into direct costs, which can easily be traced to an end-product, and indirect costs. Reviewing *Table 12–1, p. 123*, classify the following into direct or indirect costs.

Reagents: _____ Rent: _____

Testing staff salary: _____ Chemistry analyzer: _____

Proficiency testing: _____ Management staff salary: _____

Utilities: _____

• Q 2

Your laboratory currently performs 12 000 tests per month with a reagent cost of $.80 per test. Your rent is $6000 per month. What is your fixed cost per activity? *(p. 123)*

• Q 3

What percentage of the laboratory budget do salary costs typically constitute? *(p. 123)*

• Q 4

Define the term depreciation. *(p. 123)*

• Q 5

Your laboratory works under a capitation system where it receives a fixed dollar amount per member per month (PMPM) for its outpatient members. There are 1500 members in the Health Maintenance Organization (HMO) and you receive $1.65 PMPM. In the most recent fiscal year, your operating costs were $26 800. *(p. 125)* Did you make a profit or realize a loss?

• Q 6

What two health screening tests are covered by Medicare? *(Table 12–6, p. 128)*

• Q 7

The length of time required for an investment's net revenue to cover the cost of the initial investment is termed _____ *(p. 130)*

• Q 8

When the volume of sales is such that total revenue equals total costs, both fixed and variable, and profit is zero, this is termed _____ *(p. 130)*

ANSWERS

A1. Direct costs include reagents, testing staff salary/wages and other consumables. Indirect costs include rent, utilities, proficiency testing, management salaries, the equipment and its servicing, and other overhead costs.

A2. 12 000 tests × $.80 per test = $9600 for reagents. Rent is $6000, so the cost to perform these tests is $9600 + $6000 = $15 600 per month. At 12 000 tests per month the cost per test is $15 600/12 000 = $1.30 per test. This is the fixed cost per activity. If you can increase the number of tests you perform each month, you will decrease your fixed cost per activity, and increase your profit.

A3. This is usually 50–70% of the budget.

A4. Depreciation is the annual loss of a capital item's value. A capital item would be a hematology analyzer or computer system, for example.

A5. The amount your laboratory received from the HMO was 1500 members × $1.65 PMPM × 12 months = $29 700. You received more than you spent by $2900. Good job!

A6. These are the PAP test and the prostate-specific antigen (PSA).

A7. This is payback. You want your payback period to be as short as possible, as equipment depreciates over time, particularly high-end technological equipment.

A8. This is the breakeven point.

CHAPTER 13

Biological, chemical, and nuclear terrorism:
role of the laboratory

QUESTIONS

• Q 1

List four advantages of bioterrorism agents from the perspective of the terrorist. (p. 133)

• Q 2

List the three categories of the most likely biological weapons as published by the Centers for Disease Control (CDC), and the key agents in each category. (p. 133)

• Q 3

What is the cardinal responsibility of the Level A laboratory? (p. 134)

• Q 4

Your laboratory performs a blood culture on a patient who presented yesterday with acute respiratory distress after 3–4 days of malaise. The patient dies the following day in the ICU, and anthrax is suspected. Review the microbiologic characteristics you would see on the sample. Keep in mind that once you make a presumptive diagnosis, you will submit the sample to a Level B or C facility. *(Table 13–6, p. 135)*

Gram stain: _____   Morphology: _____

Growth rate: _____   Motility: _____

Catalase: _____

• Q 5

State the four criteria for 'weapons grade' anthrax. *(p. 136)*

• Q 6

What is the most likely delivery system (method of dissemination) of *Yersinia pestis* by a terrorist? *(p. 137)*

• Q 7

What is the Level A laboratory role in the work-up of a case of suspected botulinum exposure? *(Table 13–10, p. 138)*

• Q 8

What is the presumed aerosol infective dose of smallpox? How does this dose compare with that for the agents of plague and anthrax? *(p. 139)*

• Q 9

Briefly discuss the two methods of spreading smallpox and the CDC's response plan if an outbreak should occur. *(p. 139)*

• Q 10

Why are encephalitis viruses, such as St Louis, eastern and western equine, Japanese B-type and others, with the exception of Venezuelan equine encephalitis (VEE), rarely considered as a potential agent of bioterrorism? *(p. 140)*

• Q 11

What was the chemical contained in Agent Orange, and what was its tactical purpose? *(p. 141)*

• Q 12

Define dual-use technology as it applies to chemical weapons manufacturing. *(p. 141)*

• Q 13

The Level A laboratory plays mostly a supportive role in the event of a chemical weapons attack. However, an automated chemistry analyzer may have the capacity to measure increased cholinesterase activity. This would assist in the assessment and treatment of persons exposed to what class of chemical agent? *(p. 142)*

• Q 14

Describe the function of a survey instrument such as the Ludlum Model 3/Model 44-9 combo Geiger–Mueller detector. *(p. 143)*

ANSWERS

A1. Agents of bioterrorism are typically inexpensive, made with microorganisms that are easily obtained, easy to manufacture, and have the potential to wreak psychological damage in addition to the health threats.

A2. *Deadly bacteria* include the agents of anthrax, plague and tularemia. *Viruses* include the agents of smallpox and the hemorrhagic fevers. *Toxins* include agents such as botulinum, fungal toxins and ricin. Know that the CDC also categorizes biological agents/diseases according to priority of risk and the ease of ability to disseminate the agent. In this scheme, bacteria, viruses and toxins are grouped together. See *Tables 13–2, 13–3, and 13–4* to learn about the risk categories.

A3. The cardinal response of the Level A laboratory, or sentinel laboratory, is to rule out agents of bioterrorism, rather than to perform complete identification or complex analysis. These functions are performed at Level B and C facilities.

A4. Gram stain: positive
Morphology: large bacillus
Growth rate: rapid, within 24 hours
Motility: negative
Catalase: positive

A5. Criteria for the classification as weapon grade are small spore size (1–3 μm), lack of clumping, the amount of spores present and an effective delivery system.

A6. An aerosol delivery system is more likely to be effective than trying to use a flea vector.

A7. Level A laboratories should *not* manipulate, culture or attempt to identify *Clostridium botulinum*. The specimen should be submitted immediately to a Public Health laboratory.

A8. Only 10–100 organisms are thought to be enough to infect a person with smallpox. Plague has a similar infective dose of about 100 organisms. The dose for anthrax is much higher, with 8000–40000 spores as the estimated infective dose. Keep in mind that we are referring to completely different organisms here, viruses versus bacteria versus spores.

A9. The two methods of spreading smallpox are by an aerosol delivery system (the more deadly method) and by direct contact with volunteers who would physically interact with the general population to infect as many persons as possible. The CDC's response, should an outbreak occur, is to vaccinate the population in the vicinity of the outbreak. Post-exposure vaccines can be given 3 days (at least) after exposure.

A10. The attack rate of these viruses is low, so few persons would become ill upon exposure. The exception is VEE, which has an attack rate of about 100%.

A11. Agent Orange contained dioxin and was used as a defoliating agent or herbicide in the Vietnam War.

A12. Dual-use technology involves the conversion of a chemical manufacturing plant, which was built to develop pharmaceuticals or insecticides, to a chemical weapons development site.

A13. Nerve agents act on the acetylcholine/cholinesterase system.

A14. This instrument detects alpha-, beta- and gamma-emitting radionuclides and would be used to identify a nuclear event. While a hospital emergency department may have such an instrument, a clinical laboratory would not.

Part II

Clinical chemistry

CHAPTER 14

Evaluation of renal function, water, electrolytes and acid–base balance

QUESTIONS

• Q 1

Antidiuretic hormone (ADH) is a key hormonal regulator of fluid balance in the body. What is the most important regulator of ADH in persons with normal to elevated blood pressure? *(pp. 150, 158)*

• Q 2

What is the action of aldosterone? *(p. 150)*

• Q 3

Potassium typically shifts into and out of cells in the opposite direction to hydrogen ion.
Thus, in acidemia, K shifts _____ cells, and in alkalemia, K moves _____ cells *(p. 155)*

• Q 4

Give the formula for urinary clearance of a substance. *(Eq. 14–6, p. 152)*
C = _____

• Q 5

The fractional excretion tells us about the resorptive function of the tubules, so it is a useful indicator of tubular disease. What is this formula for sodium? *(Eq. 14–20, p. 154)*

FE_{Na} = _____

• Q 6

Briefly outline the Jaffé reaction and list some of the positive and negative interfering substances. *(p. 152)*

• Q 7

Complete the following table listing the primary and compensatory changes in CO_2 and HCO_3 in the main classes of acid–base disorders. *(pp. 161–166)*

Disorder	Primary change	Compensation
Resp. acidosis	_____	_____
Resp. alkalosis	_____	_____
AG met. acid.	_____	_____
Non-AG met. acid.	_____	_____
Met. alkalosis	_____	_____

• Q 8

Increases in the anion gap are typically due to replacement of _____ with the anion of _____. *(p. 164)*

• Q 9

What are the major osmotically active substances in normal plasma? *(p. 149)*

• Q 10

If the measured osmolality, measured by the colligative property of freezing point depression, exceeds the calculated osmolality determined by a formula, then an osmolal gap exists. There is another solute in the blood. List the four mood-altering substances that a person might ingest which would cause an osmolal gap, and then the one osmotically active substance clinicians sometimes use to treat cerebral edema. *(p. 149)*

• Q 11

The glomerular filtration rate (GFR) is estimated by the clearance of creatinine (CrCl). Creatinine is filtered by the glomeruli. What percentage is then reabsorbed by the proximal tubules? *(p. 152)* _____ What drug is used to block tubular secretion of creatinine when using creatinine as an estimate of glomerular filtration rate? _____

• Q 12

What is the formula for estimating GFR? *(Eq. 14–10, p. 153)*

• Q 13

Clinical Consultation: A clinician has just admitted a 15-year-old type 1 diabetic female in diabetic ketoacidosis (DKA). She has been nauseated and vomiting all day. Her plasma creatinine is 4.8 mg/dL, and BUN is 25 mg/dL. You ask your laboratory technician to recheck her admission Cr. The astute technician sees that she is in DKA, and 'gets a more accurate Cr' of 2.1 mg/dL. What did she do and why? *(p. 152)*

• Q 14

Enzymatic measurements of urea or BUN actually measure released _____ _____ *(p. 153)*

Q 15

A 25-year-old man is presented by his friends in an obtunded state to a local emergency department. His breathing is slow and shallow. Initial laboratory values are: glucose 82 mg/dL, sodium 143 mmol/L, chloride 95 mmol/L, bicarbonate 15 mmol/L and BUN 10 mg/dL. What is his anion gap (AG), what type of acid–base disorder does he have, and what are the most likely etiologies? *(Table 14–10, pp. 163–164)*

Q 16

True/False. In Type IV renal tubular acidosis (RTA), impaired renal tubular potassium secretion leads to hyperkalemia, which mimics Conn's syndrome. *(p. 163)*

Q 17

FE_{Na} is less than 1% in prerenal azotemia, due to the action of what hormone? *(p. 154)*

Q 18

What two drugs stimulate the respiratory center directly, leading to respiratory alkalosis? *(p. 165)*

Q 19

The syndrome of inappropriate antidiuretic hormone secretion (SIADH) has several causes including tumors, pulmonary tuberculosis, pneumonia and others. This term is reserved, however, for ADH secretion that occurs despite two parameters being present which would both normally inhibit ADH secretion. *(p. 160)* These two parameters are:

• Q 20

What are the electrolyte concentrations in sweat? *(p. 151)*

• Q 21

Glucose is an osmotically active substance. In hyperglycemic states, glucose in plasma will draw water out of cells and dilute the main extracellular cation, sodium. Specifically, for every 100 mg/dL of glucose above normal (for ease of calculation, call normal 100 mg/dL), the sodium will fall by *(p. 160)* _____ _____ mmol/L.

• Q 22

What is the most common cause of hypokalemia? *(p. 156)*

• Q 23

Clinical Consultation: A clinician correctly conducts a water deprivation test on a 48-year-old female. Her baseline labs were: Na 142 mmol/L, K 4.1 mmol/L, BUN 11 mg/dL, Cr 0.4 mg/dL, urine osmolality 93 mOsm/kg, plasma osmolality 293 mOsm/kg. After 4 hours, her urine remained dilute with hourly values of 90, 94, 99, and 92 mOsm/kg. At this point, pitressin was administered and two additional hourly urine samples were collected. These were 88 and 94 mOsm/kg. *(Table 14–5, pp. 159–160)*
What is the classification of her disorder? _____
What drug is likely to have caused her disorder? _____

• Q 24

How will a plasma renin activity (PRA) help you distinguish between the most common cause of aldosterone deficiency and a less common cause, namely Addison's disease? *(p. 157)*

ANSWERS

A1. Plasma osmolality. A drop in blood pressure of 5% or more can also stimulate ADH production.

A2. Aldosterone causes reabsorption of sodium in the cortical collecting duct.

A3. Acidemia – K moves out of cells as H moves into cells to lower the blood H ion concentration.
Alkalemia – K moves into cells as H moves out of cells into blood to raise blood H ion levels.

A4. $C = UV/P$
C = concentration, usually in mL/min. U = concentration of the substance in urine, in mg/dL often to match the units of P. V = volume of urine. In a typical 24-hour urine collection, we divide the total milliliters of urine by 1440 (how many minutes in 24 hours) to get V in mL/min. P = plasma concentration of substance in mg/dL. So, if we were calculating creatinine clearance, and the plasma Cr was 3.5, we would use the mg/dL units for both plasma and urine concentrations.

A5. $FE_{Na} = (U_{Na} \times P_{Cr})/(U_{Cr} \times P_{Na})$

A6. The Jaffé method is the old standard for measuring creatinine. Creatinine is treated with an alkaline picrate to yield an orange complex that absorbs light at 485 nm. Certain serum chromogens are the same color and give positive interference. These are glucose, fructose, ascorbic acid, pyruvate, and uric acid. The negative interfering agents are lipids, bilirubin, and hemoglobin.

A7. Disorder; Primary change; Compensation
Resp. acidosis; inc. P_{CO_2}; inc. HCO_3, dec. Cl
Resp. alkalosis; dec. P_{CO_2}; dec. HCO_3, inc. Cl
AG met. acid.; dec. HCO_3; dec. P_{CO_2}
Non-AG met. acid.; dec. HCO_3; dec. P_{CO_2}, inc. Cl
Met. alkalosis; inc. HCO_3; inc. P_{CO_2}, dec. Cl

A8. In an AG metabolic acidosis, bicarbonate is low. It has been replaced by the anion of an organic acid, such as lactic acid, a ketoacid, acetosalicylic acid, etc.

A9. Sodium, urea, and glucose. The calculated osmolality formula is 2Na + glu/20 + BUN/3.
Sodium gets twice the credit because it exists as sodium chloride, which dissociates into two osmotically active substances, Na and Cl, which are in equal proportions.

A10. Ethanol, methyl alcohol, isopropanol, and ethylene glycol are the mood-altering agents. Mannitol is another key cause of an osmolal gap and is used to treat cerebral edema.

A11. 0% is reabsorbed. 10% is secreted at normal creatinine levels. Cimetidine blocks tubular secretion of creatinine.

A12. Estimated GFR = $\dfrac{(140 - \text{Age})/(\text{Wt in kg})}{\text{Plasma Cr} \times 72}$

A13. She determined that the original Cr was performed by the Jaffé reaction. Acetoacetate in ketoacidosis cross-reacts with the Jaffé reaction. Fortunately, your laboratory also has the creatinase method, which will give a more accurate reading in the DKA patient, as well as for patients on cephalosporins and high-dose Lasix.

A14. Ammonia.

A15. The AG is 143 − (95 + 15) = 33. With an elevated AG, this is a metabolic acidosis (note the decreased bicarbonate). Uremia is not the cause, as his BUN is within the reference range. Slow, shallow respirations make salicylate toxicity unlikely. Methanol or ethylene glycol poisoning are the probable causes. These substances are sometimes used as substitutes for ethanol to induce intoxication.

A16. False. Conn's syndrome is due to an aldosterone-producing adrenal adenoma, which leads to potassium wasting. Type IV RTA is caused by aldosterone deficiency or tubular unresponsiveness, causing potassium retention.

A17. Aldosterone can decrease FE_{Na} down to 0.1%.

A18. These are salicylates and progesterone.

A19. Hyponatremia and a normal–increased effective vascular volume both inhibit ADH secretion.

A20. Sodium is present at 50 mEq/L and potassium at 5 mEq/L, so sweat is hypotonic.

A21. 1.5 mmol/L.

A22. The most common cause of hypokalemia is renal wasting of potassium, most often due to increased activity of aldosterone, either as a primary disorder, or secondary to increased renin secretion.

A23. This is a typical presentation of nephrogenic diabetes insipidus, often due to lithium therapy.

A24. The most common cause of aldosterone deficiency is hyporeninemic hypoaldosteronism. Here the plasma renin activity (PRA) is low, obviously. In Addison's disease, the defect is in the adrenal gland, which fails to secrete aldosterone and other hormones. The lack of negative feedback from the sick adrenal gland to the kidney leads to increased PRA.

CHAPTER 15

Biochemical markers of bone metabolism

QUESTIONS

Q 1

Calcium that is bound to plasma proteins, chiefly albumin, accounts for approximately 40% of total serum calcium. Thus, hypoalbuminemia can result in a falsely low total calcium level. If a patient has a measured total calcium of 8.2 mg/dL and an albumin of 2.6 mg/dL, what is the corrected calcium? *(p. 172)*

Q 2

What two dyes are commonly used to measure total calcium? *(p. 172)*

Q 3

If RBCs contain organic phosphate esters, and analytic techniques measure inorganic phosphate, why does hemolysis give falsely elevated phosphorus levels? *(p. 172)*

• Q 4

What method and what reagent are most commonly used to measure total magnesium? *(p. 173)*

• Q 5

Low serum levels of what two cations stimulate the parathyroid to release parathyroid hormone (PTH)? *(p. 174)*

• Q 6

Which analytic technique is used to measure PTH intraoperatively? Is this method as sensitive as the standard assay? *(p. 175)*

• Q 7

PTH-related peptide (PTH-rP) is 141 amino acids long and shows homology in only the first 13 amino acids with PTH, an 84-amino-acid peptide. How do you explain its similar biological effects? *(p. 175)*

• Q 8

Explain the finding of hypercalcemia in diseases such as sarcoidosis. *(pp. 176, 178)*

• Q 9

What two disorders account for 80–90% of cases of hypercalcemia? *(p. 176)*

Q 10

What is the most severe bone manifestation of hyperparathyroidism? *(p. 177)*

Q11

Differentiate between the pathophysiology of type I and type II vitamin D-dependent rickets. *(p. 179)*

Q 12

What is the most common cause of hyperphosphatemia? *(p. 179)*

Q 13

Clinical Consultation: A 63-year-old male alcoholic with uncontrolled diabetes and hypertension is admitted for seizures. When he is stabilized, he complains of 3 days of diarrhea, which he feels is his only problem. His wife had attempted to keep him hydrated and gave him his Lasix for his hypertension twice daily, as directed. On admission, serum glucose is 382 mg/dL and Mg is 0.38 mmol/L. What in his history contributed to his hypomagnesemia? *(p. 180)*

Q 14

Which collagen breakdown product is specific for bone and correlates well with bone turnover? *(p. 181)*

Q 15

Contrast the pathophysiology and key cell lines in osteoporosis in a 53-year-old female and an 83-year-old male? *(p. 182)*

53-year-old: _____

83-year-old: _____

ANSWERS

A1. Using the formula in the text, the additional measurement $(4.4 - 2.6) \times 0.8 = 1.44$. Add 1.44 to 8.2 to arrive at the corrected calcium of 9.64 mg/dL.

A2. Orthocresolphthalein complexone and arsenazo III are the two main dyes used in total calcium measurements.

A3. The organic esters are hydrolyzed during storage to inorganic phosphate as red cells hemolyze. A hemolyzed sample will accomplish the same thing.

A4. Photometric methods, using metallochromic dyes which bind magnesium, are commonly used. The calmagite method is key among these.

A5. Both calcium and magnesium stimulate PTH secretion when ionized levels are low.

A6. The immunochemiluminometric assay is used intraoperatively. It is less sensitive, but more than adequate to measure the large drops in PTH seen during surgery.

A7. This is the amino-terminal end, where the biologic activity of PTH is known to reside. Additionally, PTH-rP shares the same receptor as PTH, so the end-organ effect is similar.

A8. Granulomatous tissue produces $1,25(OH)_2D_3$, just as the kidney does. The increase in active vitamin D increases calcium absorption from the intestines to raise blood calcium.

A9. Primary hyperparathyroidism and malignancy are the two main causes of hypercalcemia.

A10. Osteitis fibrosa cystica.

A11. In type I rickets, patients have decreased activity of the renal enzyme 1-alpha hydroxylase, not wholly unlike patients with chronic renal failure. If given calcitriol, they respond to generate normal levels of active vitamin D.
In type II rickets, there are mutations in the receptor for $1,25(OH)_2D$. As active D cannot enter cells, serum levels are elevated. This is end-organ resistance. High doses of calcitriol raise $1,25(OH)_2D$ even higher, but do not get vitamin D into cells.

A12. Renal failure, especially chronic renal failure, is the most common cause of hyperphosphatemia.

A13. All contributed. Alcoholism is a well-known cause. Others in his history are diabetes, due to osmotic diuresis, loop diuretics, and diarrhea.

A14. The pyridinium crosslink called deoxypyridinoline (Dpyr) is a good marker. Additionally, crosslinked telopeptides may be measured by immunoassays. Hydroxyproline is not a useful marker.

A15. In the postmenopausal woman, excessive osteoclastic activity is the cause of osteoporosis. In the senile form, which occurs in men and women, there are fewer osteoblasts than are needed, and cortical bone is lost.

CHAPTER 16

Carbohydrates

QUESTIONS

• Q 1

Abnormalities in the beta cells of the pancreas in both type 1 and type 2 diabetes result in the release of this molecule, which has 10–15% of the biological activity of insulin. *(p. 186)*

• Q 2

In normal fasting individuals, the molar ratio of C-peptide to insulin in serum is 5:1. What happens to this ratio in cirrhosis and why? *(p. 187)*

• Q 3

Elevated somatostatin levels are sometimes seen in what three cancers? *(p. 187)*

• Q 4

In a person with a normal WBC, what are the rates of glucose utilization per hour at room temperature and at 4°C? *(p. 188)*

25°C: _____   4°C: _____

• Q 5

How do whole blood glucose readings compare with those from plasma? *(p. 188)*

• Q 6

What is the reference method for measuring glucose, and what is the analyte that is measured? *(p. 188)*

• Q 7

Define the diagnostic criteria for diabetes. *(p. 189, Table 16–1)*
Fasting sample: _____
Random sample: _____

• Q 8

Outline the 50-mg screening and both the 75- and 100-mg confirmatory oral glucose tolerance tests used to diagnose gestational diabetes. *(p. 189, Table 16–2)*

• Q 9

A person with low C-peptide levels, and autoantibodies to islet cell antigen 512 and glutamic acid decarboxylase, has what type of diabetes? *(p. 190)*

• Q 10

True/False. Glycosylated hemoglobin, HbA_{1c}, is the irreversibly generated product of a slow Amadori rearrangement of a Schiff base. *(p. 191)*

• Q 11

Diagnosis of an insulinoma may require a prolonged fast, with several analytes being higher than normally expected during a fast. What three analytes must meet 'greater than or equal to' criteria? *(p. 194)*

• Q 12

The Beutler fluorescent test screens for galactosemia in newborns by measuring the deficiency of what enzyme? *(p. 196)*

• Q 13

Review some of the key inborn errors of glycogen metabolism by filling in the following chart. *(Tables 16–8 and 16–9, pp. 195–196)*

Name	Number	Enzyme deficiency	Clinical features
McArdle's			
		glucose-6-phosphatase	
	IV		
			cardiomegaly, death in infancy

• Q 14

In 2000, approximately 64 million adults in the United States had three or more of the following signs, which put them at increased risk of cardiovascular disease and development of diabetes: impaired fasting glucose, high blood pressure, increased waist circumference, elevated serum triglycerides and elevated low-density lipoprotein levels. *(p. 189)* This disorder is termed _____

• Q 15

An intern admitted a 15-year-old boy with type 1 diabetes in diabetic ketoacidosis (DKA) to the hospital last night. The patient's ketones were elevated in his admission blood sample, and the intern wants to monitor ketone levels with a urine dipstick to chart the patient's improvement. *(p. 192)* You reply:

ANSWERS

A1. This is proinsulin. Different defects in the beta cells in the two types each contribute to inappropriate release of proinsulin.

A2. Cirrhotics have decreased hepatic clearance of insulin, and thus have lower ratios.

A3. Small cell lung carcinoma, medullary thyroid carcinoma, and pheochromocytoma may all show elevated somatostatin levels.

A4. At 25°C, glucose is utilized at 7 mg/dL/h. At 4°C, it is at 2 mg/dL/h.

A5. Whole blood glucose levels, such as those performed at home by diabetics, are 10–15% lower than plasma levels. However, the home glucose devices are calibrated to convert their readings to an equivalent plasma reading, so a patient's home readings should accurately reflect a reading you might obtain if you drew a plasma sample at his home.

A6. The hexokinase system assay measures NAD(P)H at 340 nm.

A7. Fasting: ≥ 126 mg/dL on at least two occasions.
Random: ≥ 200 mg/dL with symptoms of hyperglycemia, such as polyuria, polydipsia, weight loss, on at least two occasions.

A8. A 100-g oral glucose load is unpleasant, so pregnant women are screened with the more tolerable 50-g load. If the 1-hour level is ≥ 140 mg/dL, then the confirmatory test is performed.
Confirm with either a 75- or 100-g oral glucose load. If any *two* of the following four levels are noted, then the patient has gestational diabetes:
Fasting: ≥ 95 mg/dL for 75-g load (≥ 95 mg/dL for 100-g load)
One hour: ≥ 180 mg/dL (≥ 180)
Two hours: ≥ 155 mg/dL (≥ 155)
Three hours: no test at 3 hours for 75-g load (≥ 140 for 100-g load).

A9. This is type 1 diabetes. There are several antibodies one may test. Sometimes, antibodies may be present well before the onset of type 1 diabetes, but not always.

A10. True. The Schiff base is reversible, but the Amadori rearrangement results in an irreversible product – glycosylated Hb.

A11. Insulin, C-peptide, and proinsulin are all elevated in insulinomas.

A12. This is galactose-1-phosphate uridyl transferase (GALT).

A13.

Name	Number	Enzyme deficiency	Clinical features
McArdle's	V	muscle phosphorylase	myalgia after exercise, myoglobinuria
von Gierke's	I	glucose-6-phosphatase	growth retardation, hepatomegaly, dec. glucose
Andersen's	IV	1,4-α-glucan branching	HSM, cirrhosis, neurological dysfunction
Pompe's	II	α-1,4-glucosidase	cardiomegaly, death in infancy

A14. This is metabolic syndrome.

A15. This is not the optimal method for monitoring this patient. The sodium nitroprusside reagent found in strips and tablets is not useful for monitoring therapy. Sodium nitroprusside does not measure β-hydroxybutyrate (BOHB), which is proportionally elevated in DKA. BOHB levels fall with therapy, but the acetoacetic acid and acetone levels then *rise*, so the results would be confusing and misleading.

CHAPTER 17

Lipids and dyslipoproteinemia

QUESTIONS

• Q 1

Which lipoprotein causes 'milky' plasma in blood samples? *(p. 202)*

• Q 2

Which apolipoprotein is specific for chylomicrons? *(Table 17–4, p. 203)*

• Q 3

What is the predominant apolipoprotein in low-density lipoprotein (LDL)? *(p. 202)*

• Q 4

Where does high-density lipoprotein (HDL) migrate on protein electrophoresis? *(Table 17–1, pp. 200–201)*

• Q 5

Which apolipoprotein activates the enzyme lipoprotein lipase (LPL)? *(p. 204, Table 17–5)*

• Q 6

What is the role of lipoprotein lipase? *(pp. 203, 205, Table 17–6)*

• Q 7

An overnight fast ensures that which lipoprotein is cleared from plasma in a normal individual? *(p. 206)*

• Q 8

Why is EDTA the preferred anticoagulant for a cholesterol panel when cholesterol and triglyceride levels in plasma are about 3% lower in EDTA-preserved specimens than in serum samples? *(p. 207)*

• Q 9

Review the cholesterol oxidase method of measuring cholesterol and describe how ascorbic acid would result in a falsely low value. *(p. 207)*

Q 10

Enzymatic measurements of triglycerides that measure NADH or NAD as end-products involve cleaving triglycerides to generate what intermediate? *(p. 208)*

Q 11

A 31-year-old man completes a half-iron triathlon and immediately submits several blood samples for a research protocol on the effects of vigorous exercise on lipids. His triglycerides (TG) are found to be elevated at 232 mg/dL. He consumed almost no fat during the race and ate a carbohydrate-rich breakfast. How do you explain his result? *(p. 208)*

Q 12

Review the electrophoretic patterns of the lipoproteins by stating which fraction they migrate in on SPEP. *(p. 208)*

CM: _____ VLDL: _____

LDL: _____ HDL: _____

Q 13

State the Friedewald formula for estimating LDL in mg/dL, and state when a direct LDL method would be more accurate. *(Eq. 17–1, pp. 209–210)*

Q 14

A patient with dysbetalipoproteinemia has elevated levels of what lipoprotein? What electrophoretic feature helps distinguish this disorder from others? *(p. 216)*

• Q 15

According to the AFCAPS trial, which apolipoprotein was found to be the single best lipid, lipoprotein or apolipoprotein measurement to predict coronary artery disease risk? *(p. 211)*

• Q 16

What is the effect of age on cholesterol concentrations in both sexes? *(p. 206)*

• Q 17

Using the Friedewald equation for LDL on *page 209 (Eq. 17–1)*, calculate the LDL in a patient with a total cholesterol of 287 mg/dL, an HDL of 22 mg/dL, and a triglyceride of 400 mg/dL.

• Q 18

Which cholesterol is not addressed in the Fredrickson Classification scheme? *(p. 213)*

• Q 19

Premature coronary disease is most clearly associated with which types of lipoproteinemia in the Fredrickson Classification? *(Tables 17–3 and 17–14, pp. 202, 213)*

Q 20

Briefly outline the pathophysiology of familial hypercholesterolemia. *(p. 215)*

Q 21

What cholesterol ratio is used to screen for type III hyperlipoproteinemia/dysbetalipoproteinemia? *(p. 216)*

Q 22

What vitamin deficiency is most pronounced in abetalipoproteinemia and why? *(p. 216)*

Q 23

A 25-year-old male body builder has an HDL of 12 mg/dL. HEENT examination is normal. What do you suspect? *(pp. 213, 216, Table 17–15)*

ANSWERS

A1. Chylomicrons (CM) cause milky plasma;. When a sample is refrigerated, the CM will form a creamy layer at the top of the sample. VLDL causes cloudy plasma, which is distinct from the milky/creamy plasma that forms during the refrigeration test.

A2. B-48 is found only in chylomicrons.

A3. B-100 is the key apolipoprotein in LDL. It is also found in VLDL.

A4. HDL migrates in the alpha-1 fraction.

A5. This is apoC-II.

A6. LPL hydrolyzes triglycerides from CM and VLDL. The type I hyperlipoproteinemia in the Fredrickson Classification scheme is a deficiency of LPL. This is an autosomal recessive disorder. With CM poorly handled in circulation, these patients have milky plasma.

A7. CMs should be cleared by 9–12 hours of fasting.

A8. EDTA retards oxidative and enzymatic changes that can occur in lipoproteins during storage.

A9. Ascorbic acid consumes hydrogen peroxide, a reaction product, which is converted to H_2O and a dye measured at 500 nm. Less H_2O_2 would result in less final product, in this case, the dye.

A10. Glycerol is the first intermediate. Two approaches then produce glycerophosphate.

A11. Vigorous exercise can generate free glycerol in the plasma, interfering with enzymatic triglyceride measurements. To correct for this, a blanking procedure should be performed prior to measuring the subject's sample.

A12. CM – origin; it has almost no protein and does not move.
VLDL – pre-beta.
LDL – beta.
HDL – alpha-1.

A13. LDL = total cholesterol – [HDL] – TG/5
Use 5 as the denominator for the units mg/dL. If TGs are greater than 400 mg/dL, then a direct measurement of LDL is more accurate.

A14. This is beta-VLDL. On protein electrophoresis, a broad band between VLDL and LDL is present and distinctive. This is type III in the Fredrickson scheme.

A15. This is apoB.

A16. Cholesterol concentrations increase with age in both sexes starting in early adulthood.

A17. LDL = 185 mg/dL.

A18. HDL is not adequately addressed in the Fredrickson Classification scheme.

A19. Type IIa and IIb with elevations of LDL are clearly implicated in premature coronary artery disease. Type III (dysbetalipoproteinemia) is also implicated. Here though, the atherosclerotic lesions are predominantly in the abdominal and femoral arteries. Apparently, they have enough disease in the heart to suffer coronary artery disease as well.

A20. One of several hundred mutations of the LDL-receptor gene on chromosome 19 causes a defect in receptor synthesis, transport or function. The defective receptor cannot effectively bind or clear LDL from the circulation. Elevated LDL levels lead to premature coronary artery disease and other stigmata.

A21. A useful screening test is the ratio VLDL/TG. The normal ratio is 0.2. In the dysbetalipoproteinemic patients, this ratio is >0.3 with all their excess VLDL.

A22. Vitamin E requires CM for absorption, VLDL for transport, and LDL for delivery into the cells. Without the apoB proteins, there is no B-48 (recall that this is the major protein in CM – no B-48, no CM-based absorption of vitamin E). These patients also are deficient in B-100, a key protein in both LDL and VLDL, so these proteins cannot be properly synthesized. Patients can develop retinal and peripheral nerve deficits if vitamin E is not replaced.

A23. This is a classic case of anabolic steroid use. The normal HEENT examination ruled out the orange tonsils of Tangier disease.

CHAPTER 18

Evaluation of cardiac injury and function

QUESTIONS

Q 1

What lipoprotein is taken up by macrophages, which then invade the coronary endothelium to initiate plaque formation? *(p. 220)*

Q 2

What is the characteristic lactate dehydrogenase isoenzyme pattern in acute myocardial infarction (AMI)? *(p. 221)*

Q 3

What relative index (RI) of creatine kinase MB antigen mass (CK-MB) to total CK activity is suggestive of AMI? *(p. 221)*

Q 4

What is currently the most important laboratory test for acute coronary syndrome (ACS)? *(p. 221)*

• Q 5

Give two reasons for the high specificity of cardiac troponin I and T (cTnI, cTnT). *(p. 221)*

• Q 6

How long after an AMI does cTn peak? *(p. 221)*

• Q 7

A 63-year-old male is admitted to the intensive care unit (ICU) with chest pain and ECG changes consistent with AMI. The day after admission, his cTnI is 3.8 mg/dL (0–0.6 mg/dL). Twelve hours later the level has dropped to 1.3 mg/dL, but then sequential Q24-hour (every 24 hours) cTnI levels begin to gradually rise again. The patient denies chest pain, and the ECG shows no new changes, apart from those seen on admission. Do these findings represent a second, silent AMI? *(p. 221)*

• Q 8

What is the window of opportunity (timeline) for using myoglobin as a marker for cardiac injury? *(p. 222)*

• Q 9

True/False. According to the American Heart Association and Centers for Disease Control, universal screening of the adult population for increased risk of coronary heart disease (CHD) with high-sensitivity C-reactive protein (hs-CRP) is recommended. *(Table 18–3, p. 225)*

• Q 10

In what clinical situation would a homocysteine measurement be warranted? *(p. 225)*

• Q 11

Brain natriuretic peptide (BNP) is a biomarker for heart failure (HF) measured by automated immunoassay platforms. However, it has limitations as an analyte for HF. Briefly discuss its shortcomings. *(p. 227)*

ANSWERS

A1. This is oxidized low-density lipoprotein.

A2. The typical pattern in AMI has LD_1 in greater concentration than LD_2. The testing methodology has largely been supplanted by other, more specific, assays, such as the troponins.

A3. At least 2% is necessary for the suggestion of AMI.

A4. This is cardiac troponin (cTn). Both cTnI and cTnT are in use.

A5. One reason is that the forms of both TnI and TnT are different in cardiac muscle compared to those in skeletal muscle. The assays are specific for the cardiac forms.
A second reason is that both these compounds are essentially absent from normal serum. Any elevation is very likely to represent cardiac damage.

A6. The peak occurs at about 24 hours, similar to that for CK-MB.

A7. No. The initial release of cTn comes from the free cytosolic portion, which leaks readily from damaged myocytes. The majority of cTn is bound to muscle fibers and is released more slowly in the week-plus after the AMI.

A8. Elevated serum levels are apparent within 2–3 hours after an AMI, but return to baseline by 24 hours.

A9. False. While hs-CRP is the current analyte of choice as an inflammatory marker for risk assessment of CHD, universal screening is not recommended.

A10. If a person who is at low risk of CHD, based on traditional risk factors, develops CHD, then a homocysteine level may provide some useful data.

A11. BNP is not an especially specific marker, as it is elevated in other conditions of fluid imbalance, such as renal failure. Secondly, chronic HF patients with stable disease may have values within the reference range. Thirdly, intra-individual variation can be as great as 30–40% in chronic HF patients with stable disease.

CHAPTER 19

Specific proteins

QUESTIONS

• Q 1

Define endosmosis. Which proteins are weakly anionic and are swept up in endosmotic flow? *(p. 233)*

• Q 2

What electrophoretic technique resolves various forms of a single protein, and is used in clinical laboratories? *(p. 233)*

• Q 3

What is the most common analyte measured by affinity chromatography, and what chemical is used to bind the molecule of interest? *(p. 234)*

• Q 4–9

Match the method of protein quantitation to its description. *(pp. 234–235)*

Q4 _____ Kjeldahl technique   A. A drop of serum is placed on a refractometer

Q5 _____ Specific gravity   B. Acid digestion releases ammonium ions which are then quantitated using iodides

Q6 _____ Turbidimetry   C. Copper salts in alkaline solution form a purple complex with substances with two or more peptide bonds

Q7 _____ Biuret method   D. Most common dye-binding method to quantitate albumin

Q8 _____ Ninhydrin   E. Used often to detect peptides after paper chromotography or ion exchange

Q9 _____ Bromcresol green   F. An acid such as trichloroacetic forms a precipitate which clouds the solution

• Q 10

What is the chief physiologic function of prealbumin? *(p. 235)*

• Q 11

What is the clinical significance of a prealbumin band in CSF? *(p. 236)*

• Q 12

Do patients with analbuminemia suffer from ascites and edema, as do cirrhotics? *(p. 236)*

• Q 13

What methods are used to screen patients suspected of having the ZZ phenotype of AAT deficiency? *(p. 237)*

• Q 14

In what disease state is alpha-2-macroglobulin most increased? *(p. 237)*

• Q 15

Does haptoglobin bind myoglobin in cases of rhabdomyolysis? *(p. 238)*

• Q 16

Clinical Consultation: A 17-year-old male admitted after a motor vehicle accident has a small amount of clear fluid draining from his left nasal passage. Describe how you can determine if this fluid is CSF. *(p. 238)*

• Q 17

Clinical Consultation: A 38-year-old female on oral contraceptives being treated with heparin for a pulmonary embolism has blood drawn in a red top tube for serum protein electrophoresis (SPEP). A distinct band is noted just anodal to the gamma fraction. How will you explore this result more thoroughly before assuming that it is a monoclonal band? *(p. 239)*

• Q 18

Which acute phase reactant rises most quickly and returns to normal most quickly in inflammatory states? *(p. 241)*

• Q 19–25

Using Figure 19.1, match the protein electrophoresis pattern with the most appropriate history. All samples are serum, except C, which is urine. Use the letters A–G on the SPEP for your answers. *(p. 241–242)*

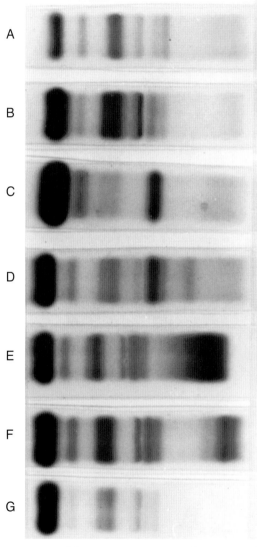

Q19 _____ A 23-year-old pregnant woman with an iron of 27 μg/dL and iron-binding capacity of 603 μg/dL

Q20 _____ A 1-year-old boy with recurrent infections and no CD19-positive lymphocytes on a peripheral blood flow cytometry

Q21 _____ A 28-year-old HIV-positive male with marked peripheral edema
(urine sample)

Q22 _____ Same patient as in Question 21 (serum sample)

Q23 _____ A 30-year-old type 1 diabetic who had a kidney transplant
1 year ago

Q24 _____ A 60-year-old male alcoholic with a total protein of
9.4 g/dL and an albumin of 3.1 g/dL

Q25 _____ An 83-year-old female living alone, subsisting on tea
and toast

ANSWERS

A1. The buffer solutions used in electrophoresis contain positively charged ions.
When a current is applied, these ions are carried toward the negatively charged
cathode in a sort of sweeping fashion. Proteins that are weakly negative, such as
globulins, poorly resist the sweeping action and are swept toward the cathode.
Strongly negative proteins, such as albumin, move straight for the positively
charged anode.

A2. This is isoelectric focusing. SDS–PAGE is an alternative method, but it is used
chiefly in research laboratories.

A3. Quantitation of glycosylated hemoglobin is a very common test with the large
diabetic population. The affinity matrix utilizes dihydroxyboronate.

A4. B

A5. A

A6. F

A7. C

A8. E

A9. D

A10. Although we refer to prealbumin as thyroxine-binding prealbumin, it actually
contributes little to the physiology of thyroxine transport. More important is its
role in vitamin A metabolism. It binds to vitamin A along with retinol-binding
protein to transport vitamin A throughout the body.

A11. This is a normal finding. As a compact molecule, prealbumin crosses the
CSF barrier more readily than do other proteins, and it shows up on CSF
electrophoresis.

A12. No. These patients engage in compensatory mechanisms to maintain their
oncotic pressure.

A13. Both nephelometry and serum protein electrophoresis are used in screening. Confirmation must be performed with ancillary tests in order to rule out other alleles, however. The ZZ phenotype shows markedly decreased levels of AAT.

A14. Nephrotic syndrome. As a particularly large molecule, alpha-2-macroglobulin (AMG) is not lost through the glomerulus as are other, smaller proteins. There may also be enhanced synthesis of AMG during nephrotic syndromes as well.

A15. No. Haptoglobin scavenges hemoglobin in times of hemolysis, but not myoglobin. One may use serum haptoglobin levels to distinguish between hemolysis and rhabdomyolysis when one is confronted with a positive urine dipstick for blood, which could be either hemoglobin or myoglobin. The dipstick will not distinguish the two.

A16. There is a variant of transferrin found in normal CSF. This manifests as a double band on CSF electrophoresis. One can run a parallel set of electrophoreses on this patient – one on the nasal fluid, one on his serum. If the serum has a single band, showing that he has normal monotypic serum transferrin, and the CSF shows the expected double band, then you may diagnose the fluid as coming from the CSF.

A17. This unexpected band is fibrinogen. Heparinized patients' blood does not always clot completely, even when blood is drawn in a red top tube. Unclotted blood will demonstrate fibrinogen on an SPEP, and as this as an acute phase reactant, and as this patient has just had an event (her PE), her fibrinogen may be elevated and even more prominent than it would otherwise be. It would be helpful to redraw the blood in another red top, and observe for more complete clotting before running the SPEP. An alternative technique is to add thrombin to the sample to cause clotting.

A18. This is C-reactive protein.

A19. D

A20. G

A21. C

A22. B

A23. F

A24. E

A25. A

CHAPTER 20
Clinical enzymology

QUESTIONS

• Q 1

Electrophoretic migration of isoenzymes forms the basis of standard nomenclature. Any isoenzyme designated '1' has what migration pattern? *(p. 246)*

• Q 2

Write the Michaelis–Menten equation. *(Eq. 20–13, p. 249)*

• Q 3

In the Michaelis–Menten equation, what is the velocity of a reaction when $K_M = S$? *(Eq. 20–18, p. 249)*

• Q 4–6

Match the pattern of inhibition with its definitions. (*Figs. 20–8–20–11, pp. 250–251*)

Q4 _____ Competitive

Q5 _____ Noncompetitive

Q6 _____ Uncompetitive

A. Inhibitor binds to a site on the enzyme apart from the active site.

B. Inhibitor binds to the enzyme's catalytic site.

C. Inhibitor binds to enzyme–substrate complex and prevents it from dissociating.

D. K_M and V_{max} are both reduced.

E. K_M increases, V_{max} is unchanged.

F. K_M is unchanged, V_{max} decreases.

• Q 7

When enzyme activity is measured in a sample, the reaction rate, V, is set to proceed at maximum velocity, V_{max}. Using the Michaelis–Menten equation, what substrate concentration will allow the reaction to proceed at V_{max}? (*Eq. 20–21, p. 249*)

• Q 8

In clinical laboratory reactions that measure enzyme activity, what order kinetics is occurring? (*p. 254*)

• Q 9

What is the utility of acid phosphatase (ACP) in screening for and monitoring prostate cancer? (*p. 255*)

• Q 10

A 38-year-old woman who is blood group O demonstrates an increase in her alkaline phosphatase (ALP) level of 26 IU/L from her baseline in a sample taken immediately after a meal. When will her ALP return to her baseline? How about in the woman's 31-year-old, group O sister who just delivered a baby and has increased ALP due to the placental contribution? *(p. 256)*

• Q 11

An overweight black male smoker who takes phenobarbital for a seizure disorder has an ALP of 147 IU/L. Give four reasons for this individual having an ALP above the upper reference limit. *(p. 256)*

• Q 12

A 59-year-old woman who takes Prempro and smokes 1/2–1 pack of cigarettes per day has an angiotensin-converting enzyme (ACE) level of 25 IU/L. Her twin sister, a nonsmoker who takes no medications, has an ACE level of 52 IU/L. How do you explain these results? *(p. 257)*

• Q 13

True/False. While angiotensin-converting enzyme (ACE) levels are not specific for sarcoidosis, they are fairly sensitive indicators of disease activity. *(p. 257)*

• Q 14

Clinical Consultation: A military medical officer is deploying with a unit which may be exposed to organophosphates as a chemical weapon. Although the soldiers will take prophylaxis, the medical officer is preparing for the event of exposure. Before the unit deploys, what laboratory test do you recommend and why? *(p. 258)*

• Q 15

For the following disorders, give the lactate dehydrogenase isoenzyme that is typically elevated. *(Table 20–8, pp. 258–259)*
Skeletal muscle injury: _____
Leukemia: _____
Hemolytic anemia: _____
Toxic hepatic injury: _____

• Q 16

How useful are myoglobin assays compared to other tests in diagnosing rhabdomyolysis? *(p. 260)*

· ·

ANSWERS

A1. The number '1' isoenzyme is the one that migrates the farthest toward the anode. Recall that the anode is positively charged, so the protein that migrates farthest toward it will be the one which is most negatively charged.

A2. $v_{o} = \dfrac{V_{max}\,[S]}{([S] + K_{M})}$

A3. This is $1/2 V_{max}$

A4. B, E.

A5. A, F.

A6. C, D.

A7. A substrate concentration much, much greater than the K_M will achieve this: $S >>> K_M$.

A8. This is zero-order kinetics. Any reaction can be pushed to zero-order kinetics by increasing the substrate concentration high enough.

A9. ACP is less sensitive than prostate-specific antigen (PSA) in screening and lacks specificity, being elevated in benign prostatic hyperplasia. However, it is unaffected by androgen levels and may be used to monitor for recurrence in men on androgen deprivation therapy.

A10. The 38-year-old woman's ALP will return to baseline in a short time (within an hour), as the $t_{1/2}$ of intestinal ALP is just minutes. Her sister will take a few weeks to normalize, as the $t_{1/2}$ of placental ALP is 7 days.

A11. Black males have about 15% higher ALP than white males. Obesity and smoking both increase total ALP. Tobacco contributes via pulmonary placenta-like ALP. In patients on phenobarbital, the liver fraction is elevated.

A12. Smokers have ACE levels which are roughly 30% lower than those in nonsmokers. Also, postmenopausal estrogen replacement lowers the ACE levels by 20%.

A13. True. If a sarcoidosis patient is known to have an elevated ACE level, then it may be useful as a monitor of granuloma activity.

A14. The members of the unit should have a baseline pseudocholinesterase level. There is significant inter-individual variation, and symptomatic persons may have levels which are technically within the reference range. However, a fall from one's baseline, or significant intra-individual variation, can be documented and is clinically useful in anticipating symptoms.

A15. Skeletal muscle injury – LD_5
Leukemia – LD_3
Hemolytic anemia – LD_1
Toxic hepatic injury – LD_5

A16. Not very useful. This is due to the insensitivity of assays for myoglobin and its short half-life. A very high CK (some suggest 20 times the upper reference limit), coupled with markers of cell lysis such as potassium and phosphate, is a better approach.

CHAPTER 21

Evaluation of liver function

QUESTIONS

Q 1

What is the most important test of hepatic metabolic function? *(p. 263)*

Q 2

What cellular organelle conjugates bilirubin in the liver? *(Fig. 21–2, p. 264)*

Q 3

What enzyme is responsible for conjugation of bilirubin, and what two diseases are due to mutations in the gene for this enzyme? *(Fig. 21–2, pp. 264–265)*

Q 4

Clay-colored stool is due to the absence of what pigment? *(p. 264)*

Q 5

Review the congenital causes of hyperbilirubinemia by completing the following chart. *(Fig. 21–2, pp. 264–265)*

Disease	Elevated bilirubin fraction	Enzyme/protein defect	Prognosis
Dubin–Johnson			
Crigler–Najjar I			
Crigler–Najjar II			
Gilbert's			

Q 6

What reagents are used to measure total bilirubin? Include the main reagent as well as the accelerants used to speed up the reaction of the slow unconjugated bilirubin. *(p. 265)*

Q 7

Is arterial or venous blood the preferred specimen for measurement of ammonia in cases of hepatic encephalopathy? *(p. 266)*

Q 8

Explain the etiology of hypertriglyceridemia in a cirrhotic patient who does not have a congenital enzyme deficiency and has provided a fasting sample. *(p. 266)*

Q 9

What is the role of ceruloplasmin in iron metabolism? *(p. 267)*

Q 10

Describe the likely patterns of elevated AST vs. ALT in acute hepatocellular injury over time by stating which is higher. *(p. 269)*

First 24 hours: _____

After 24–48 hours: _____

Q 11

List three medications that increase gamma-glutamyl transferase levels. *(p. 270)*

Q 12

What subtype of antimitochondrial antibody is specific for primary biliary cirrhosis (PBC)? *(p. 271)*

Q 13

Compare and contrast type 1 and type 2 autoimmune hepatitis. *(p. 271)*

	Antibodies (common)	Age	Seen in USA?
Type 1			
Type 2			

Q 14

What is the incubation period of hepatitis A virus (HAV)? *(Fig. 21–4, p. 271)*

Q 15

What is the incubation period of hepatitis B virus (HBV)? *(Fig. 21–5, pp. 271–272)*

• Q 16

What is the first serologic marker of HBV infection, and how soon after exposure is it detectable in most cases? *(p. 271)*

• Q 17

What antibody is useful in assessing recovery and clearance of HBV? *(p. 272)*

• Q 18

What HBV marker correlates well with the amount of HBV DNA? *(p. 272)*

• Q 19–22

Using Table 21.1 *(Table 21–1, p. 272)* interpret the HBV serology patterns.

Pattern	IGM anti-HBc	Total anti-HBc	HBsAg	Anti-HBs	HBeAg	Anti-HBe
1	–	–	+	–	–	–
2	+	+	+	–	+	–
3	+	+	–	+	–	+
4	+	+	–	–	–	–
5	–	+	+	–	+	–
6	–	+	+	–	–	+
7	–	+	–	+	–	+
8	–	–	–	+	–	–

Q19 Which pattern indicates a resolved HBV infection? _____

Q20 What is the interpretation of pattern #2? _____

Q21 Is the person with pattern #5 infectious to others? _____

Q22 How likely is an elevation of ALT in patient #1?_____

• Q 23

What confirmatory tests are used for hepatitis C virus (HCV) in the following situations? *(p. 273)*

Blood donor with positive anti-HCV: _____

Chronically infected HCV patient: _____

Q 24

Which HCV genotypes are most responsive to treatment? Which type(s) is/are most common in the USA? *(p. 273)*

Q 25

What is the cardinal laboratory finding in acute hepatitis? *(p. 274)*

Q 26

What is the most common molecular defect in hemochromatosis, and where is the *HFE* gene located? *(p. 274)*

ANSWERS

A1. This is bilirubin.

A2. Conjugation occurs in the smooth endoplasmic reticulum.

A3. The conjugation enzyme is uridine diphosphate (UDP) glucuronyl transferase. Different mutations result in Gilbert's and Crigler–Najjar syndromes.

A4. This is stercobilin.

A5.

Disease	Elevated bilirubin fraction	Enzyme/protein defect	Prognosis
Dubin–Johnson	conjugated	canalicular anion transporter	good
Crigler– Najjar I	unconjugated	UDP-glucuronyl trn'ase	poor
Crigler– Najjar II	unconjugated	UDP-glucuronyl trn'ase	fair
Gilbert's	unconjugated	UDP-glucuronyl trn'ase	good

A6. Diazolized sulfanilic acid is the main reagent. The accelerants are caffeine or methanol.
Direct bilirubin is the measurement of bilirubin without the accelerants.

A7. Arterial blood levels correlate with clinical symptoms better than do venous levels. Ammonia is a product of cellular metabolism. Specimens should be kept in ice water until separation of plasma can be performed to limit excess generation of ammonia.

A8. The damaged liver produces decreased amounts of lipoprotein lipase, so TG are not removed from the bloodstream, and measured levels are increased.

A9. Ceruloplasmin converts iron from the ferrous to the ferric state, which allows it to bind to transferrin.

A10. In the first 24 hours, AST is greater than ALT due to the higher activity of AST in the hepatocytes. After 24–48 hours, the longer half-life of ALT makes it the predominant enzyme in serum.

A11. Phenytoin, carbamazepine, and acetaminophen all raise GGT.

A12. This is AMA M2. Other subtypes are associated with other diseases.

A13. In type 1, antinuclear (ANA) and anti-smooth muscle (ASMA) antibodies are commonly seen. This type is seen in adults and is the predominant type seen in the USA.
In type 2, ANA and ASMA are rare, but the anti-liver-kidney microsomal antibodies are seen. This type is seen in children and is much more common in Europe than in the USA.

A14. HAV usually incubates 2–3 weeks, a month and a half at the most.

A15. HBV incubates 1–3 months.

A16. The first marker, seen in most infected persons, is the surface antigen, HBsAg. It shows up 2–3 months after exposure.

A17. Anti-HBs is a good indicator of clearance of the virus.

A18. This is HBeAg.

A19. Pattern #7.

A20. This is acute HBV infection. Note that IgM is still present.

A21. Yes. This is active chronic hepatitis B. Some argue that HBeAg correlates well with infectivity, particularly in pregnant women.

A22. Unlikely. This is the incubation period, and the person is probably asymptomatic and without transaminasemia.

A23. For blood donors, the recombinant immunoassay and nucleic acid test are used. In high-risk populations, a confirmatory test is unnecessary, as the PPV is high. For the chronically infected, HCV RNA is used to monitor disease and assess response to treatment.

A24. Genotypes 2 and 3 respond best to the treatment modalities available. Unfortunately, 65% of white people and 90–95% of black people in the USA are infected with genotype 1, which does not respond as well to treatment.

A25. An elevation of the aminotransferases, frequently to levels greater than 500 IU/L is characteristic of acute hepatitis. Other parameters are often increased as well.

A26. At amino acid 282 in the gene product, tyrosine is substituted for cysteine (C282Y). The *HFE* gene is located on chromosome 6p.

CHAPTER 22

Laboratory diagnosis of gastrointestinal and pancreatic disorders

QUESTIONS

• Q 1

Clinical Consultation: A 34-year-old female has severe gastric ulcers and her clinician wants to rule out gastrinoma. After an overnight fast, her serum gastrin is 550 pg/mL. Describe for the clinician how to perform the secretin test. *(p. 280)*

_____
_____
_____

The clinician performs the test, and at 10 minutes, her gastrin level is 900 pg/mL.
Your diagnosis: _____

• Q 2

What molecules make up the macroamylase complex? *(p. 280)*

• Q 3

What is the predominant form of P-amylase? *(p. 288)* _____
What change in the P2/P1 or P3/P1 ratio strongly suggests a pancreatic pseudocyst?
_____

• Q 4

Clinical Consultation: A remorseful intern brings you a red top tube on Monday morning for serum amylase and lipase measurements. The blood was drawn on Friday afternoon and has been sitting in his lab coat pocket over the weekend. There is some evidence of gross hemolysis. Can you get an accurate reading for these analytes? *(pp. 287–288)*

• Q 5

What is the method of stimulating sweat gland secretion in the sweat chloride test? *(p. 290)*

• Q 6

In a patient with diarrhea and a known carcinoid tumor, what two related analytes will be elevated, and what method is used to measure them? *(Table 22–3, p. 284)*

• Q 7

Which antibody offers the best sensitivity and specificity for diagnosing celiac sprue and is detected by immunofluorescence? *(p. 286)*

• Q 8

What test is the gold standard for fat malabsorption? *(pp. 285, 291)*

How much fat is consumed daily in this test? _____

Q 9

Clinical Consultation: An 8-year-old girl with a history suggestive of cystic fibrosis, but not clearly established, presents for a D-xylose test. She weighs 38 kg. For children, the dose of D-xylose is 0.5 g/kg body weight. A full dose is dissolved in 250 mL of water, and smaller doses are given in proportionately smaller volumes of water. Assist her pediatrician in administering the test. You may need a calculator for this question. *(p. 291)*

What is the dose of D-xylose for this patient? _____

In what volume of water should it be administered? _____

Over 5 hours, she excretes 1.2 g of D-xylose. Does this reflect enteric malabsorption?

_____

What amount should she excrete based on her dose? _____

What is your diagnosis? *(pp. 285, 291)* _____

Q 10

What clinical sequelae, in addition to the expected diabetes, are associated with a glucagonoma? *(Table 22–7, p. 287)*

Q 11

What is the Apt test, and how sensitive is it? *(pp. 290–291)*

ANSWERS

A1. Give 2 U/kg secretin intravenously and measure the serum gastrin at 2, 5, 10, 15, and 20 minutes. An increase by 100 pg/mL supports a diagnosis of Zollinger–Ellison syndrome, and in this patient the increase was 350 pg/mL, so she has a gastrinoma.

A2. Normal amylase is linked to either IgA or IgG in most cases, or to a polysaccharide in some cases.

A3. P1 is the predominant form, accounting for 80–90% of amylase activity. In 90% of patients with a pseudocyst, the ratio of P2/P1 or P3/P1 increases.

A4. Yes. Room temperature is fine for 1 week with both of these analytes. Hemolysis does not interfere with either analyte as long as the turbidimetric method is used. Peroxidase methods would show interference because of the peroxidase activity of hemoglobin.

A5. Pilocarpine is introduced into the skin by iontophoresis.

A6. Urine 5-hydroxyindoleacetic acid and blood serotonin are measured by HPLC.

A7. IgA endomysial activity.

A8. A 72-hour stool collection on high-fat diet with quantitation of fecal fat per 24 hours. Patients consume 100 g of fat daily.

A9. For children, the amount of D-xylose is 0.5 g/kg body weight, so she would ingest 19 g. The full dose is dissolved in 250 mL water, and is adjusted for the lower children's doses. At 19 g, this would be 190 mL water. Urine is saved for 5 hours. Normal excretion of a full dose of D-xylose is 3 gm; for her dose she should excrete 2.28 g. She excretes only 1.2 g, which is consistent with enteric malabsorption. Pancreatic enzymes are not needed for the absorption of D-xylose; yet, she could not absorb it normally. She certainly has enteric maldigestion, not cystic fibrosis.

A10. Other manifestations of this rare neuroendocrine tumor are necrolytic migratory erythema, weight loss, depression, and deep venous thromboses.

A11. The Apt test determines if blood in a newborn's stool is of maternal or neonatal origin. It uses the same principle of alkali denaturation as the Kleihauer test. It has a relatively low sensitivity.

CHAPTER 23

Toxicology and therapeutic drug monitoring

QUESTIONS

• Q 1

In the fluorescence polarization method of detecting a drug in serum, is an *increase* or *decrease* in fluorescence indicative of the presence of the drug? *(Fig. 23–1B, pp. 298–299)*

• Q 2

What technique is considered the gold standard for detection and quantitation of volatile drugs and poisons? *(p. 298)*

• Q 3

Drugs of abuse are usually _____ derivatives, with the exception of barbiturates, which are acids. *(p. 298)*

• Q 4

What advantages does high-performance liquid chromatography (HPLC) offer over traditional thin-layer chromatography (TLC) in the detection of tricyclic antidepressants (TCAs)? *(pp. 298, 300)*

• Q 5

Briefly state the principle of mass spectroscopy. *(p. 302)*

• Q 6

What is the common chemical structure of morphine, codeine, and heroin? *(p. 303)*

• Q 7

What is the less active metabolite of cocaine which may be detected in the urine up to 24–48 hours after cocaine use, depending on the method of testing? *(Fig. 23–7, pp. 303–306)*

• Q 8

True/False. Both heroin and methadone act by binding to μ-receptors in the central nervous system and have a similar chemical structure. *(Fig. 23–7, pp. 304, 306)*

• Q 9

Benzodiazepines appear to work by inducing the secretion of what neurotransmitter? *(p. 306)*

• Q 10

What receptor, newly discovered, does phencyclidine bind to, possibly accounting for the psychosis seen in many users? *(p. 307)*

• Q 11

Why is naloxone an effective antidote for propoxyphene toxicity? *(p. 307)*

• Q 12

What are the two major metabolites of cannabis detected in urine? *(p. 307)*

• Q 13

To what chemical class does lysergic acid diethylamide belong? *(p. 308)*

• Q 14

A steady state of drug concentration is reached in _____ half-lives. *(Fig. 23–9, pp. 308–309)*

• Q 15

What is the mechanism by which procainamide causes a lupus-like syndrome? *(p. 310)*

• Q 16

Why is phenobarbital contraindicated in patients with acute intermittent porphyria? *(p. 311; also Fig. 30–12, p. 492)*

• Q 17

What is the clinical implication of the serum half-life of phenytoin being dose-dependent? *(p. 312)*

• Q 18

True/False. The half-life of theophylline is shorter in smokers than nonsmokers, and shorter still in children. *(Table 23–6, pp. 314–315)*

• Q 19

Clinical Consultation: A 16-year-old female presents to the ER remorseful about a suicide attempt by acetominophen overdose 12 hours ago. She weighs 60 kg and said she took 20 extra-strength (500 mg) tablets. How likely is it that this represents a toxic dose? *(p. 316)*

Her dose: _____

Toxic dose at her weight: _____

Likelihood: _____

• Q 20

Clinical Consultation: Twelve hours after ingesting an unknown quantity of aspirin tablets, a child has a serum salicylate concentration of 62 mg/dL. Using the nomogram, what level of toxicity is this? *(Fig. 23–14, p. 316)*

• Q 21

The optimal trough levels for cyclosporin are 50–300 ng/mL. What kind of toxicity is often seen at trough levels greater than 500 ng/dL? *(p. 317)*

• Q 22

Hyperactive deep tendon reflexes, choreoathetoid movements, and persistent vomiting in a patient with bipolar disorder who states that his last dose of lithium was about 12 hours ago probably has (give qualitative estimate) _____

_____ to _____ toxicity and a lithium level of roughly _____

_____ to _____ mEq/L. *(p. 318)*

Q 23

What are the two cardinal signs of TCA overdose? *(p. 319)*

Q 24

What is the role of the oxidants amyl nitrite or sodium nitrite in treatment of cyanide poisoning? *(pp. 320–321)*

Q 25

What metabolite of ethylene glycol correlates directly with symptomatology and mortality and is the major contributor to the characterisitc high anion gap seen in toxic ingestions? *(p. 321)*

Q 26

Clinical Consultation: 45 minutes after ingesting ant poison, a 6-year-old boy complains of burning in his mouth and throat. He is vomiting and passes bloody stool. An odor of garlic is present on his breath. What toxin did he ingest? *(p. 322)*

Q 27

Which of the four chemical forms of mercury is well absorbed after oral ingestion and typically causes GI symptoms and kidney damage, including acute tubular necrosis? *(p. 322)*

Q 28

What form of iron is toxic to hepatic cells and results in shock and lactic acidosis? *(p. 322)*

Q 29

List the four enzymes in the heme synthetic pathway that are inhibited by lead. *(p. 323)*

Q 30

In cases of *chronic* lead poisoning, what technique allows for the determination of cumulative lead burden? *(p. 323)*

. . . .

ANSWERS

A1. A decrease of fluorescence indicates the presence of drug in the sample. Fluorescence, which arises from immobilized antibody–reagent drug–fluorescent probe complexes, decreases when patient drug binds to the reagent antibodies and frees up reagent drug bound to a fluorescent probe molecule to tumble in solution.

A2. This is gas–chromatography–mass spectroscopy (GC–MS).

A3. Most drugs of abuse are amine derivatives and are basic, except barbiturates.

A4. HPLC is quantitative and allows for a sharp separation of similar compounds, such as parent compounds and their metabolites. However, capillary electrophoresis, a variation of TLC, now offers some of the advantages of HPLC.

A5. High temperatures or electron bombardment of a molecular species will cause the molecules to lose electrons, becoming ionized into cations. These molecule-ions will decompose into characteristic fragments, and these fragments are present in characteristic ratios, resulting in a fingerprint pattern unique to a particular compound.

A6. All are basic, tertiary amines containing a benzene ring.

A7. This is benzoylecgonine.

A8. False. Methadone is a nonbicyclic drug, but both act on the μ-receptor.

A9. This is gamma-aminobutyric acid (GABA).

A10. This is the sigma-receptor.

A11. Propoxyphene has pharmacologic properties similar to those of the opiates, although it is structurally quite different.

A12. These are delta-9-carboxytetrahydrocannabinol (δ-9-carboxy-THC) and 11-hydroxy-delta-9-THC.

A13. LSD is a semisynthetic indolalkylamine.

A14. Steady state is four-plus half-lives.

A15. WBCs convert procainamide to a metabolite which can covalently bind to the membrane proteins of monocytes and macrophages. This then stimulates the production of antibodies. Also, this metabolite can mimic a portion of the histone protein, leading to the production of antihistone antinuclear antibodies.

A16. Barbiturates enhance the synthesis of delta-aminolevulinc acid synthetase. Since AIP patients cannot readily continue in the heme synthetic pathway past porphobilinogen because they lack PBG deaminase, they accumulate both ALA and PBG when given barbiturates.

A17. Excretion does not follow first-order kinetics. Thus, small increases in dosage can result in great increases in serum concentration, causing toxicity.

A18. True. The text in this edition does not address the half-life in children, but it is shorter than in adults, no matter their habits.

A19. Quite likely. She ingested 10 000 mg and a toxic dose for her weight is 8400 mg.

A20. Using the nomogram, this would be mild-moderate toxicity.

A21. Nephrotoxicity occurs at this high level.

A22. These signs constitute moderate to severe toxicity. It is likely that his lithium level is between 2.5–3.5 mEq/L. Note, though, that Henry stresses that lithium levels do not correlate all that well with clinical presentations.

A23. Dry skin and, in particular, dilated pupils are the two key signs.

A24. Either of these agents will convert hemoglobin (Fe^{2+}) to methemoglobin (Fe^{3+}). The cyanide ion CN^- binds reversibly to cytochrome A_3 to inhibit cellular respiration, but it can be removed with methemoglobin. Methemoglobin competes with ferricytochrome A_3 to form a complex with the CN^- ion, cyanomethemoglobin, which can then be converted to thiocyanate and excreted in the urine.

A25. This is glycolic acid.

A26. This is arsenic. If the garlic odor is not given as a clue, then the history of insecticides/ant poison is a helpful clue to arsenic as the agent.

A27. This is mercuric salt, in the Hg^{2+} form. This is one of the inorganic forms of mercury.

A28. Elemental iron, Fe, is very toxic when free in the body. A high enough dose overwhelms the transferrin sites.

A29. These are ALA synthetase, ALA dehydratase, coproporphyrinogen decarboxylase, and ferrochelatase.

A30. As 96% of the total body burden of lead is in bone, a fluorescence X-ray is more useful than blood lead levels. Lead does not stay in the blood very long, so serum levels are really helpful in acute exposures rather than chronic exposures.

CHAPTER 24

Evaluation of endocrine function

QUESTIONS

• Q 1

Clinical Consultation: A 30-year-old male has been showing the physical manifestations of acromegaly over a 2-year period. A random insulin-like growth factor-1 (IGF-1) is elevated at 1650 ng/mL (four times the upper reference limit). *(p. 330)*

What test do you recommend to confirm the clinician's suspicion, in addition to an MRI of the brain?

_____

_____

After a surgical resection of a pituitary adenoma, what two tests may be used to monitor this patient?

_____

_____

• Q 2

What is the most common hormone secreted by a pituitary adenoma? *(Table 24–3, p. 328)*

● Q 3

Clinical Consultation: A 67-year-old female with small cell carcinoma of the lung is suspected of having syndrome of inappropriate antidiuretic hormone (SIADH). Her serum sodium today is 132 mmol/L, Cr is 1.0 mg/dL. She weighs 60 kg. Assist the clinician in performing a water load test. *(Table 24–8, pp. 333–334)*

The clinician says that the patient completed chemotherapy 3 months ago. What other medications do you want to know about, as they can cause SIADH?

_____

She takes no medications at this time. Her water load should be _____ mL, to be consumed within _____ minutes. The clinician should collect urine every _____ for the next _____ hours.

The woman does as you instruct, and passes a total of 610 mL of urine over 5 hours. Your diagnosis: _____

● Q 4

What is the first test to perform in determining thyroid dysfunction, because of its high sensitivity? *(p. 337)*

● Q 5

T_3 thyrotoxicosis, due to elevated serum triiodothyronine, has what laboratory values (high, normal, or low)? *(p. 338)*

T_4: _____

Free T_4: _____

T_3: _____

TSH: _____

● Q 6

Clinical Consultation: A 28-year-old female is found to have lost 15 lb on a routine physical examination and has a mild tremor. The clinician suspects Graves' disease and finds that her TSH is very low and T_4 is elevated. Upon further questioning, he finds that she seems unconcerned with her abnormal results and reluctant to pursue any more studies. He then wonders if she is taking thyroxine surreptitiously. What two tests can you recommend to distinguish these two disorders? *(p. 339)*

Q 7

If plasma free metanephrine and normetanephrine are not available, then what methodology of what test is the most sensitive urine screening test for pheochromocytoma? *(p. 342)*

Q 8

Which test has the greatest sensitivity (90% of patients positive) in children with suspected neuroblastoma? *(p. 344)*

Q 9

Most inborn errors of adrenal cortical steroid metabolism involve what type of enzyme? *(p. 344)*

Q 10

What is the most common congenital enzyme deficiency of the adrenal cortex? *(p. 346)*

Q 11

What are the genes responsible for 21-hydroxylase and 11β-hydroxylase deficiencies? *(pp. 346, 348)*
21-hydroxylase: _____
11β-hydroxylase: _____

Q 12

What is the substrate for 21-hydroxylase, which is present in excess in the plasma of persons with the enzyme deficiency? *(Fig. 24–11, pp. 346–347)*

Q 13

Why do persons with 11β-hydroxylase deficiency have hypertension when the pathway to aldosterone is blocked? *(Fig. 24–11, p. 347)*

Q 14

In 17-hydroxylase deficiency, testosterone levels are low, because progesterone cannot be converted to the precursor of the sex steroids, which is: *(Fig. 24–11, pp. 347–348)*

Q 15

ACTH levels can discriminate between primary and secondary adrenal insufficiency, without the need for a stimulation test. What levels of ACTH are useful cutoffs? *(p. 355)*

Primary: _____

Secondary: _____

Q 16

Which methodology offers high specificity for both serum cortisol and urinary free cortisol measurements? *(pp. 351–352)*

Q 17

What is the most common endogenous disorder of glucocorticoid excess? *(p. 353)*

Q 18

What will be the effect of the high-dose dexamethasone suppression test on a patient with adrenal adenoma or adrenal carcinoma? *(Table 24–22 and Fig. 24–17, pp. 354–355)*

With adrenal adenoma: _____

With adrenal carcinoma: _____

• Q 19

How specific is the overnight dexamethasone suppression test in hospitalized patients? *(p. 353)*

• Q 20

Outline the principle of the metyrapone test to assess for pituitary insufficiency. What is the major risk in performing this test? *(p. 355)*

• Q 21

What are the typical changes in these laboratory parameters in primary hyperaldosteronism? *(pp. 357–358)*

Serum K: _____

Urine K: _____

Plasma renin: _____

Urine aldosterone: _____

· ·

ANSWERS

A1. The oral glucose tolerance test (OGTT) should be performed. An acromegalic patient will fail to suppress GH to less than 1 ng/mL and may show a paradoxical rise in GH with the glucose load. These patients are usually monitored with insulin-like growth hormone (IGF-1) after surgical removal of their pituitary tumor, although the OGGT may also be used.

A2. Prolactin-secreting adenomas are the most common adenoma of the pituitary.

A3. A person with such a devastating malignancy may be on antidepressants; both tricyclics and monoamine oxidase inhibitors, as well as nicotine can cause SIADH. At 60 kg, this woman should drink 20 × 60 = 1200 mL of water over 30 minutes. Urine is collected hourly for 5 hours, and volume and osmolality are tested on each sample. She passed less than 80% of the water load in

5 hours, excreting only 51%. This, in the absence of other causative factors, is sufficient for the diagnosis of SIADH.

A4. This is thyroid-stimulating hormone (TSH).

A5. In T_3 thyrotoxicosis, T_4 and free T_4 are normal, while T_3 is elevated. TSH is suppressed and low.

A6. Thyroglobulin is a key test here. It will be undetectable in thyrotoxicosis factitia, but will be elevated in Graves' disease. Another option is the TSH receptor antibodies, which are present in Graves', but would be absent in a factitious disorder.

A7. A 24-hour urinary total metanephrine assay, measured by high-performance liquid chromatography (HPLC), would be best. A 24-hour sample will pick up the intermittent release of metanephrines, and a total metanephrines is preferred over individual metanephrines in a screening test. Additionally, urinary catecholamines are a sensitive test. VMA lacks sensitivity, with 10–30% false negatives.

A8. This is urinary homovanillic acid (HVA). Additionally, urinary vanillymandelic acid is present in 75% of cases of neuroblastoma.

A9. This is a hydroxylase enzyme in the steroid biosynthesis pathway.

A10. 21-hydroxylase deficiency is by far the most common, accounting for 95% of cases.

A11. 21-OH is *CYP21*. 11β-OH is *CYP11B 1* and *2*.

A12. This is 17α-hydroxyprogesterone.

A13. Deoxycorticosterone (DOC) has mineralocorticoid activity. This is one of the steroids in excess in these patients.

A14. This is 17α-hydroxyprogesterone.

A15. In primary adrenal insufficiency, levels are elevated, usually above 50–100 pg/mL, as the pituitary tries to whip the adrenal into action. In secondary adrenal insufficiency, levels are decreased, often to less than 10 pg/mL.

A16. This is HPLC.

A17. This is Cushing's disease, due to an ACTH-producing tumor of the pituitary.

A18. Patients with adrenal adenomas or carcinomas usually do not suppress with high-dose dexamethasone.

A19. Not very specific. There is a 30% false-positive rate. Patients in hospital frequently have excess cortisol, because they are stressed.

A20. Metyrapone is taken orally at midnight. It is an inhibitor of 11-hydroxylase and thus blocks cortisol production. This should stimulate the pituitary to release ACTH to increase cortisol levels. Plasma 11-deoxycortisol and cortisol are measured the following morning at 8 a.m. to assess the response. The major drawback is that patients with inadequate pituitary function may suffer acute adrenal insufficiency during the test when you shut off what little cortisol they have.

A21. Serum K is low, as it is lost in the urine, so urine K is high. Plasma renin is low, as it is suppressed by the high levels of aldosterone. Urine aldosterone is high as the person excretes the excess.

CHAPTER 25

Reproductive function and pregnancy

QUESTIONS

Q 1

List three key indications for performing semen analysis. *(p. 368)*

Q 2

A patient collecting semen should remain abstinent for a fairly strict period of
_____ to _____ days, and he should transport
his semen sample to the laboratory within _____ hour(s) of
collection. *(p. 368)*

Q 3

What is the normal pH of semen? *(p. 368)*

Q 4

Normal sperm motility is considered to be greater than _____%. *(p. 368)*

• Q 5

What are the two methods to detect sperm antibodies, and what type of antibody is clinically most significant? *(p. 369)*

• Q 6

Which common subunit is found in follicle-stimulating hormone (FSH), luteinizing hormone (LH) and thyroid-stimulating hormone (TSH), and which subunit confers functional specificity? *(p. 366)*

• Q 7

What is the typical laboratory profile (which hormones are increased or decreased) in an infertile male with a 47, XXY karyotype? *(p. 369)*

• Q 8

What subunits do most immunometric assays for human chorionic gonadotropin (HCG) measure, and when does HCG reach a maximum in a normal pregnancy? *(p. 372)*

• Q 9

A blighted ovum is indicated by what levels of estradiol and progesterone? *(p. 373)*

• Q 10

Assisted reproductive technology (ART) involves the administration of several hormones to stimulate specific physiologic processes. State the function of the following medications. *(p. 371)*

GnRH analog: _____

Human menopausal gonadotropin (HMG): _____

HCG bolus: _____

• Q 11

Fetal serum α-fetoprotein (AFP) concentrations peak at 12–14 weeks' gestation, yet maternal screening is performed in the *second* trimester. *(p. 373)* Why is this?

• Q 12

What anticonvulsant is associated with an increased risk of neural tube defects? *(p. 373)*

• Q 13

State the five clinical factors that are taken into account in determining the maternal serum α-fetoprotein (MSAFP) multiples of the median (MoM) and how each affects the MSAFP. *(p. 373)*

• Q 14

What is the profile of maternal serum markers in fetal Down syndrome? *(p. 374)*

MSAFP: _____

Unconjugated estriol (uE3): _____

HCG: _____

• Q 15

A 23-year-old woman who has taken no prenatal vitamins has an MSAFP of her singleton fetus that is 6.8 multiples of the mean (MoM). The ultrasound is abnormal. What is the most likely diagnosis? *(p. 374)*

• Q 16

What lecithin/sphingomyelin (L/S) ratio indicates fetal lung maturity? *(p. 376)*

• Q 17

True/False. The primary risk to the fetus in hemolytic disease of the newborn is the accumulation of unconjugated bilirubin in the central nervous system (kernicterus). *(p. 374)*

• Q 18

Interpret the Liley graph in Figure 25.1. *(p. 375 Also Figure 25.10, p. 375)*

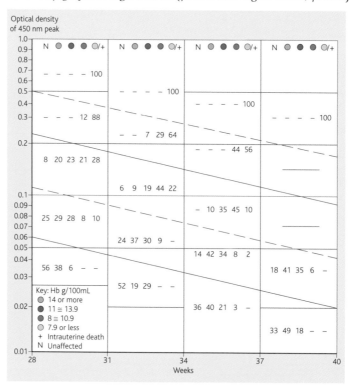

Fig. 25.1
(From Liley AW: Am J Obstet Gynecol 1963; 86:485, with permission.)

At 31–34 weeks of gestation, an absorbance at 450 nm of 0.1 is associated with a hemoglobin of 7.9 g/dL or less and/or fetal demise in what percent of cases?

At 37–40 weeks' gestation, what percent of fetuses with an absorbance of 0.035 have a Hb of 11–13.9 g/dL? _____

• Q 19

Briefly outline the commonly used test for diagnosing premature rupture of membranes. *(p. 376)*

• Q 20

Although the lecithin/sphingomyelin (L/S) ratio is frequently measured by thin-layer chromatography to assess fetal lung maturity, this method has several disadvantages. Briefly list them, including the pre-analytic variables affecting its accuracy. *(p. 376)*

. . . .

ANSWERS

A1. Semen analysis is used in the evaluation of male infertility, to select donors for therapeutic insemination, and to monitor the success of surgical procedures such as varicocelectomy and vasectomy.

A2. Semen for analysis should be collected after 3 days, but not more than 5 days from the last intercourse, and should be transported to the laboratory within 1 hour of collection.

A3. Normal pH is 7.2–7.8. Acute prostatitis or epididymitis may raise the pH above 8.0, and urine contamination can lower it below 7.0.

A4. Normally more than 50% of sperm are motile. There is a grading scale from 0–4 for assessing motility, and a score of 2 is considered normal.

A5. Sperm antibodies can be detected by a direct or indirect mixed agglutination reaction, or by an immunobead assay. The agglutination reaction can pick up IgG or IgA, and the immunobead assay can pick up IgG, IgA, or IgM. IgA is the most clinically significant.

A6. The α-subunit is common, while the β-subunit confers specificity.

A7. The 47, XXY karyotype is termed Klinefelter's syndrome. The pathophysiology is characterized by primary testicular failure. Thus, testosterone is decreased, and the normal pituitary gland secretes excess FSH and LH because it receives no negative feedback in the form of inhibin from the testes.

A8. These 'sandwich' assays usually measure both the free β-subunit, which is specific for HCG, and intact HCG, which contains both the α- and β-subunits. The maximum HCG level is usually reached at 10 weeks' gestation.

A9. An estradiol of <200 ng/mL and a progesterone of <15 ng/mL indicate a blighted ovum.

A10. The GnRH analog suppresses normal FSH and LH synthesis and secretion. HMG has predominantly FSH activity, so it will stimulate follicular growth of several follicles simultaneously. The HCG bolus acts as the LH surge of midcycle and stimulates ovulation.

A11. Fetal serum AFP diffuses across the amniotic membrane into the amniotic fluid (AF) and then from the AF into maternal serum (MS). The AFAFP levels peak at 13–14 weeks' gestation, but due to changes in the transfer to MS and maternal clearance of AFP, the MSAFP levels increase by approximately 15% per gestational week in the second trimester.

A12. This is valproate.

A13. Maternal weight – MSAFP decreases with increasing weight.
Race – black people have levels 10–15% higher than white people.
IDDM – levels are 20% lower than in the general population.
Multiple gestation – MSAFP is proportional to the number of fetuses.
Gestational age – MSAFP increases 15% per week in the second trimester.

A14. MSAFP is low, by about 25%. uE3 is low. HCG is high, usually 2.0 MoM.

A15. With an MoM of 6.8, this is very likely to be anencephaly.

A16. An L/S ratio of 2.0 is indicative of fetal lung maturity.

A17. False. The placenta normally removes unconjugated bilirubin, and it thus appears in the AF. Anemia is the primary risk to the fetus. *After delivery*, both anemia and kernicterus threaten the neonate.

A18. 31–34 weeks, 0.1 transmittance – 22% are in poor outcome category.
37–40 weeks, 0.035 transmittance – 35% should have a Hb of 11–13.9 g/dL.

A19. To detect amniotic fluid (AF) in the posterior vaginal pool, a sample of fluid is aspirated and placed on nitrazine-impregnated paper. An alkaline pH of 7.0–7.5 (recall that AF is an alkaline fluid, while vaginal secretions are acidic) will turn the paper a blue color and indicate rupture of the amniotic membranes.

A20. The L/S ratio method is slow, labor intense, and only 25% sensitive in predicting respiratory distress syndrome at the level of 2.0. Vaginal secretions and meconium both interfere with measurement.

CHAPTER 26

Vitamins and trace elements

QUESTIONS

• Q 1

The human body depends on dietary intake for all of the vitamins except _____
_____ *(p. 380)*

• Q 2

Strict vegetarians who consume no animal products may become deficient in these vitamins if they do not supplement it into their diet. *(p. 382)*

• Q 3

If corn is rich in niacin, why is pellagra (niacin deficiency) prevalent in regions of the world where corn is a staple food in the diet? *(p. 382)*

• Q 4

An alcoholic presents to a local emergency department in a confused state and has an epileptic seizure. Alcohol withdrawal and hypoglycemia are certainly likely causes, but in this case, a plasma pyridoxal 5′-phosphate (PLP) level is decreased. *(p. 383)* What vitamin deficiency explains these findings?

• Q 5

What is the most common cause of cobalamine deficiency? *(p. 383)*

• Q 6

True/False. A 22-year-old woman eats three to four carrots daily and manifests yellow-orange discoloration of her skin. This represents vitamin A toxicity, and she should be counseled to restrict her intake of carrots. *(p. 384)*

• Q 7

A 31-year-old male with celiac sprue has been noncompliant with his diet and has suffered a 15-pound weight loss since his last check-up 4 months ago. He reports easy bruising, but denies gum bleeding. What laboratory test can you perform to quickly evaluate his vitamin K status? *(p. 384)* _____

• Q 8

What is the method of choice for determination of serum, plasma, or urine copper levels? *(p. 385)*

• Q 9

How useful is a serum copper level in the assessment of the following patients? *(p.387)*
14-year-old female with early stage anorexia: _____
4-month-old male with kinky hair and poor mental development: _____
21-year-old with acute hepatitis and neuropsychiatric symptoms: _____

• Q 10

True/False. While zinc is a cofactor for almost 300 enzymes, it exists only in a divalent state in the body and thus cannot participate in oxidation–reduction reactions. *(p. 387)*

• Q 11

You are on a mission to evaluate zinc deficiency in a third-world country. You draw whole blood samples into red top tubes on 20 children in a small village early in the morning before they have eaten breakfast and transport the tubes 100 miles back to the city hospital, where flame atomic absorption spectrometry is performed the following day. None of the children has a low zinc level; in fact, many have significantly elevated levels. What happened? *(p. 388)*

ANSWERS

A1. This is vitamin D, which is synthesized in the skin from a cholesterol precursor.

A2. These are cobalamine, or vitamin B_{12} and vitamin D.

A3. The niacin in corn is bound to protein and is poorly bioavailable. Other grains, and meat, eggs and milk, are superior sources of niacin.

A4. This is vitamin B_6, or pyridoxine, deficiency.

A5. Atrophy of the gastric mucosa, with inadequate intrinsic factor and subsequent malabsorption, is the most common cause.

A6. False. Excessive carotene intake, from eating carrots, is benign. Most vitamin A toxicity results from intake of supplement capsules.

A7. A prothrombin time will provide a functional assessment of his vitamin K stores.

A8. Atomic absorption spectrometry is the method of choice for copper levels, as it is for most metals.

A9. Serum copper is a useful test in the assessment of Menkes' kinky hair syndrome, where serum copper is decreased. In Wilson's disease and in all but the most severe cases of malnutrition, this is not a useful test. Ceruloplasmin would be a better test for Wilson's disease, and a simple serum albumin for the anorexic patient.

A10. True.

A11. Zinc is present in 10 times the concentration in erythrocytes as compared to serum. Hemolysis, as occurred in the plain red top tubes, falsely increased the results.

Part III

Urine and other body fluids

CHAPTER 27

Basic examination of urine

QUESTIONS

Q 1

What are the three essential labeling requirements for a urine specimen? *(p. 394)*

Q 2

What is the typical color of urine in lead porphyrinuria? *(p. 394)*

Q 3

Describe the foam test to distinguish normal concentrated urine from bilirubinuria. *(p. 394)*

Q 4

A patient with ulcerative colitis taking sulfasalazine might have what color of urine at pH 7.5? *(Table 27–3, p. 395)*

Q 5

What is the characteristic odor of urine in a patient with tyrosinemia? *(p. 396)*

Q 6

Define specific gravity and osmolality and state which parameter would be affected more in the following situations. *(p. 396)*
Specific gravity: _____
Osmolality: _____
Patient with hyperaldosteronism (kaliuria): _____
Patient with nephrotic syndrome: _____

Q 7

Briefly state the principle of the reagent strip method of measuring urine specific gravity. *(p. 397)*

Q 8

Will the following persons have acidic or alkaline urine? *(p. 398)*
Postprandial – citrus fruit salad: _____
Postprandial – turkey with cranberry sauce: _____
Proximal renal tubular acidosis: _____
Person taking acetazolamide: _____

Q 9

How sensitive is each of the following methods in detecting Bence Jones proteins? *(p. 400)*
Tetrabromphenol blue at pH 3: _____
Sulfosalicylic acid: _____
Electrophoresis with Coomassie brilliant blue: _____

Q 10

Reinforce the fact that reagent strip methods for determining glucose in urine are specific for glucose by writing out the double sequential enzyme reaction. *(p. 401)*

Q 11

What method would you use to estimate the fructose in urine in a neonate with hereditary fructose intolerance? The previous day, fructose was noted to be 5 g/dL. Thin-layer chromatography and the resorcinol test are not available at your laboratory. *(pp. 401–402)*

Q 12

Which is the most abundant ketone in the urine in ketonuria? *(p. 402)*

Q 13

Which ketones are measured by the nitroprusside strip (Rothera method)? *(p. 403)*

Q 14

True/False. Both hemoglobin and myoglobin have peroxidase-like activity and thus will both liberate oxygen from H_2O_2 to give a positive result on reagent strips. *(p. 404)*

Q 15

An ammonium sulfate test is performed on urine to distinguish hemoglobin from myoglobin, and the supernatant is colored. What is the presumptive diagnosis? *(p. 405)*

Q 16

An increase in indirect bilirubin is usually associated with what levels of bilirubin and urobilinogen in urine? *(Table 27–10, pp. 405–406)*

Bilirubin: _____ Urobilinogen: _____

Q 17

What reagent is used to confirm bilirubinuria in the diazo tablet method? *(p. 406)*

Q 18

Clinical Consultation: A 34-year-old female presents with abdominal pain, blood pressure of 190/100, and bizarre behavior. She is admitted, and on urinalysis she is found to have 4 mg/dL of urobilinogen using the Multistix method. What disease should you consider, why is her urobilinogen elevated, and what alternate reagent strip will clarify her apparent urobilinogenuria? *(pp. 406–407)*

Q 19

What common etiologic agent of urinary tract infections does not reduce nitrate to nitrite and will give a negative nitrite reaction? *(p. 407)*

Q 20

What sexually transmitted disease may result in a false-positive leukocyte esterase reaction? *(p. 407)*

Q 21

What reagent strip reactions may be inhibited by large quantities of ascorbic acid? *(p. 407)*

Q 22

The patient from Question 18 had a false-positive test for urobilinogen due to porphobilinogens in her urine. In the Watson–Schwartz test, describe the aqueous phase after addition of chloroform, assuming she has minimal urobilinogen. *(Fig. 27–3, pp. 408–409)*

Aqueous phase: _____

After addition of butanol, what are the colors of the upper and lower phases?

Upper: _____ Lower: _____

Where is the porphobilinogen? _____

If this woman was taking high doses of methyldopa for her hypertension, what test could confirm the positive Watson–Schwartz test?

Q 23

Erythrocytes with membrane blebs or fragmented cells suggest what source of bleeding? *(p. 410)*

Q 24

What is the use of the Hansel stain for urine sediment? *(p. 411)*

Q 25

Increased numbers of epithelial cells of collecting duct origin may be seen following what toxic ingestion? *(pp. 411–412)*

_____

What stain will highlight these cells to aid in distinguishing them from WBCs?

_____

Q 26

What protein forms the matrix of all casts? *(p. 412)*

Q 27

Clinical Consultation: A 28-year-old woman who completes a marathon provides a urine sample for a research study. Present in her urine 1 hour after the race are 2+ glucose, 1+ protein, 1+ myoglobin, 2+ hemoglobin, 6 RBCs/hpf, and several hyaline casts. Which of these findings cannot be attributed to her recent exercise? *(pp. 398–413)*

Q 28

Patients with chronic renal failure may have what characteristic cast? *(p. 413)*

Q 29

Fatty casts are seen in what renal disease? *(p. 414)*

Q 30

A few uric acid crystals are seen in normal urine, but markedly increased numbers may be seen in what X-linked disorder of purine metabolism? *(p. 415)*

Q 31

Sulfonamides and ampicillin may both precipitate as crystals in urine. Describe how you would differentiate between the two morphologically. *(Figs. 27–41 & 27–42, pp. 417–418)*

Q 32

Reviewing the illustrations of urine crystals, sulfonamide crystals could easily be confused with what normal crystal found in alkaline urine? *(Figs 27–27 to 27–49, pp. 415–418)* _____

At what pH are sulfonamide crystals seen? *(p. 417)* _____

Q 33

What is the common morphologic feature of starch granules and cholesterol droplets, and how are the two distinguished? *(pp. 418–419)*

Q 34

What is the most common chemical component of urinary calculi? *(p. 420)*

_____

At what pH does this chemical precipitate? _____

Q 35

Why would a person with Crohn's disease be discouraged from drinking caffeinated beverages? *(p. 421)*

Q 36–40

Match the inherited metabolic disease with the results of the test used in screening urine samples. *(pp. 423–424)*

Q36 _____ Phenylketonuria

Q37 _____ Alkaptonuria

Q38 _____ Tyrosinuria

Q39 _____ Maple syrup urine disease

Q40 _____ Cystinuria

A. Two drops of 10% ferric chloride solution turn the urine blue

B. Commercially available reagent strips impregnated with ferric ammonium sulfate turn gray-green in 30 seconds after immersion in urine

C. 10 minutes after adding dinitrophenyl-hydrazine, a chalky white precipitate forms

D. The cyanide–nitroprusside test produces a red-purple color

E. A soluble red complex forms with nitrosonaphthol and is confirmed with a serum assay of the same amino acid

ANSWERS

A1. The patient's name, the date, and the time of collection must all be on the label.

A2. This urine is normal in color. It does not have a red pigment.

A3. Bilirubin will manifest as a yellow foam, while normal urine will have white foam.

A4. Sulfasalazine can cause an orange-yellow pigment.

A5. Tyrosinemia causes a rancid odor to the urine.

A6. The specific gravity is the relative proportion of dissolved solids to the total volume of the specimen. Osmolality is the number of particles of solute per unit of solution. A patient with hyperaldosteronism with lots of potassium ions in his urine would have a high osmolality, while a urine sample with lots of protein would have a higher specific gravity than would be suggested just by its osmolality.

A7. Ions in urine will decrease the pK_a of a pretreated polyelectrolyte, and this will then change the color of an indicator substance relative to the ionic concentration of the urine.
Various colors correspond to different specific gravities.

A8. Citrus foods – alkaline.
Meats and cranberry – acid.
Any renal tubular acidosis – alkaline urine.
Acetazolamide – alkaline.

A9. Tetrabromphenol blue is the indicator dye for the standard reagent strip, which is insensitive to Bence Jones proteins. Both the sulfosalicylic acid and electrophoresis methods are sensitive to Bence Jones proteins.

A10. $$\text{Glucose} + O_2 \xrightarrow{\text{Glucose oxidase}} \text{Gluconic acid} + H_2O_2$$
$$H_2O_2 + \text{Chromogen} \xrightarrow{\text{Peroxidase}} \text{Oxidized chromogen} + H_2O$$
Note that the first enzyme is *glucose* oxidase.

A11. The two-drop Clinitest copper reduction method is best for high concentrations of reducing sugars.

A12. The most abundant ketone is 3-hydroxybutyrate. Unfortunately, most methods do not detect it.

A13. The nitroprusside strip measures the other ketones – acetoacetic acid and acetone.

A14. True. The reagent strip does not distinguish between the two, but it picks up both.

A15. Myoglobinuria is picked up by the ammonium sulfate test if the supernatant is colored.

A16. Recall that indirect bilirubin is *insoluble*. Thus, there is no bilirubin in urine in indirect bilirubinemia. Urobilinogen is increased. Hemolysis is a classic example in this situation.

A17. Most routine bilirubin methods use a diazonium salt. The confirmatory test uses *p*-nitrobenzene diazonium *p*-toluene.

A18. She has acute intermittent porphyria and is having an acute attack. She is passing porphobilinogen in her urine. This is detected by the Erlich's reagent used in Multistix. Chemstrips are specific for urobilinogen and will be negative in this patient. There are also methods to test specifically for porphobilinogen, as we shall see in Question 22.

A19. This is *Enteroccocus*.

A20. This is *Trichomonas vaginalis*.

A21. Many analytes are inhibited by ascorbic acid: glucose, blood, bilirubin, nitrite, and leukocyte esterase.

A22. Chloroform, aqueous phase – color is present.
Butanol, upper phase – clear
Butanol, lower phase – pink, rose red; this is where the porphobilinogen is.
The Hoesch test can confirm a questionable Watson–Schwartz test.

A23. Renal glomerular bleeding.

A24. The Hansel stain highlights eosinophils, as might be present in acute interstitial nephritis.

A25. Salicylate intoxication can result in many epithelial cells of collecting duct origin. The Papanicolaou stain will highlight these nicely.

A26. This is the Tamm–Horsfall protein, a glycoprotein secreted by the thick ascending loop of Henle.

A27. Glycosuria would not be expected after strenuous exercise. Perhaps this woman is diabetic, but exercising to maintain her health.

A28. Waxy casts are often seen in patients with chronic renal failure.

A29. Fatty casts suggest nephrotic syndrome.

A30. Patients with Lesch–Nyhan syndrome may have many uric acid crystals.

A31. Sulfonamide crystals are typically yellow-brown and appear as sheaves of wheat with a central binding in many cases, although there are other morphologies seen at times. Ampicillin crystals are colorless, long and fine unless refrigerated; cold coarsens the crystals.

A32. Calcium phosphate resembles the sulfonamide crystal, but sulfonamide crystals are seen in acid urine, so this should help distinguish the two.

A33. Both demonstrate a Maltese cross on polarization. Starch granules are much larger than cholesterol droplets.

A34. Calcium oxalate is the most common component of urinary calculi. It is an acidic crystal, precipitating at pH 6.0–6.5.

A35. Many common caffeinated beverages, such as tea, coffee, and cola, contain oxalates. Crohn's patients often show increased absorption of oxalates and may develop calcium oxalate stones.

A36. B

A37. A

A38. E

A39. C

A40. D

CHAPTER 28

Cerebrospinal, synovial, and serous body fluids

QUESTIONS

Q 1

What substances freely diffuse into the cerebrospinal fluid (CSF)? *(p. 426)*

Q 2

An elevated opening pressure of >180 mmH$_2$O may be the only abnormality in what two disorders? *(p. 427)*

Q 3

What are the three tubes of a CSF specimen used for? *(p. 427)*
Tube 1: _____
Tube 2: _____
Tube 3: _____

Q 4

Xanthochromia due to subarachnoid hemorrhage may be seen as early as _____ _____ hours after a bleed. *(p. 428)*

Q 5

State the normal WBC count in CSF for adult and neonates. *(p. 428)*
Adults: _____ Neonates: _____
_____

Q 6–10

Analyze the following cerebrospinal fluids. A calculator is necessary for some of the cases. *(pp. 428–437)*

Q 6

A 25-year-old female complains of episodes of urinary incontinence as well as hesitancy for the past year. She now reports visual impairment in her left eye. CSF results are: WBC: 98/µL. Differential: 90% lymphocytes (?plasma cells), 8% monocytes, 2% PMNs. RBCs: 50/µL. Protein: 90 mg/dL. Glucose: 57 mg/dL. Albumin: 28 mg/dL. CSF IgG: 55 mg/dL. Serum total protein: 7.2 g/dL. Serum albumin: 3.9 g/dL.

What is your leading diagnosis? _____

Calculate the CSF/serum albumin index. *(p. 432)* _____

_____

Is this normal? _____ Can her increased protein be explained by impairment of the blood–brain barrier? _____

Calculate the IgG index. Assume that all of the serum nonalbumin protein is globulin and that it is predominantly IgG. *(p. 432)* _____

_____

Is this normal? _____

A protein electrophoresis stained with paragon violet shows some blurred bands in the gamma region which are not seen on a concurrent SPEP. What two procedures might clarify these bands?

_____

_____

One of these two procedures is performed and oligoclonal bands are now clearly present. Is this definitive evidence for multiple sclerosis?

_____

Q 7

A 21-year-old male with a history of acute myelogenous leukemia (M4), status post-chemotherapy (failed twice), complains of headaches and feeling vaguely disoriented for 3 weeks. CSF results are: opening pressure: 200 mmH$_2$O. WBC: 275/µL. Differential: 85% lymphocytes, 10% PMNs, 5% monocytes. Protein: 110 mg/dL. Glucose: 34 mg/dL. Gram stain: negative for bacteria. AFB stain: negative. India ink stain: negative. No blasts seen. What classes of microorganisms are still likely? Think carefully and do not be too quick to rule anything out.

_____

A polymerase chain reaction (PCR) for *M. tuberculosis* DNA is performed and is negative. What is the sensitivity of India ink on a single CSF specimen? _____

_____

What other test can be performed on the CSF to explore *Cryptococcus neoformans*? __

_____

This test is performed and is negative. What modification of this test can you make to improve its sensitivity? _____

This modification yields a positive result for *Cryptococcus* antigen. What was his risk factor for cryptococcal meningitis? _____

Q 8

A 4-year-old boy presents with marked mental status changes and acute hepatic failure following a seemingly mild viral illness for which he was treated with children's aspirin. Plasma ammonia levels are 137 μg/dL by the enzymatic method. *(Table A5–4, p. 1405)*

What is your leading diagnosis? _____

What do you expect as a range for CSF ammonia, given the plasma level? _____

_____

Your laboratory technician performs a CSF ammonia, and it is 18 mg/dL. What is the explanation? _____

What analyte can you measure to assess for ammonia in the CSF? _____

_____

This analyte is measured and is 48 mg/dL. What is your diagnosis? _____

_____

Q 9

An 18-year-old male presents after 1 day of headache and confusion. He is now obtunded, but his brother reports that the only activity they did out of the ordinary was to swim in a local reservoir earlier that week. What is your leading diagnosis?

_____

CSF results are: opening pressure: 205 mmH₂O. WBC: 18 000/μL. Differential: 96% PMNs, 4% monocytes. Protein: 950 mg/dL. Glucose: 50 mg/dL. Cytospin stained with Giemsa shows cells which look like macrophages.

What stain will help differentiate between amebae and macrophages? _____

_____

What will you likely see on a wet preparation? _____

What does the acute inflammatory response suggest in terms of an etiologic agent once you have narrowed the field down to ameba? _____

Q 10

A 21-year-old female presents after 1 day of malaise, fever, and headache. Her temperature is 40.4°C (104.7°F), and she complains of photophobia in the ER. CSF results are: WBC: 7500/μL. Differential: 95% PMNs, 3% lymphocytes, 2% monocytes. Protein: 320 mg/dL. Glucose 11 mg/dL.

What class of microorganisms is most likely? _____

In her age group, what etiologic agent is most likely? _____

What is the sensitivity of a Gram stain in this case? _____

A Gram stain is performed and shows many PMNs with Gram-negative diplococci. Your diagnosis: _____

Would a rapid bacterial antigen test (BAT) improve sensitivity over a negative Gram stain? _____

• Q 11

Why is powdered EDTA unacceptable for synovial fluid (SF) specimens? *(p. 437)*

_____

Is liquid EDTA acceptable? _____

• Q 12

What procedure can reduce viscosity in synovial fluid (SF) if an automated cell count is to be performed, to avoid sludging in the cell counter? *(p. 438)*

• Q 13

What is a normal WBC count and differential in SF? *(p. 438)*

• Q 14

Describe the appearance of monosodium urate crystals under polarized light. *(p. 439)*

• Q 15

Calcium pyrophosphate dihydrate crystals are seen in degenerative arthritis, but also in arthritis associated with what disorders? *(p. 439)*

• Q 16

How useful are synovial fluid analyses of rheumatoid factor (RF) and antinuclear antigen (ANA) in the diagnosis of rheumatoid arthritis? *(p. 440)*

Q 17

Describe the specimen containers which should be used for a pleural fluid specimen. *(p. 441)*

Q 18

State the Light's criteria for discriminating between transudates and exudates in serous body fluids. *(pp. 441–442)*

Q 19

Clinical Consultation: A 36-year-old HIV-positive male has a bilateral pleural effusion. It has a milky consistency with a slight gold metallic sheen. How will analysis of the lipid content help you distinguish between a chylous and a pseudochylous effusion? *(Table 28–20, pp. 442–444)*

Triglycerides are measured at 32 mg/dL, and electrophoresis shows no chylomicrons. What kind of effusion is this, and what is the likely etiologic agent?

Q 20

Which analyte is particularly useful in diagnosing an infectious pleuritis when levels are >90 mg/dL? *(p. 443)*

Q 21

What enzyme activity test is associated with a tuberculous effusion? *(pp. 443–444)*

• Q 22

What is the serum–ascites albumin gradient used for? *(p. 446)*

• Q 23

How are the total WBC count and differential used to diagnose spontaneous bacterial peritonitis? *(p. 447)*

• Q 24

What level of amylase in ascitic fluid is good evidence of an ascites due to pancreatic disease? *(p. 448)*

ANSWERS

A1. Glucose, urea, and creatinine all diffuse freely.

A2. In cryptococcal meningitis and pseudotumor cerebri, this may be the only positive finding.

A3. Tube 1 – chemistries and serologies.
Tube 2 – microbiology.
Tube 3 – cell count, differential.

A4. Two to four hours is the earliest typically.

A5. Adults have 0–5 WBCs/µL, while neonates can have more, 0–30/µL.

A6. This is a typical story for multiple sclerosis. The CSF/serum albumin index is 7.18, which is within the reference range, so one cannot account for her increased protein by an impaired blood–brain barrier. The IgG index is 2.32, which is increased, indicating production of immunoglobulins in the CSF.

Either a silver stain or immunofixation electrophoresis would resolve these bands.

The diagnosis of multiple sclerosis rests on a combination of laboratory, clinical, and radiological findings. MS is not the only disorder causing oligoclonal bands.

A7. With a subacute onset and a low glucose, both tubercular and fungal meningitis are possibilities. Bacterial etiologies are less likely with a subacute course, and viral causes are not so probable with the low glucose.

The sensitivity of India ink on just a single sample is only 25%, so the negative finding should not dissuade us from this diagnosis. Latex agglutination is a useful adjunct for cryptococcal antigen. It is sometimes negative when the antibody concentration is high; this is the prozone effect, and that's what is happening here. Diluting the CSF 1 : 10 and running the latex agglutination again should resolve this.

His risk factor is immunosuppression from his leukemia.

A8. This case is a classic presentation of hepatic encephalopathy due to Reye's syndrome, thought to be associated with aspirin ingestion. The CSF ammonia should be one-third to one-half of the plasma ammonia. However, in the brain, α-ketoglutarate combines with ammonia to form glutamine in order to protect the brain from excess ammonia. Thus, ammonia levels can be deceptively low, as is the case here. Glutamine measurements in the CSF are useful, and the level here of 48 mg/dL is consistent with hepatic encephalopathy.

A9. Freshwater exposure and a clinical picture of encephalopathy suggest primary amebic meningoencephalitis. Trophozoites of *Naegleria fowleri* can look like macrophages in CSF. The acridine orange stain can help; it stains amebae brick red and WBCs bright green. The presence of an acute inflammatory response, seen here with the high WBC and predominance of PMNs, also suggests *Naegleria* over *Acanthamoeba*.

A10. An acute onset, high protein and very low glucose all suggest a bacterial etiology here. In her age group, *Neisseria meningitidis* is a likely candidate. The sensitivity of Gram's stain is 60–90% in experienced hands, and in this case it is diagnostic for *Neisseria*. The BAT does not improve sensitivity over Gram stain. These latex agglutination tests are most useful in partially treated meningitis cases.

A11. Powdered EDTA may form crystals which would confound specimen evaluation. Liquid EDTA and sodium heparin are acceptable.

A12. Incubation with hyaluronidase to break down hyaluronic acid.

A13. WBC: 0–200/μL. Differential: 20% PMNs, 15% lymphocytes, 65% monocytes/macrophages, 2% eosinophils.

A14. These crystals are needle-shaped classically, usually 5–20 μm long. They are yellow when parallel to the compensator, and blue when perpendicular.

A15. Hypomagnesemia, hemochromatosis, hyperparathyroidism, and hypothroidism all may cause pseudogout.

A16. Neither of these assays is specific enough for routine use. RF is found in the synovia of 60% of RA patients, and ANA in just 20%.

A17. EDTA should be used for the cell counts, and heparin for the other tubes to prevent clotting.

A18. 1. Pleural/serum protein ratio >0.5.
2. Pleural/serum LDH ratio >0.6.
3. Pleural fluid LDH >2/3 of upper reference limit.
An exudate meets any one of these criteria.

A19. Chylous effusions usually have triglycerides (TG) > 110 mg/dL and chylomicrons (CM) present on lipoprotein electrophoresis. In pseudochylous effusion, TGs are less than 50 mg/dL, and CMs are absent on electrophoresis. In this case, the patient has a pseudochylous effusion and it is likely due to tuberculosis, seen in the HIV-positive population.

A20. A high lactate suggests an infectious etiology for pleuritis.

A21. This is adenosine deaminase, particularly the isoenzyme ADA-2.

A22. A serum–ascites albumin gradient of >1.1 g/dL is consistent with portal hypertension, while a value of <1.1 g/dL suggests an alternative etiology.

A23. The vast majority of spontaneous bacterial peritonitis patients have a WBC >500/μL with >50% PMNs. Alternatively, the absolute neutrophil count can be used, with either 250 or 500/μL as a cutoff.

A24. An ascitic value three times the serum value suggests a pancreatic etiology.

Part IV

Hematology

CHAPTER 29

Basic examination of blood and bone marrow

QUESTIONS

• Q 1

In the body, iron is found in the ferric and ferrous states. In oxyhemoglobin, iron is _____, while in methemoglobin it is in the _____ _____ state. *(p. 457)*

• Q 2

The hemiglobincyanide (HiCN) method of determining hemoglobin (Hb) involves the generation of an intermediate Hb, called _____, and measures HiCN at a wavelength of _____ nm on a spectrophotometer. *(p. 458)*

• Q 3

Clinical Consultation: A 64-year-old male presents to his internist with complaints of fatigue. A CBC reveals a Hb of 16 g/dL, a hematocrit (Hct) of 30%, and white cell count (WBC) of 7300/μL. A recent lipid profile was within the reference range. How do the WBC and lipid profile help you rule out causes of a falsely elevated Hb? What is a likely cause for the erroneous Hb in this case? *(p. 459)*

• Q 4

Describe the two categories of hereditary methemoglobinemia. *(pp. 457–458)*

• Q 5

A patient with sickle cell anemia has 1.5 mL of whole blood drawn into a 3.0-mL vacutainer tube with tripotassium EDTA as the anticoagulant. What are three potential sources of error in determining this patient's Hct? *(p. 460)*

• Q 6

Briefly describe the Coulter principle of electronic counting of RBCs. *(Fig. 29–6, p. 466)*

• Q 7

Give the formulas for mean cell volume (MCV), mean cell hemoglobin (MCH), and mean cell hemoglobin concentration (MCHC). *(p. 460)*

MCV =

MCH =

MCHC =

• Q 8

Give the equation for correcting a WBC for nucleated red cells (NRBC). *(p. 462)*

• Q 9

What is the effect of EDTA on mean platelet volume (MPV)? *(p. 462)*

• Q 10

Define field error as it applies to the hemocytometer method of cell counting. How significant is field error in manual platelet counts? *(p. 463)*

• Q 11

On the Coulter analyzer, how is hematocrit determined? *(p. 459)*

• Q 12

All major multichannel analyzers utilize light scattering to determine cell counts and white cell differentials. The Abbott Cell Dyn uses four simultaneous measurements. State what parameter is determined with each scattering measurement. *(p. 467)*

Zero-degree: _____   Ninety-degree: _____

Ten-degree: _____   Depolarized ninety-degree: _____

• Q 13

How useful is the erythrocyte sedimentation rate (ESR) in the diagnosis of rheumatoid arthritis? How about for monitoring disease activity? *(p. 466)*

• Q 14

What is the normal reticulocyte percentage in newborns, and when does this value approach 'adult' levels? *(p. 463)*

• Q 15

What dye can be used to demonstrate reticulocytes? *(p. 461)*

• Q 16

Clinical Consultation: A clinician calls about a report of anisochromia in a 32-year-old female he is treating for iron deficiency anemia, who began iron supplementation 3 weeks ago. You explain: *(p. 470)*

• Q 17

Acanthocytes on a peripheral blood smear suggest what two disorders, in addition to the McLeod phenotype, which is not discussed in this section? *(p. 471)*
_____ and _____

• Q 18

The correct name for inorganic iron granules within erythrocytes on a Wright-stained peripheral blood smear is *(p. 472)*

• Q 19

Clinical Consultation: A neonatal intensive care unit resident calls you about the significance of a normoblast count of 185/µL in the peripheral blood of a 33-week gestational age twin, now 1 day old, with a Hb of 15.0g/dL, indirect bilirubin of 1.0mg/dL. You reply: *(p. 463)*

• Q 20

Cytoplasmic vacuolization is a characteristic feature of what type of normal leukocyte? *(p. 475)*

Q 21

Clinical Consultation: A 15-month-old white male has a Hct of 38%, RBC of 5.2×10^6, and a MCV of 73 fL. Iron studies are within the reference range. The clinician wants to perform a hemoglobin electrophoresis to explore a diagnosis of thalassemia. You reply: (p. 464)

Q 22

Which patient in each of the following pairs will have a higher erythrocyte sedimentation rate (ESR)? (p. 465)

Hct of 22% vs. 37%: _____

Hereditary spherocytosis vs. megaloblastic anemia (both have Hct of 34%): _____

_____

Fibrinogen of 200 mg/dL vs. 120 mg/dL: _____

Q 23

What is an advantage of convenience with the modified Westergren method of determining ESR? (p. 465)

Q 24

Why is heparin unacceptable as an anticoagulant in determining ESR? (p. 465)

ANSWERS

A1. Oxyhemoglobin is ferrous, or Fe^{2+}. Methemoglobin contains oxidized iron (ferric), or Fe^{3+}.

A2. The intermediate is methemoglobin. HiCN is measured at 540 nm.

A3. Clearly, the Hb does not correlate with the Hct, and since the patient is fatigued, the Hct of 30% is more likely to be accurate. Causes of falsely elevated Hb by the HiCN method include hyperlipemia and leukocytosis, not seen here, and abnormal plasma proteins. This patient could well have multiple myeloma, and this should be explored.

A4. The first is a deficiency of NADH-cytochrome-b_5 reductase. This is an autosomal recessive condition resulting in the inability of the RBC to reduce Hi back to Hb.

   HbM is an autosomal dominant condition causing asymptomatic cyanosis. The patients cannot reduce their Hb because of its structural abnormality, so they show an increase in oxidized Hb. Oxidized Hb (methemoglobin, or Hi) cannot combine with oxygen, but it can be measured by the HiCN method. The iron in HiCN is in the ferric state.

A5. Sickle cells can trap plasma, giving a falsely elevated Hct.
Tripotassium EDTA causes red cell shrinkage, giving a falsely low Hct.
Dilution with the liquid tripotassium EDTA, due to inadequate volume of blood, gives a falsely low Hct.

A6. Blood cells are suspended in a liquid contained in two chambers connected by a small aperture. Electrodes measure the current in each chamber. As cells pass through from one chamber to the other, they generate resistance, which is measurable as voltage pulses.

A7. All three of these RBC indices are calculated; none is measured.

   MCV = (Hct/RBC) × 10. Use the Hct as a percent (45%), and the RBC in million/μL.

   MCH = (Hb/RBC) × 10. Use g/dL as the units for Hb, RBC in million/μL.

   MCHC = (Hb/Hct). Use Hb as g/dL, and Hct as a decimal.

A8. Corrected WBC = (total WBC × 100)/(100 + NRBC). By total WBC, Henry means the original WBC.

A9. EDTA increases MPV by inducing a shape change in the platelets from discoid to spherical.

A10. Field error is the statistical error due to counting a limited number of cells in the hemocytometer chamber. It is higher for platelets than for red or white cells.

A11. Hematocrit is calculated on the Coulter, using estimates from the histogram of MCV and RBC. The equation just reviewed for calculating the MCV is turned around, and the Hct is calculated instead.

A12. Zero-degree – cell size
Ninety-degree – lobularity
Ten-degree – cell structure, complexity
Depolarized ninety-degree – granularity

A13. The ESR is a nonspecific test, so it has little value in diagnosis, but it can be used to monitor patients with an established diagnosis.

A14. Newborns have a higher reticulocyte percentage, 3–7%, than adults, but this quickly falls to adult levels, 1–3%, by the seventh day of life. Adult levels are 1%.

A15. New methylene blue and brilliant cresyl blue (not mentioned in the text) are both supravital stains which bind to ribonucleoprotein, making a visible precipitate.

A16. Anisochromia means that some cells are hypochromic and some are normochromic. This is an expected finding in treatment of iron deficiency, where the hypochromic cells are joined by cells with a normal Hb content.

A17. Acanthocytes are seen in abetalipoproteinemia, either hereditary or acquired, and some forms of liver disease.

A18. These are Pappenheimer bodies. When an iron stain is used, the term is siderocytes for those cells.

A19. This is within the reference range. There is no evidence of hemolysis from the indirect bilirubin, and the Hb is also within the reference range. Normoblasts are seen in the fetus and very young infants. They are *not* normal in children and adults.

A20. This is the monocyte. Vacuoles may be more prominent in the tissue form, the macrophage.

A21. The MCV is typically lower in children than in adults. In boys age 1–15 years, it rises gradually from 70 to 76 fL. Also, thalassemia is unlikely in a white person. Electrophoresis is not indicated here.

A22. Hct of 22%. Anemia increases the ESR.

Megaloblastic anemia. Macrocytes have a decreased surface/volume ratio, which increases the rate of falling.

Most plasma proteins, fibrinogen to a greater extent than the others, increase the ESR, so the patient with a fibrinogen of 200 mg/dL would have the higher ESR.

A23. EDTA can be used as the anticoagulant in the modified Westergren method, and this is the anticoagulant in routine hematology studies to begin with.

A24. Heparin alters the zeta potential of red cells. The zeta potential is the diffuse positive charge around the surface of red cells that naturally inhibits them from aggregating. Red cells have many sialic acid residues sitting in their surface which are negatively charged, and which attract positively charged ions in the plasma to create this ion cloud that we call the zeta potential. Anything that decreases the positive charge around the red cells will increase the ESR, as the cells will aggregate more readily.

CHAPTER 30
Hematopoiesis

QUESTIONS

Q 1

The pluripotential stem cell gives rise to two major progenitors, the _____
_____ and _____ stem cells. *(p. 485)*

Q 2

The earliest hematopoietic precursor cells, which can differentiate into either
hematopoietic or marrow stromal cells, have the following cell surface marker:
(p. 485)

Which key markers are not yet present?

Q 3

What cell surface marker denotes erythroid differentiation in progenitor cells?
(p. 485)

Q 4

Which cytokine is the ligand for the proto-oncogene *c-mpl*? What is its role in
hematopoiesis? *(p. 486)*

Q 5

Which cytokine stimulates eosinophils? *(p. 486)*

Q 6

Which cytokine is referred to as 'stem cell factor' or 'steel factor' and act synergistically with GM-CSF and IL-3 to stimulate myeloid, erythroid and lymphoid progenitors? *(p. 486)*

Q 7

True/False. In megaloblastic erythroid maturation, nuclear maturation lags behind cytoplasmic maturation, and karyorrhexis may be seen in erythroid nuclei. *(p. 488)*

Q 8

Use Figure 30–8 to answer the following question. A person with a 2,3-DPG level of 4.4 µmol/g is noted to have a Hb O_2 saturation of 70% at a P_{O_2} of 40 mmHg. He is given 2,3-DPG to raise his level to 11.6 µmol/g. At a P_{O_2} of 40 mmHg, what is his new Hb saturation? *(Fig. 30–8, pp. 488–489)*

_____ Can he offload oxygen to his tissues more readily at this level? _____

Q 9

The synthesis of heme is a multistep process involving several intermediates, but two reactions are key, as they are affected in the fairly common disorders acute intermittent porphyria and iron deficiency. Write out the reactions which form porphobilinogen and the final product, heme. *(Figs 30–9, 30–10, pp. 489–490)*

Q 10

What is the normal mechanism by which senescent erythrocytes are culled from circulation, i.e., what biochemical change takes place? *(p. 491)*

Q 11

The corrected reticulocyte index, or reticulocyte production index (RPI) as it is sometimes called, gives a clinically useful assessment of a patient's response to anemia because it accounts for the degree of anemia as well as the expected maturation time of reticulocytes released early from the marrow into the peripheral blood. Give the formula for the RPI. *(p. 492)*

Q 12

Azurophilic granules mark the transition in neutrophilic maturation from the
_____ cell to the _____ cell. What is contained in these granules? *(p. 494)*

Q 13

How do eosinophils contribute to fibrosis in Hodgkin's lymphoma? *(p. 496)*

Q 14

What are the actions of eosinophilic cationic protein (ECP)? *(p. 496)*

Q 15

Basophils and mast cells are related cell types, but have different origins, and they are stimulated by different growth factors. What is the principal growth factor for basophils and for mast cells? *(p. 497)*

Basophils: _____

Mast cells: _____

• Q 16

List three cell surface markers found on monocytes and macrophages which are often screened for in flow cytometry. *(p. 498)*

_____, _____ and _____

• Q 17

Define endomitosis as it applies to megakaryocyte maturation. *(p. 498)*

• Q 18

What are the cell markers of the progenitor (pro) B cell? *(p. 499)*

_____ and _____

• Q 19

Intracytoplasmic μ heavy chains without surface immunoglobulin are characteristic of what phase of B cell development? *(p. 500)*

• Q 20

What two key events in T cell functional development occur in the thymic medulla? *(Table 30–8, p. 501)*

• Q 21

What cell surface markers are helpful in differentiating NK cells from T cells? *(p. 502)*

• Q 22

Where in the heme biosynthetic pathway is zinc protoporphyrin synthesized, and why does this occur in iron deficiency? *(Fig. 30–10, pp. 490, 492)*

• Q 23

What analytical technique has replaced the Watson–Schwartz test and is now used to screen for porphobilinogen in cases of suspected porphyria? *(p. 493)*

• Q 24

Prior to your role as a consultant at your hospital's porphyria clinic, review the major features of the following porphyrias. *(Table 30–2, pp. 493–494)*

Inheritance	Def. enzyme	ALA (U)	PBG (U)	UP (U)	PP (RBC)	PP (F)
AIP						
VP						
CEP						
PCT						

• Q 25–28

Which of the four porphyrias reviewed above is suggested by each of the following case presentations? *(Table 30–2, pp. 493–494)*

• Q 25

John is a 53-year-old chronic alcoholic who has had longstanding porphyria. Minor trauma has caused several erosions on his forearms, and sun exposure has led to vesicle formation on his face. A full laboratory panel is performed. The only abnormality is a urine uroporphyrin (UP) of 200 µg in 24 hours.

Q 26

Susan is a 4-year-old wearing long sleeves and a large sun hat on a warm day. She smiles at you, displaying pink-red teeth and provides a red-pigmented 24-hour urine sample which has 2000 μg of urine UP.

Q 27

Leonard is a 14-year-old holding his stomach and acting in an agitated way in the waiting room. His mother is with him. She had a tubal ligation after he was born because she could not tolerate oral contraceptives. His 24-hour urine amino levulinic acid is 500 mg, and porphobilinogen is 205 mg. Total bilirubin today is 3.5 mg/dL, and alkaline phosphatase is 130 IU/L. Fecal protoporphyrin is 600 μg over 24 hours.

Q 28

Carol is a 32-year-old white female from South Africa. She has a few skin lesions on her forearms and face. She has required tranquilizers twice in her life during acute attacks. She is at the clinic today because she has been feeling 'suspicious' for the past couple of days. Fecal protoporphyrin (PP) is 10 000 μg over 24 hours, and 24-hour UP is 420 μg. Carol has:

· ·

ANSWERS

A1. Lymphoid and myeloid. Recall that the myeloid stem cell gives rise to erythroid, platelet, and monocytic precursors as well as granulocytic cells.

A2. These earliest cells are CD34+, CD38−, and HLA-DR−.

A3. CD71 is an early erythroid marker.

A4. This is thrombopoietin, the primary regulator of platelet production. It is required for full maturation of megakaryocytes.

A5. IL-5. GM-CSF and IL-3 help out as well, but IL-5 is the key cytokine for eosinophils.

A6. This is kit ligand, the ligand for the tyrosine kinase receptor *c-kit*.

A7. True.

A8. At this higher 2,3-DPG level, the Hb saturation is 55%. This is helping him offload oxygen to his tissues.

A9. 2δ-Aminolevulinic acid $\xrightarrow{\text{ALA-dehydrase}}$ Porphobilinogen

Protoporphyrin IX + Fe^{2+} $\xrightarrow{\text{Ferrochelatase}}$ Heme

A10. The sialic acid residue on the glycophorin molecule is lost, and asialoglycophorin is seen as an antigen. Autoantibodies bind to the red cell and process it for removal.

A11. $RPI = \dfrac{\text{Pt retic. \%} \times \text{Pt Hct} \times 1}{\text{Nl retic. \%} \times \text{Nl Hct} \times \text{Mat. time}}$

Nl retic. = 1%; Nl Hct = 0.45; Mat. time = maturation time.

A12. Azurophilic granules mark the transition from myeloblast to promyelocyte. These granules contain several lysosomal enzymes, such as acid hydrolases, acid phosphatase, and β-glucuronidase. They also contain peroxidase (this is why we use the MPO stain for AML leukemias and why M0 does not stain more than 3%), muraminidase, and cationic antibacterial protein.

A13. Eosinophils secrete tumor necrosis factor (TNF), which promotes fibrosis.

A14. ECP shortens the coagulation time and alters fibrinolysis, inhibits lymphocyte proliferation, and acts as a potent neurotoxin.

A15. Basophils are stimulated by IL-3. Mast cells respond to the *c-kit* ligand.

A16. Monocytes have several markers, but CD14, CD64 and CD68 are the three used to identify cells as being of monocyte lineage. Other less-specific markers are HLA-DR, CD4, and CD11.

A17. Endomitosis is nuclear division without accompanying cytoplasmic division. In megakaryocytes, it results in ploidies from 2N up to 64N.

A18. The pro-B cell is CD19 and TdT positive.

A19. This is the pre-B cell. Mature B cells have surface immunoglobulin.

A20. In the thymic medulla, self-reactive T cells are culled out so they will not attack in an autoimmune fashion. Also, the T cell receptor (TCR) rearranges to generate diversity.

A21. CD16 and CD56 are helpful markers in identifying NK cells.

A22. Zinc protoporphyrin is synthesized at the end of the heme biosynthetic pathway, from protoporphyrin IX, by the action of ferrochelatase. If no, or limited, iron is available, ferrochelatase will substitute zinc in its place.

A23. Chromatographic techniques are now used to screen for PBG in cases of suspected porphyries. The old Watson–Schwartz test lacked sufficient sensitivity to be used reliably.

A24.

	Inheritance	Def. enzyme	ALA (U)	PBG (U)	UP (U)	PP (RBC)	PP (F)
AIP	auto. dom.	PBG deaminase	inc.	inc.	inc.	N	N
VP	auto. dom.	protopor. oxidase	inc.	inc.	N–inc.	N	inc.
CEP	auto. rec.	uro. III synthase	N	N	inc.	inc.	N
PCT	auto. dom. acq.	uro. decarboxylase	N	N	inc.	N	N–inc.

A25. John has porphyria cutanea tarda, acquired, and exacerbated, by his drinking.

A26. Susan has congenital erythropoietic porphyria.

A27. Leonard has acute intermittent porphyria, currently exacerbated by the hormones of puberty (not discussed in Henry).

A28. Carol has variegate porphyria.

CHAPTER 31

Erythrocytic disorders

QUESTIONS

• Q 1

What is the role of CD71 in erythroid precursor cells in the marrow? *(p. 504)*

• Q 2

True/False. Ascorbic acid facilitates iron absorption, while tannins inhibit it. *(p. 505)*

• Q 3

Clinical Consultation: A clinician is preparing to treat a 24-year-old female with marked iron deficiency anemia (Hb = 6.3 g/dL, serum Fe = 12 µg/dL). You advise her that the best test for monitoring a response is *(p. 507)* _____, and that the earliest she might check for a response is after the _____ _____ day. After the first week, the Hb can be expected to rise by _____ _____ per day for the next 3 weeks.

• Q 4

Describe how a zinc protoporphyrin (ZPP) level is used to distinguish between iron deficiency and thalassemia. *(p. 507)*

Q 5

What changes are found in the marrow in megaloblastic anemia? *(p. 507)*
Marrow cellularity: _____
Number of erythroid precursors: _____
Myeloid : erythroid ratio: _____

Q 6

What molecule serves as the chief transport protein for cobalamin and is lacking in severe megaloblastic anemia of infancy? *(p. 508)*

Q 7

Describe the two types of antibodies to intrinsic factor (IF) seen in pernicious anemia. *(p. 509)*

Q 8

A 39-year-old male immigrant from Finland has recently been diagnosed with megaloblastic anemia. Serologic tests for autoantibodies are negative. What parasite could cause his anemia? *(p. 509)* _____
If he does have this parasite, will assays for cobalamin be elevated, decreased or normal? _____ For urine methylmalonic acid?_____

Q 9

Clinical Consultation: A clinician is treating a 27-year-old male with celiac disease. The patient is receiving monthly injections of vitamin B_{12} and oral folate, among other supplements. His serum B_{12} level is 327 pg/mL (160–950), and serum folate is 5.1 ng/mL (>3.5). Is a red cell folate indicated? *(Table 31–2, p. 511)*

Q 10

What is a likely red cell and iron studies profile in a 62-year-old female with an acute flare of her rheumatoid arthritis? *(p. 511)* Respond with high, low, or normal.

MCV: _____ MCH: _____ RDW: _____

Serum Fe: _____ TIBC: _____ % Iron sat: _____

Ferritin: _____ Free erythrocyte porphyrin: _____

Q 11

A percentage of patients taking chloramphenicol develop reticulocytopenic anemia, neutropenia, and thrombocytopenia, as well as morphologic changes in the marrow. What is the outcome for most of these patients? *(p. 514)*

Q 12

Several of the viral hepatitides have been associated with aplastic anemia (AA). Does serology identify the specific hepatitis virus for most cases of AA? What are the demographics of the typical patient? *(p. 514)*

Q 13

True/False. Thymomas are associated with acquired pure red cell aplasia in 10–15% of cases, but are not associated with aplastic anemia. *(p. 514)*

Q 14

What types of chemical agents stimulate chromosomal breaks and rearrangements in Fanconi's anemia? *(p. 514)*

Q 15

What hemoglobin anomaly is shared by patients with Fanconi's anemia and Diamond–Blackfan syndrome? *(pp. 514–515)*

• Q 16

What is the most common cause of reversible acquired sideroblastic anemia? *(p. 515)*

Other, less common, causes include some drugs and an environmental toxin. List these. *(p. 515)*

• Q 17

What two laboratory tests are used to diagnose congenital dyserythropoietic anemia type II (CDA-II)? Give the result of each. *(p. 516)*

• Q 18

Patients with hereditary spherocytosis (HS) have an increased osmotic fragility. Studying Figure 31.1 *(Fig. 31–11, p. 518)*, which patient, a, b, or c, has increased fragility?

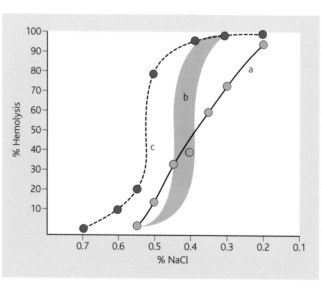

• Q 19

A 12-year-old girl whose father has HS has an osmotic fragility test performed immediately on drawing her blood. The result is within the reference range, but at the high (borderline increased fragility) end. A 24-hour incubation test is performed to explore this further. Reviewing Figure 31.2 *(Fig. 31–12, p. 518)*, which patient, 1 or 2, demonstrates HS?

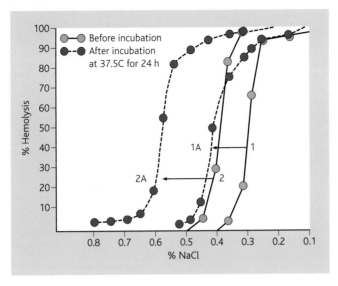

• Q 20

Several red cell membrane proteins which defend against the body's own complement system are decreased or absent in paroxysmal nocturnal hemoglobinuria (PNH). Two key proteins are CD55 and CD59. What are their functions? *(p. 519)*

• Q 21

Name the three hemoglobins that are normally present in the first trimester of gestation. *(Figs 31–13, 31–14, p. 520)*

• Q 22

A 20-month-old female has 8% Hb F on electrophoresis. Is this diagnostic of a hemoglobinopathy? *(p. 520)*

• Q 23

Hb A_2 quantitation is most often used to identify individuals with what common hemoglobinopathy? *(p. 520)*

• Q 24

Contrast the results of the acid elution slide test for Hb F in persons with hereditary persistence of fetal hemoglobin (HPFH) and thalassemia. *(p. 521)*

• Q 25

What two hemoglobins migrate with Hb S at alkaline electrophoresis? *(Fig 31-19, pp. 521, 525)*

_____ and _____

At acid pH, these two migrate with Hb _____ and _____

• Q 26

Give the levels of the following hemoglobins in sickle cell disease, Hb AS, Hb C disease, Hb SC, Hb AC. *(pp. 524–527)*

	Hb A%	Hb S%	Hb C%	Hb F%	Hb A_2%
Hb SS					
Hb AS					
Hb C					
Hb SC					
Hb AC					

• Q 27

Homozygotes for Hb D, E, and G are all usually asymptomatic. What laboratory result is abnormal in one of these hemoglobinopathies, giving a clue to its presence? *(p. 527)*

• Q 28

In Cooley's anemia, what is the predominant Hb? *(p. 530)*

• Q 29

Double heterozygotes for the sickle cell mutation and β-thalassemia have more Hb S than Hb A. This is useful in the distinction of Hb S/β⁺-thalassemia from Hb AS. How is the distinction between Hb S disease and Hb S/β⁰-thalassemia made? *(p. 529)*

• Q 30

Review the phenotypes seen in α-thalassemia with the following gene deletions. *(Table 31–9, p. 531–532)*
One gene deletion: _____
Two genes deleted: _____
Three genes deleted: _____
Four genes deleted: _____

• Q 31

After the neonatal period, Hb Bart's is seen only in what disorder? *(Table 31–9, p. 532)*

• Q 32

True/False. Reticulocytes are preferentially destroyed in glucose-6-phosphate dehydrogenase (G6PD) deficiency. *(p. 533)*

• Q 33

After receiving primaquine, a person with which G6PD variant would be likely to have the most severe hemolysis? (circle correct choice) *(p. 534)*

Variant A–   Variant B   Variant Mediterranean

• Q 34

True/False. Heinz bodies may be found in the red cells in the most common red cell enzyme deficiency involving the glycolytic pathway. *(p. 534)*

• Q 35

Some patients with thrombotic thrombocytopenic purpura (TTP) are deficient in a particular enzyme, and this deficiency contributes to their disease process. Describe the enzyme and the pathophysiology. *(p. 536)*

• Q 36

What is the bacterial agent responsible for the hemolytic anemia Oroya fever? *(p. 536)*

• Q 37

Warm autoimmune hemolytic anemia is usually due to an IgG antibody. The most common subclass of IgG is _____, and hemolysis is absent with subclasses _____ and _____ . *(p. 537)*

• Q 38

A patient has chronic paroxysmal cold hemoglobinuria (PCH). What class of immunoglobulin is involved in PCH? *(p. 538)*
_____ What disease might his mother have had? _____

• Q 39

Explain the disparity between the percentage of patients taking methyldopa who have a positive direct antiglobulin test (DAT) and the percentage with a hemolytic anemia. *(p. 539)*

Q 40

Give a physical description of a person with Gaisböck's syndrome (spurious polycythemia). *(p. 540)*

Q 41

List three disorders of the kidney which are associated with inappropriate erythropoietin production. *(p. 541)*

• •

ANSWERS

A1. CD71 is the transferrin receptor. It allows the erythroid precursor to receive iron from the recycling pool.

A2. True.

A3. The best test for monitoring response to iron therapy is the hemoglobin level. The 5th day is the earliest you would expect to see a response, and the Hb should rise 0.1–0.2 g/dL per day for 3 weeks after a week of treatment.

A4. ZPP is elevated (>99 μg/dL) in iron deficiency and normal (10–99 μg/dL) in thalassemia.

A5. Hyperplastic marrow, increased number of erythroid precursors, and a decreased M:E ratio.

A6. Transcobalamin II (TC II). Remember that TC II is an acute phase reactant.

A7. The blocking antibodies block the binding of cobalamin to IF in the stomach. The binding antibodies bind to the cobalamin–IF complex, preventing it from binding to the ileal receptors in the small bowel.

A8. The broad fish tapeworm, *Diphyllabothrium latum*, is a well-described cause of vitamin B_{12} deficiency. It is rare in the US, but is seen in Finland. This patient's serum cobalamin will be decreased, and his urine methylmalonic acid will be increased.

A9. No. Vitamin B_{12} is required for folate to gain entry into the red cells, but both B_{12} and serum folate are within the reference range, so it is unlikely that red cell folate would be abnormal. Vitamin replenishment therapy is successful in this patient.

A10. In anemias of chronic disease (ACD), the MCV and MCH may be either normal or somewhat low. The RDW is usually normal with little anisocytosis. Serum iron is low. TIBC is normal or low, and the saturation of transferrin is low. Both ferritin, an acute phase reactant, and FEP are high.

A11. A transient pancytopenia occurs in about half of patients taking chloramphenicol, but only a small percentage of these go on to develop the catastrophic irreversible aplastic anemia associated with this antibiotic. These two syndromes are unrelated to each other.

A12. No, most cases are seronegative for hepatitis A, B, C and G. The patients are usually male under 20 years of age.

A13. False. Thymomas are associated with both pure red cell aplasia and aplastic anemia.

A14. Both alkylating agents and DNA crosslinking agents readily cause breaks in the DNA of Fanconi's patients.

A15. Both Fanconi's and Diamond–Blackfan patients have increased Hb F.

A16. Ethanol is the number one cause. These siderocytes resolve promptly (few days) with abstinence. The antitubercular drugs isoniazid, cycloserine, and pyrazinamide lead to SA in some patients, and lead is a key toxin to be considered in patients with SA of unknown etiology.

A17. The acidified serum hemolysis test is positive.
The sucrose hemolysis test is negative.
CDA-II red cells react strongly with anti-I and anti-i.

A18. Patient c shows increased fragility.

A19. Patient 2 has a more prominent fragility which is characteristic of HS.

A20. CD55 is decay accelerating factor (DAF). It antagonizes the convertase complexes of complement. CD59 is membrane inhibitor of reactive lysis (MIRL). It controls and inhibits the membrane attack complex (C5b–C9).

A21. Hbs Gower 1, Portland, and Gower 2. These can roughly be thought of as the first attempt at Hbs A, F and A_2, only using the zeta and epsilon chains which are analogs of the fetal and adult chains alpha, beta, delta, and gamma.

A22. No. About 20% of toddlers ages 12–24 months have a Hb F levels of 3–10%.

A23. Persons with β-thalassemia trait may have Hb A_2 levels up to 7%; 3.5% is usually the high end of the reference range.

A24. In HPFH, Hb F is evenly distributed among the red cells. In thalassemia and other hemoglobinopathies where Hb F is increased, the Hb F is unevenly distributed.

A25. Hbs D and G migrate with Hb S on alkaline electrophoresis and may cause some confusion if Hb S has not already been identified in the patient. At acid pH, both Hbs D and G migrate with Hb A and thus distinguish themselves from Hb S.

A26.

	Hb A%	Hb S%	Hb C%	Hb F%	Hb A$_2$%
Hb SS	0	>80	0	1–20	2.0–4.5
Hb AS	50–65	35–45	0	0–1	2.0–4.5
Hb C	0	0	>90	2–4	~2
Hb SC	0	50	<50	<2	~2
Hb AC	55	0	~40	<7	~2

A27. Hb E is abnormal. Persons with both Hb E disease and trait have a low MCV. This may suggest thalassemia trait until explored more thoroughly.

A28. Hb F is the predominant Hb in homozygotes for β-thalassemia. In β^0-thalassemia, Hb F can be as high as 98%. In β$^+$-thalassemia, a slightly less debilitating form of homozygosity for β-thalassemia, Hb F is 60–95%.

A29. Hb S/β^0-thalassemia double heterozygotes have a lower MCV and MCH, and an increased Hb A$_2$ due to their thalassemia, compared to sickle cell disease patients.

A30. One gene deleted – silent carrier
Two genes – α-thalassemia trait
Three genes – Hb H disease
Four genes – hydrops fetalis

A31. This is Hb H disease in which three of the four alpha-globin genes are deleted. These patients have 5–30% Hb H and just a trace of Hb Bart's as adults.

A32. False. It is the senescent red cells, with less G6PD activity to begin with, that are at greatest risk of hemolysis.

A33. The Mediterranean variant patient may have as little as 1% G6PD activity and is at risk for greater hemolysis than the black person with variant A, who has 5–15% activity. Variant B is the most common of the 300-plus G6PD variants and is normal.

A34. False. No Heinz bodies are seen in pyruvate kinase deficiency.

A35. A von Willebrand factor (vWF)-cleaving protease, present in normal individuals, cleaves the ultra-large vWF multimers which are secreted by endothelial cells. A person deficient in this protease fails to cleave these multimers, which are highly adhesive and induce platelet clumping throughout the circulation. The gene coding for this enzymes is *ADAMTS13*, and the enzyme itself is frequently referred to by the same name.

A36. This is *Bartonella bacilliformis*.

A37. IgG1 is the most common subclass associated with hemolysis. IgGs2 and 4 do not cause hemolysis.

A38. The Donath–Landsteiner antibody is a biphasic IgG. Chronic PCH is associated with congenital syphilis.

A39. In addition to causing a positive DAT in up to one-third of patients taking the drug, methyldopa also decreases mononuclear phagocytic activity, and this may explain the lower than expected percentage of persons with hemolysis.

A40. This would be an obese, male smoker. He would also be hypertensive.

A41. Renal tumors, especially renal cell carcinoma. Renal cysts. Hydronephrosis.

CHAPTER 32

Leukocytic disorders

QUESTIONS

Q 1

A 35-year-old woman successfully completes a 50-mile ultramarathon. What will be the effect on her neutrophil count? *(p. 547)*

Q 2

What type(s) of neutrophil predominate(s) in the marrow in Kostmann's disease? *(p. 548)*

Q 3

True/False. Patients with May–Hegglin anomaly have increased numbers of Döhle bodies. *(Table 32–4, pp. 549–550)*

Q 4

How do the neutrophils of Pelger–Huët anomaly compare functionally with those in Alder–Reilly anomaly? How about with those in Chédiak–Higashi syndrome? *(pp. 550–551)*

Q 5

Review the features of tropical pulmonary eosinophilia. *(p. 553)*
Peripheral blood eosinophils: _____
Serum IgE level: _____
Sex predilection: _____
Geography: _____
Likely causative agent: _____

Q 6

Both basophilia and monocytosis should prompt a search for what possible disorder? *(p. 553)*

Q 7

How does the cellular immune function in neonates compare with that in normal adults? *(p. 554)*

Q 8

List four viruses associated with acute infectious lymphocytosis (AIL). *(p. 554)*

Q 9

What is the typical peripheral blood profile in human T lymphotropic leukemia virus 1 (HTLV-1) infection? *(p. 555)*

Q 10

What is the site of Epstein–Barr virus (EBV) attachment to B cells? *(p. 555)*

Q 11

Describe briefly the principle underlying the heterophil antibody test for infectious mononucleosis (IM). *(p. 556)*

_____ RBCs will preferentially absorb heterophil antibodies in IM, while Forssman's antigen, found in _____, will absorb non-IM heterophil antibodies.

Q 12

What are three peripheral blood features that favor a diagnosis of chronic myelogenous leukemia (CML) over a leukemoid reaction? *(p. 558)*

Q 13

The French–American–British (FAB) criteria for a diagnosis of acute myeloid leukemia (AML) required that 30% of nucleated cells in the marrow or blood are blasts. The current WHO criteria requires what percentage of blasts? *(p. 565)*

Q 14

What three cell surface markers typically distinguish AML with minimal differentiation (M0) from a lymphoid malignancy? *(p. 565)*

_____, _____ and _____

Q 15

The translocation t(8;21)(q22;q22) is associated with which genes? What is the prognostic significance of this translocation compared to other types of AML? *(p. 567)*

Q 16

What translocation is seen in most cases of the acute promyelocytic leukemia (APL), hypergranular variant? *(p. 567)*

_____

Are Auer rods seen in M3V? _____

• Q 17

True/False. The nonspecific esterase stains alpha-naphthyl acetate and alpha-naphthyl butyrate are specific for the acute leukemias of monocytic lineage, AML-M4 and -M5. *(pp. 568–569)*

• Q 18

What is the prognostic significance of inv(16)(p13q22)? *(p. 567)*

_____

What leukemia is it seen in? _____

• Q 19

What is the usual immunophenotypic profile in acute megakaryoblastic leukemia? *(p. 569)*

• Q 20

What is the prognostic significance of a chromosome band 11q23 abnormality in AML? *(p. 567)*

• Q 21

In CML, there is a marked increase in the number of cells of the neutrophil line. In most cases, how are the other cell lines affected? *(p. 559)*

Basophils: _____ Eosinophils: _____ Monocytes: _____

RBCs: _____ Platelets: _____

• Q 22

In polycythemia vera (PV), all three cell lines are proliferative, and there is a moderate neutrophilia. What is the neutrophil alkaline phosphatase level? *(p. 560)*

• Q 23

Which of the myeloproliferative disorders (MPDs) may progress to an acute leukemia? *(pp. 560–562)*

• Q 24

Essential thrombocythemia (ET) is a diagnosis of exclusion, particularly exclusion of other MPDs. What laboratory and biopsy findings are required for the diagnosis? *(p. 562)*

PV: _____

CML: _____

CIM: _____

• Q 25

What clinical feature, as might be assessed on physical examination, typically distinguishes the myelodysplastic syndromes (MDS) from the MPDs? *(p. 562)*

• Q 26

The MDS subcategories are based chiefly on the percentage of blasts present in the marrow and peripheral blood. Review these blast percentages below. *(Table 32–13, pp. 564–565)*

Refractory anemia (RA): _____ BM _____ PB

Refractory anemia with ring sideroblasts (RARS): _____ BM _____

_____ PB (the percentage of ring sideroblasts in the BM is: _____)

Refractory anemia with excess blasts: _____ BM _____ PB

• Q 27

Immunohistochemistry was used prior to flow cytometry to distinguish the blasts of acute lymphoblastic leukemia (ALL) from those of AML. It is still a useful adjunct today. *(p. 571)*

In ALL blasts are consistently negative for _____ and _____

_____.

They are generally negative for_____.

They exhibit coarse block positivity for _____.

• Q 28

The most frequent translocation in adults with ALL is _____

_____ and is associated with a poor prognosis. *(p. 571)*

• Q 29

Clinical Consultation: An 8-year-old girl has an acute leukemia which appears to be lymphoid in origin, based on morphology. Your flow cytometry technician performs a TdT, HLA-DR, CD10, CD19, CD20, and SIg. Of these, which three will be most useful in distinguishing between early pre-B ALL and Burkitt lymphoma? *(pp. 571, 581)*

• Q 30

Compare and contrast B cell chronic lymphocytic leukemia (CLL) with prolymphocytic leukemia (PLL). *(Table 32–17, p. 573)*

	CLL	PLL
Lymphadenopathy		
WBC		
Gender bias		
Prognosis		
Percent prolymphs		

• Q 31

What immunophenotypic differences distinguish CLL from PLL? *(Table 32–17, p.573)*

CLL: _____

PLL: _____

• Q 32

In Sézary syndrome, what is the characteristic immunophenotype? *(Table 32–20, p.582)*

• Q 33

What are the two common chromosomal abnormalities seen in small lymphocytic lymphoma (SLL)? *(Table 32–17, p. 573)*

_____ and _____

• Q 34

Does a negative test for t(11;14) or a lack of overexpression of cyclin-D1 rule out mantle cell lymphoma? *(p. 579)*

• Q 35

What is the most common lymphoma of the CNS? *(p. 579)*

• Q 36

Helicobacter pylori is associated with what type of lymphoma? *(p. 577)*

_____

What is its immunophenotype? _____

• Q 37

Clinical Consultation: A clinician is treating a 9-year-old boy for Burkitt lymphoma. He wants to perform an EBV test. Which types of Burkitt lymphoma are associated with EBV? *(p. 581)*

• Q 38

In what way might T lymphoblastic lymphoma present as a medical emergency? *(p. 572)*

• Q 39

Anaplastic large cell lymphoma (ALCL) is a disease of adolescents and young adults, as is Hodgkin's lymphoma, and the malignant cells of ALCL can mimic Reed–Sternberg cells, both morphologically and by immunohistochemistry, as both are CD30 positive. What cytogenetic study enables confident diagnosis of ALCL? *(p. 586)*

• Q 40

Classic Hodgkin's disease (HD), now Hodgkin's lymphoma (HL) by WHO, is diagnosed by the presence of Reed–Sternberg cells which are positive for what cell surface markers? *(pp. 587–588)* _____

By contrast, nodular lymphocytic predominance HD demonstrates lymphocytic and histiocytic (L&H) cells which are positive for _____
_____ .

• Q 41

Lacunar cells in a mediastinal lymphoid neoplasm in a 23-year-old female would have an immunophenotype of: *(p. 588)*

• Q 42

Briefly discuss the etiologies of renal failure in multiple myeloma. *(p. 576)*

• Q 43

Clinical Consultation: Using an Ostwald viscometer, a technician measures the relative serum viscosity of a patient with Waldenström's macroglobulinemia as 6.3. The normal control, run at the same time, is read as 3.4. How do you interpret these results for the clinician? *(p. 575)*

• Q 44

Clinical Consultation: A 34-year-old woman, a recent immigrant from a rural region of Italy, presents to her internist for new-onset diarrhea with fatty stools and recurrent colds. A biopsy of the intestine shows a marked lymphoplasmacytic infiltrate. You helpfully suggest an SPEP and UPEP, and find a faint band in the beta-gamma region. What is your diagnosis? *(p. 575)*

ANSWERS

A1. She will have an increase in her neutrophil count due to severe exercise.

A2. Immature precursors, the myeloblasts and promyelocytes will be present. More mature forms, such as myelocytes, are absent.

A3. False. The structures in May–Hegglin resemble Döhle bodies, but are probably altered RNA.

A4. Both Pelger–Huët and Alder–Reilly neutrophils are normal. The term anomaly is a helpful clue. By contrast, those in Chédiak–Higashi syndrome are functionally impaired.

A5. Peripheral blood eosinophils and serum IgE are increased. This disorder is more common in males, and is seen in India, Southeast Asia, and the South Pacific. It is believed to be a reaction to a microfilaria.

A6. Basophilia may be seen in allergic reaction, and monocytosis in patients who are recovering from an infection, but both of these are also seen in a variety of hematologic malignancies. If either is found unexpectedly, a work-up is indicated.

A7. The cellular immunity of infants is comparable to that of adults.

A8. Coxsackieviruses A and B6, echoviruses, and adenovirus 12.

A9. The lymphocyte count is less than 20 000/μL, and 10–40% of the lymphocytes are immature. Recall that very few of the persons infected with HTLV-1 go on to develop adult T cell leukemia/lymphoma.

A10. EBV attaches to the C3d complement receptor, which is CD21.

A11. Beef RBCs will absorb heterophil antibodies. We can make a variety of heterophil antibodies which can cause horse RBCs to agglutinate. If a person has a disease that might be IM, we would like to know if it is really the IM-induced antibodies causing the agglutination. Beef RBC stroma will absorb the heterophil antibodies of IM; then there is nothing to cause the horse RBCs to agglutinate. So here, a *negative result* suggests IM.
     Forssman's antigen is found on guinea pig kidney. As a parallel test, we can incubate patient serum, guinea pig kidney, and horse RBCs. The guinea pig kidney will absorb all those nonspecific antibodies, and the IM antibodies will cause the horse RBCs to agglutinate. Here, a *positive result* suggests IM.

A12. CML is associated with a myelocyte peak (most cells are myelocytes), basophilia, and eosinophilia. The leukemoid reaction lacks these features.

A13. 20% blasts.

A14. The CD13, CD33 and CD117 markers are characteristic of the AMLs. They are variably expressed in M0 through M7.

A15. The genes are *AML1* and *ETO*. This translocation is seen in only 25% of cases of AML-M2, but is associated with a more favorable prognosis than if it is absent.

A16. The hypergranular variant demonstrates the (15;17)(q22;q21) that is also seen in the less common AML-M3V, and Auer rods are also seen in this variant.

A17. False.

A18. The inv(16)(p13q22) is seen in the eosinophilic variant of AML M4, called AML M4EO, and is associated with a favorable prognosis. In this variant, there may not be an abundance of eosinophils, only 1% in some cases.

A19. These are CD13, CD41, CD61.

A20. Abnormalities in 11q23 may be seen in several of the AMLs and are associated with an unfavorable prognosis. The 11q23 abnormalities are seen in a variety of translocations, including t(9;11), t(6;11), t(10;11), t(11;17), and t(11;19). They are also associated with leukemias secondary to chemotherapy for a previous malignancy.

A21. Several other cell lines are proliferative, including basophils, eosinophils, monocytes, and platelets. Patients are usually anemic, and a small percentage are thrombocytopenic rather than having increased platelets.

A22. Neutrophil alkaline phosphatase and leukocyte alkaline phosphatase are equivalent terms. Neutrophil alkaline phosphatase is markedly elevated in PV. This is a contrast to its absence in CML.

A23. All four of the MPDs may progress to acute leukemia: CML, PV, myelofibrosis with myeloid metaplasia (MMM), and essential thrombocythemia (ET).

A24. Other MPDs must be ruled out, and this is the teaching point. WHO requires a Hb of less than 13 g/dL for the diagnosis of ET. It requires an absence of the Philadelphia chromosome to rule out CML. Finally, there must be no marrow fibrosis; this rules out CIM.

A25. Lack of organomegaly is characteristic of the MDS.

A26. RA: <5% BM, <1% PB
RARS: <5% BM, <1% PB; >15% RS in BM
RAEB: 5–20% BM, <5% PB
Remember that the WHO has eliminated the category of Refractory Anemia with Excess Blasts in Transformation (RAEB-T), and moved these patients into AML.

A27. ALL blasts are consistently negative for MPO and naphthyl ASD CAE, and generally negative for SBB, although occasional staining occurs. PAS gives a block positivity.

A28. In adults with ALL, the t(9;22) translocation is the most common and contributes to the poorer prognosis in adults compared to children with this leukemia.

A29. TdT will be positive in early pre-B ALL and negative in Burkitt. CD20 and SIg will be negative in early pre-B ALL and positive in Burkitt.

A30. In CLL, lymphadenopathy may well be the presenting complaint, the WBC is variable from $30–200 \times 10^3/\mu L$, males are more commonly affected, and the prognosis is fair with an indolent course and common longer-term survival. Prolymphocytes constitute less than 10% of the lymphocyte population in peripheral blood.

In PLL, the lymph nodes are inconspicuous; the WBC is extremely high, averaging $> 100 \times 10^3/\mu L$, the male bias is present as it is in CLL, and the prognosis is poor. Prolymphocytes make up more than 55% of lymphocytes in the blood.

A31. CLL is weakly positive for surface immunoglobulin (SIg), is positive for CD5, occasionally for CD11c, CD23 and CD25 (this might be confusing for hairy cell leukemia if it were not for CD5 and TRAP).

PLL, in contrast, is strongly positive for SIg, and is typically negative for CD5 and CD23.

A32. Sézary syndrome is a T cell malignancy usually with T-helper differentiation (CD4). It often loses the pan-T cell marker CD7. CD3 is positive.

A33. Trisomy 12 is seen in 20% of cases, and 13q abnormalities are seen in 50%.

A34. No. There are false negatives with this translocation, so it is specific but not sensitive.

A35. Diffuse large B cell lymphoma.

A36. This is marginal zone lymphoma. Its phenotype is CD19, CD20, CD22, and CD79a positive; and CD5, CD10 and CD23 negative. It is sometimes driven to remission by treatment for the *Helicobacter*.

A37. The endemic form, seen in African children, and the HIV-associated forms are EBV-related. The sporadic form seen worldwide is not EBV-related. If this child is HIV-positive, it may be of interest to know if the Burkitt lymphoma is EBV positive.

A38. T lymphoblastic lymphoma often presents as a mediastinal mass, especially in young men, and it may cause airway compromise or superior vena cava syndrome.

A39. The t(2;5)(p23;q35) translocation, which results in a fusion protein, NPM-ALK, that combines a tyrosine kinase with a nucleolar shuttle protein, helps seal the diagnosis of ALCL.

A40. Classic HD Reed–Sternberg cells are positive for CD15 and CD30. The L&H popcorn cells of nodular lymphocyte predominant HD are positive for CD20 and CD45, but negative for CD15 and CD30.

A41. This is nodular sclerosis HD and is one of the classic Hodgkin's. The lacunar variant of the Reed–Sternberg cells are CD15 and CD30 positive.

A42. Light chains may cause obstruction with a resultant loss of nephrons. Also, amyloid deposits in the glomeruli contribute to renal failure.

A43. The control is abnormal. It should be 1.4–1.8. The viscometer must be recalibrated and the patient's sample retested before the result can be released to the clinician.

A44. This is alpha heavy chain disease. Routine SPEP and UPEP may be normal, hindering the diagnostic efforts, but sometimes show faint alpha-chain bands. An immunofixation electrophoresis (IFE) would show just the heavy chain, without a kappa or lambda component.

CHAPTER 33

The flow cytometric evaluation of hematopoietic neoplasia

QUESTIONS

Q 1

State the key advantage offered by flow cytometry over the older method of immunohistochemistry. *(p. 599)*

Q 2

Briefly outline the basic principle of flow cytometry. *(p. 599)*

Q 3

Define a compensation coefficient. Should this coefficient be recalculated with each new lot of reagents, or only if a new manufacturer's reagents are being introduced? *(pp. 600–601)*

● Q 4

A new hematology fellow is working up a patient with lymphadenopathy and abnormal white blood cells on a routine peripheral blood smear. He submits peripheral blood in an EDTA tube, a marrow aspirate in a heparin tube and a section of lymph node in RPMI. All of the specimens have been sitting at room temperature for 2 hours. Are these acceptable specimens for flow cytometry? *(p. 602)*

● Q 5

List the four antigens commonly used for blast identification in acute leukemia. *(p. 603)*

● Q 6

True/False. The diagnosis of acute leukemia requires greater than 20% blasts in the peripheral blood or bone marrow, and flow cytometry provides the tool for the precise enumeration of blasts needed at initial diagnosis. *(p. 604)*

● Q 7

The flow cytometry panel below (Fig. 33.1) is from a 5-year-old girl with fatigue and an elevated WBC. The population of interest is labeled in red. What is the most likely diagnosis? *(Fig. 33–12, Table 33–2, pp. 605–606)*

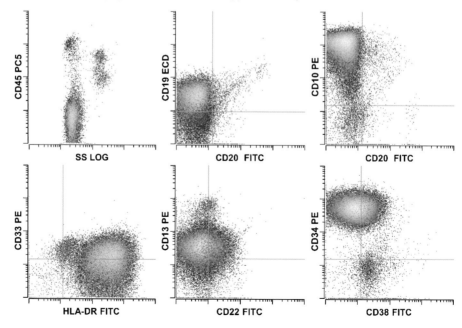

Q 8

This flow cytometry panel (Fig. 33.2) is from a 73-year-old man with diffuse moderate lymphadenopathy that has been present for 9 months. The population of interest is labeled in yellow. What is the most likely diagnosis? *(Fig. 33–16, pp. 608, 610)*

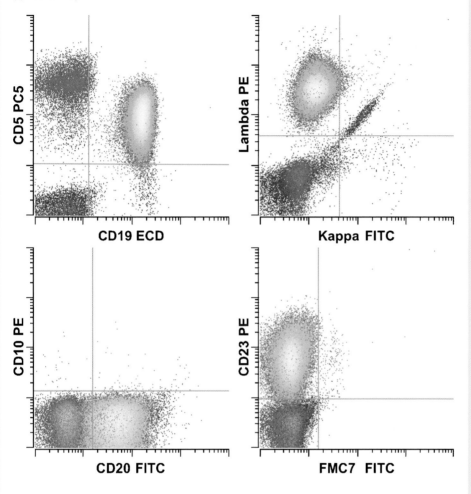

Q 9

This flow cytometry panel (Fig. 33.3) is from a 52-year-old man with an enlarged spleen, neutropenia and fatigue. The population of interest is labeled in red. What is the most likely diagnosis? *(Fig. 33–18, pp. 608, 611)*

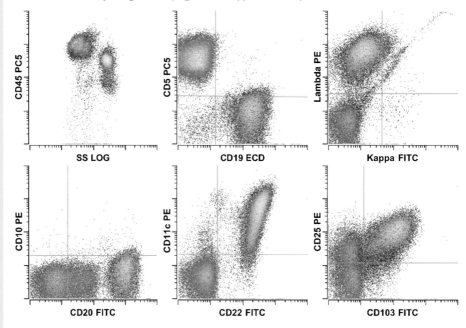

Q 10

Briefly discuss the typical cell surface marker profile in mycosis fungoides/Sézary syndrome. How specific are these markers to this disorder? *(p. 609)*

Q 11

CLL usually follows an indolent course, and survival of many years is not uncommon. However, some patients suffer an aggressive course with a poorer prognosis. What two markers, when increased on neoplastic cells, are associated with a worse outcome? *(p. 609)*

Q 12

What two key cell surface markers are used to identify plasma cells? *(p. 609)*

ANSWERS

A1. Flow cytometry performs multiparametric analysis on individual cells. The key application of this analysis is identifying dual expression of CD antigens on a cell, such as CD5 and CD19 together in CLL/SLL.

A2. Cells from a clinical specimen (blood, marrow, tissue) are suspended in fluid and injected as a monodispersed (single-file) suspension into the center of a flowing stream of fluid which passes through a quartz capillary tube. The cells may be illuminated by laser beams, which yields information about cell size and complexity; or fluorochromes may be attached to the cells and produce a fluorescent emission when excited by incident light, giving data on cell surface markers.

A3. The use of multiple fluorochromes requires that the overlapping emission spectra of each fluorochrome be resolved. Specifically, the contribution of the other fluorochromes to the signal must be subtracted to isolate the fluorescence from the desired fluorochrome. This subtraction is termed compensation, a complex mathematical process achieved with computer software. Because the spectral characteristics of fluorochromes may vary from lot to lot and between manufacturers, controls must be run with each new lot of reagents.

A4. Yes. Either blood or bone marrow may be anticoagulated with EDTA, heparin or acid citrate dextrose. Tissue is transported in RPMI.

A5. CD34, CD117, CD133 and TdT are the key markers for blasts.

A6. False: 20% blasts *are* required for the diagnosis of acute leukemia, but flow cytometry is imperfect as a tool for enumerating blasts. Bone marrow aspirates may be diluted with peripheral blood, falsely decreasing the percentage of blasts. Alternatively, lysis of the erythroid precursors may result in a falsely elevated blast percentage when nonblast nucleated cells (erythroids) are not counted. Finally, some leukemias consist of cells further along the maturational spectrum, such as the promyelocytes of APL; these cells are 'blast equivalents', but are identified by their morphology and unique cell surface markers.

A7. This is pre-B ALL.

A8. This is CLL/SLL.

A9. This is hairy cell leukemia.

A10. This lymphoproliferative disorder is *typically* CD4-positive and shows aberrant loss of CD7. However, not all cases follow this pattern, so the clinical history and cell morphology play key roles in making this challenging diagnosis.

A11. These are CD38 and ZAP70.

A12. These are CD38 and CD138.

CHAPTER 34
Immunohematology

QUESTIONS

• Q 1

Define immunogenicity and list the three characteristics of antigens that determine immunogenicity. *(p. 618)*

• Q 2

The number of antigen sites on the red cell membrane contributes to the antigenic strength of the immunogenic response. What two antigens have the greatest number of antigenic sites? *(Table 34–2, p. 618)*
_____ and _____

• Q 3

Intravascular hemolysis is seen with what two red cell antigens? *(p. 619)*
_____ and _____

• Q 4

The initial direct antiglobulin test (DAT) detects immunoglobulin or complement binding in vivo with both polyspecific antihuman globulin and anticomplement antibodies. What class of immunoglobulin and what complement component are the targets? *(p. 648)*
_____ and _____

Q 5

What is the lectin used to identify the A_1 subtype of A? *(p. 620)*

Q 6

Differentiate between the B(A) phenotype and the acquired B phenotype. *(p. 620)*

B(A): _____

Acq. B: _____

Q 7

Describe the serology of a classic Bombay individual with se/se. *(p. 620)*

Antibodies present: _____

ABH antigens in secretions: _____

ABH antigens on red cells: _____

Q 8

The H antigen, formed by adding fucose to a terminal galactose on the type 1 or 2 chain precursor, is the building block of both the A and B antigens. Both the A and B genes code for glycosyltransferases. What molecule does each glycosyltransferase add to the H antigen? *(p. 621)*

To create A: _____

To create B: _____

Q 9

Review the Wiener vs. Fisher–Race nomenclatures for Rh haplotypes. *(Table 34–16, p. 628)*

R indicates _____ and r indicates _____.

The superscript 0 or lack of a superscript indicates that both _____

and _____ are present.

The superscript 1 or ' indicates _____ and _____.

The superscript 2 or " indicates _____ and _____.

The superscript Z or y indicates _____ and _____.

Q 10

The most common Rh haplotype in African Americans is _____ in the Fisher–Race system, or _____ in the Wiener system. *(Table 34–16, p. 628)*

Q 11

In US Caucasians, the most common Rh haplotype is _____ in the Fisher–Race system, or _____ in Wiener. *(Table 34–16, p. 628)*

Q 12

What is the most common cause of the weak D phenotype? *(p. 630)*

Q 13

Why are persons with partial D more likely to make anti-D antibodies than those with weak D? *(p. 630)*

Q 14

The Rh_{null} phenotype is extremely rare. Review its laboratory features. *(p. 632)*
Morphology of red cells: _____
Osmotic fragility: _____
Fy^5, LW antigens: _____
SsU antigens: _____

Q 15

The type 1 chain is the precursor molecule for all Lewis antigens. It is the precursor substrate for both the Lewis and _____ genes, both of which are fucosyl transferases. *(p. 636)*

Q 16

To generate a Le (a+b−) phenotype, one must have at least one _____ gene, but lack the _____ gene. By contrast, the Le (a−b+) phenotype requires both the _____ and _____ genes. *(Table 34–23, p. 636)*

Q 17

Give two reasons why anti-Lewis antibodies are not associated with hemolytic disease of the newborn (HDN). *(p. 636)*

Q 18

The Lewis, P and I groups or collections of antigens have several features in common. *(pp. 625–647)*
Biochemical class: _____
Antibody isotype: _____
HDN capacity: _____
Clinical significance of antibodies: _____
Antibody reaction temperature: _____

Q 19

One exception to the rules in Question 18 is the occurrence of cold autoimmune hemolytic anemia. This occurs in association with *Mycoplasma pneumoniae* with antibodies to _____. *(p. 647)*

Q 20

The MNSs blood group system demonstrates some variation in terms of the clinical significance of antibodies to its antigens. *(p. 625)*
Which antibodies are always significant? _____
When is anti-N significant? _____

Q 21

What is the biological role of the Lutheran antigen, and in what population/disease can increased expression result in circulatory stasis? *(p. 633)*

Q 22

In the US, 9% of Caucasians are K+k+ and 91% are K–k+. What are these frequencies in African Americans? *(Table 34–22, p. 635)*
K+k+ _____   K–k+ _____

Q 23

The Kell antigen is covalently linked to the XK protein on the red cell surface, a complex integral membrane protein whose function is not yet clear. Absence of the XK protein is associated with decreased expression of the Kell antigen. This is called *(pp. 633, 636)* _____. Describe the red cell lifespan and morphology.

• Q 24

What X-linked disease is associated with the McLeod phenotype? *(p. 636)*

• Q 25

What is the evolutionary advantage of the Fy (a–b–) phenotype? *(p. 638)*

• Q 26

Clinical Consultation: A 53 year-old male who is Jk (a+b–) received several units of RBCs for a GI bleed 6 months ago. Now, he is back with another GI bleed and requires RBCs. The antibody screen is negative, and a crossmatch is compatible with Jk (a+b+) RBCs. One week after receiving the transfusion, the man's hematocrit falls from 34% to 27% in one day and his indirect bilirubin is 3.2 mg/dL. Schistocytes are seen on his peripheral smear. Explain this event. *(p. 639)*

• Q 27

The Colton blood group antigens reside on which integral membrane protein? *(p. 642)*

• Q 28

True/False. LW antigens might be absent in a person with stomatocytes. *(p. 643)*

• Q 29

What is the purpose of the immediate spin crossmatch? *(p. 657)*

Q 30

How do enzymes such as papain or ficin enhance agglutination in general? *(p. 660)*

Why are the M and N antigens destroyed by these enzymes?

Q 31

What autoimmune hemolytic anemias are usually positive only in the C3d phase of a direct antiglobulin test (DAT)? *(pp. 663–664)*

Q 32

State the American Association of Blood Banks (AABB) standard for the age of a sample for compatibility testing. *(p. 651)*

Q 33

True/False. By AABB standards, donors testing Rh-negative must be confirmed with a weak D test, but weak D testing of recipients is optional. *(pp. 653–654)*

Q 34–39

Antibody Identification Panel. For these questions, use the sample panel in *Figure 34–24*. *(pp. 656–657)*

Q 34

What is suggested by the fact that there are different reactions seen in different phases (37°C vs. AHG)? _____

What does the 2+ CC in panels 3 and 5–7 indicate? _____

What does the negative autocontrol suggest about the patient's transfusion history?

_____

• Q 35

Four cells, 3, 5, 6, and 7, show no reaction in either phase. They may be used to rule out certain antigens. The homozygous rule states that in order to rule out an antigen, it must be homozygous in that cell. Observe that e is homozygous in cell 1 (E is not present), but that it is heterozygous in cell 4 (E is present). Using the homozygous rule, what 18 antigens can be ruled out?

_____ _____ _____ _____
_____ _____ _____ _____
_____ _____ _____ _____
_____ _____ _____ _____
_____ _____

• Q 36

What antigens are left as possibilities?

_____ _____ _____ _____
_____ _____ _____ _____

• Q 37

Which two cells show a reaction in the 37°C phase with a stronger reaction in the AHG phase? _____ and _____ This is a common pattern in the Rh system. Which of the Rh antigens is left, and is it positive in these two cells? _____

• Q 38

Which two cells show a strong reaction in the AHG phase only? _____ _____
Which of the remaining antigens is positive in these two cells? _____

• Q 39

Cells 1, 9, and 11 all give a 1+ reaction only in the AHG phase, and this may be due to a single, third antigen. Which of the remaining antigens is positive in all three of these cells?

• Q 40

What is the immunoglobulin class in warm autoimmune hemolytic anemia? ____
_____ What is the optimal temperature of reaction? _____ Are these antibodies always specific for a particular antigen? _____ (p. 662)

A1. Immunogenicity is the ability of an antigen to elicit an immune response. Three characteristics contributing to immunogenicity are degree of foreignness, molecular size and configuration, and complexity.

A2. A and B. This is why they are so immunogenic.

A3. Intravascular hemolysis is seen with ABO and Kidd.

A4. IgG is the immunoglobulin, and C3d and C3b are the chief complement component.

A5. *Dolichos biflorus*.

A6. In B(A), the person is naturally type B, but he synthesizes a trace amount of A antigen. This is an autosomal dominant condition.
    In acquired B, bacteria or a colon cancer (possibly damaging the integrity of the bowel wall and allowing bacteria into the bloodstream) induces the deacetylation of the A antigen to form a B-like antigen.

A7. Bombay persons have antibodies to A, B and H. They lack all three of these antigens on their red cells. As classic Bombay persons also have the *se/se* genes, they also lack any secretions of A, B or H.

A8. The A antigen has an *N*-acetylgalactosamine. The B has a galactose at the end of the type 1 chain.

A9. Start with the basic concept that R = D and r = d. Understand that the order in Fisher–Race is always DCE whether it is upper or lower case. The C/c is the second position, and the E/e is the third position. A 0 or lack of superscript indicates that the *second and third* positions are lower case, so R^0 is Dce, and r is dce. A superscript of 1, or ′, means that the second position only is upper case, so R^1 is DCe and r′ is dCe. Now, it seems easier to grasp that the superscript 2 or ″ means that the third position is upper case, but not the second position, so R^2 is DcE, and r″ is dcE. The Z or y superscript means that both the second and third position are upper case, so R^Z is DCE and r^y is dCE.

A10. In African Americans, Dce in the Fisher–Race, or R^0 in the Weiner nomenclature, is most common.

A11. In US Caucasians, DCe or R^1 is most common.

A12. Weak D is most frequently caused by an autosomal recessive RhD mutant allele.

A13. Individuals with partial D lack certain epitopes on their D antigens. If transfused with D-positive blood, they may make antibodies to those D epitopes which they lack but which the donor has. Individuals with weak D, in contrast, usually have normal *extracellular* loops of D with normal D epitopes. They do not see anything foreign in donor D.

A14. Rh_{null} persons have spherocytes (due to mild reticuloendothelial culling) and stomatocytes (fairly characteristic), increased osmotic fragility, absent Fy^5 and LW antigens, and markedly decreased SsU antigens. The LW antigens are expressed best with RhD.

A15. Secretor.

A16. The Le a+b− individuals have at least one Le gene, but lack Se. You need Se to make Le b. The Le a−b+ individuals have both Le and Se, at least one of each.

A17. Antibodies to Lewis are IgM, and thus do not cross the placenta. Also, fetal RBCs lack Lewis antigens, so there is nothing foreign for the mother to see.

A18. The Lewis, P and I system antigens are all glycosphingolipids. I has other carbohydrate forms as well. They elicit IgM antibodies, do not cause HDN, are usually benign, and react at room temperature.

A19. Anti-I is associated with *Mycoplasma pneumoniae*, and also malignancy.

A20. Anti-S, s or U is always very clinically significant. For most individuals, anti-N is not significant, but in those rare persons who are SsU− because they lack the glycophorin B molecule, anti-N can be quite serious. The amino-terminal end of the glycophorin B molecule is identical to the amino-terminus of the N-antigen in the first 5 amino acids. The S−s−U− and N− persons who lack the entire glycophorin B molecule lack that 5-amino-acid sequence, so any N-antigen they might see in a transfusion looks *completely* foreign to them, and they make anti-N that is clinically significant.

A21. The Lutheran antigen is a receptor for laminin and is thought to mediate cell adhesion. In sickle cell disease patients, Lutheran is believed to mediate adherence of red cells to the vessel walls, causing stasis.

A22. Only 2% of African Americans are K+k+; 98% are K−k+.

A23. This is the McLeod phenotype. Keep in mind that the defect is with the XK protein, not with the Kell antigen per se. Red cells have shortened survival; some are acanthocytes.

A24. The gene for chronic granulomatous disease (CGD) is on the X chromosome, near the gene for the XK protein. Seven percent of CGD patients have the McLeod phenotype, suggesting a two-gene insult.

A25. The Fy (a−b−) phenotype offers protection against *Plasmodium vivax*. The binding site for *P. vivax* is the integral membrane protein where the Duffy antigens reside.

A26. This is a delayed hemolytic transfusion reaction, and is classic with Kidd. The recipient received Jk (b+) RBCs with his earlier transfusion, made antibodies to Jk (b), but had a fall in his antibody titer over the 6 months since he was last seen, making it undetectable in the current screen. With the current transfusion, he had an anamnestic response with both intravascular and extravascular hemolysis.

A27. This is the aquaporin 1 (*AQP-1*), a water-selective membrane channel found on red cells and several renal epithelial cells. It facilitates urine concentration in the kidney, but interestingly, Colton-null persons show no ill-effects in terms of renal function.

A28. True. The Rh null phenotype is associated with stomatocytes, and RhD antigen is linked to LW expression.

A29. The immediate spin crosssmatch is used to detect ABO incompatibility. It is the last chance to detect a potentially fatal ABO incompatibility error before a unit of red cells leaves the blood bank to be transfused to a patient.

A30. Enzymes remove sialic acid residues on the surface of red cells, reducing their negative charge. Recall that the M and N antigens sit right on those sialic acid residues, so they are removed as well.

A31. These are cold hemaglutinin disease (CHD) and paroxysmal cold hemoglobinuria (PCH). CHD is typically due to anti-I, while PCH is due to anti-P.

A32. If a patient has had a transfusion or has been pregnant in the past 3 months, then a 72-hour clock starts ticking any time he or she has a blood sample drawn for compatibility testing. Any crossmatch and/or transfusion must take place within 72 hours of that sample being drawn.

A33. True. If a recipient is assumed to be D-negative, but is actually D-positive, and gets D-negative blood, no harm is done, except that valuable D-negative blood is used when D-positive would have been alright.

A34. Multiple antibodies are suggested when you have a mixed picture in the reaction columns. The CC are the check cells. These are cells which are coated with IgG and C3 and used to confirm negative results. If there is a problem with the IgG, a patient may react as negative, falsely. If the IgG is working appropriately, then the check cells should be positive. A negative autocontrol helps rule out autoantibodies. It suggests an alloantibody, and thus a positive transfusion history.

A35. The rule-outs are: anti-D, C, c, e, f, V, M, N, s, P_1, Le^a, Le^b, Lu^b, k, Fy^b, Jk^a, Jk^b, and Xg^a.

A36. The remaining antigens are: E, Cw, S, Lu^a, K, Kp^a, Js^a, and Fy^a.

A37. Cells 4 and 10 are positive at 37°C and stronger at AHG. The only Rh antigen left is E. It is positive in cells 4 and 10 only, so this is a good fit. Anti-E is the first antibody.

A38. Cells 2 and 8 are positive in AHG only. This is characteristic of Kell, and K is positive in 2 and 8 only, so that fits. Anti-K is the second antibody.

A39. Cells 1, 9, and 11 all have the same pattern, and of the antigens left, only Fy-a is positive in all three of these cells. Anti-Fy-a is the third antibody.

A40. Warm autoantibodies are usually IgG, most often IgG1 or IgG3, react at 37°C, and are broadly reactive rather than specific to a single red cell antigen.

CHAPTER 35

Transfusion medicine

QUESTIONS

• Q 1

Review the basic qualifications for blood donors, including the maximum whole blood volume which can be collected, vital signs and Hb or Hct. *(Table 35–1, p. 670)*

Donation volume maximum for all donors: _____

Temperature: _____   Systolic blood pressure: _____

Diastolic blood pressure: _____   Hb/Hct: _____

• Q 2

There are several medications used to treat psoriasis, with similar sounding names and different deferral periods for persons wishing to donate blood. Give the deferral period for each. *(Table 35–1, p. 670)*

Isotretinoin: _____

Acitretin: _____

Etretinate: _____

• Q 3

State the deferrals for the following infectious diseases and exposures *(Table 35–1, p. 670)*:

History of Chagas' disease: _____

Needlestick (accidental): _____

Syphilis: _____

Malaria, confirmed infection: _____

• Q 4

How long may red blood cells be stored if they are preserved with CPDA-1? _____

_____ If an additive solution is used? _____

(p. 671)

Q 5

Cryoprecipitate was once used to treat hemophilia A, as it contains factor VIII. Although it may still be used for this purpose today if no factor concentrate is available, its most common use is as a source of _____. *(p. 671)*

Q 6

With current testing methods, the risk of transmission of hepatitis B virus (HBV) is _____ and the risk of transmission of hepatitis C virus (HCV) is _____. *(Table 35–10, p. 681)*

Q 7

What is the current risk of transmission of HIV?
What demographic group cannot be safely screened with the current EIA test?

Q 8

Give two particular clinical clues (vital signs) seen in a recipient, to bacterial contamination of a unit of blood. *(p. 678)*

Q 9

Clinical consultation: A 28-year-old group O-pos male who has never been transfused is receiving a unit of red blood cells. Fifteen minutes into the transfusion, his temperature increases from 36.8°C to 38.9°C, his blood pressure falls from 110/75 to 90/40, and he complains of nausea and chills. The transfusion is stopped, and the patient is treated with aggressive i.v. fluids. The anxious intern on the ward asks what laboratory tests he should order. The unit is returned to the blood bank, and it is labeled 'Group A RBCs'. Briefly outline what tests you will perform in the blood bank and what tests should be ordered on the patient. *(p. 678)*

Q 10

What medication may prevent a mild allergic reaction, such as urticaria? *(p. 677)*

Q 11

Glycerolization of red cells allows them to be frozen and stored for up to 10 years at −65°C. Once thawed and deglycerolized, the shelf life and storage requirements are: *(p. 672)*

Q 12

Leukocyte-reduced RBCs contain less than _____ WBCs per unit. *(p. 672)*

Q 13

What are the shelf life and storage temperature for fresh frozen plasma (FFP) that is still frozen? *(p. 671)*

Q 14

Outline the storage parameters for platelets. *(p. 671)*

Q 15

How does anemia affect cardiac output, red cell 2,3-DPG concentration and the oxygen–hemoglobin dissociation curve? *(p. 674)*

Q 16

What are the radiation parameters (cGy) for irradiated blood products, and what is achieved by irradiation? *(p. 672)*

• Q 17

What is the required platelet count for random-donor platelets? How about for apheresis platelets? *(p. 671)*

• Q 18

Give the formula for the corrected count increment (CCI) used to assess the response to a platelet transfusion, and the value for an 'adequate' response. *(p. 675)*

Adequate = _____

• Q 19

What are the goals for the HbS level and Hct after a red cell exchange transfusion in a sickle cell disease patient? *(p. 675)*

• Q 20

Assess the benefit of plasma transfusions in the following clinical scenarios: *(p. 676)*

A 56-year-old woman with PT 1.4 times the midpoint of the reference range, scheduled for thoracentesis: _____

A 71-year-old man on warfarin with INR of 5.3, hit his head in a fall at home: _____
_____

A 33-year-old woman with thrombotic thrombocytopenic purpura, starting therapeutic plasma exchange: _____

• Q 21

What is the definition of massive transfusion? *(p. 676)*

• Q 22

How long can a pretransfusion blood sample be used in a patient who has been pregnant or transfused in the past 3 months? *(p. 673)*

• Q 23

Briefly explain why there has been a reduction in febrile nonhemolytic transfusion reactions since the advent of universal leukocyte reduction. *(p. 677)*

• Q 24

What are the two mechanisms of pathogenesis in transfusion-related acute lung injury? *(p. 679)*

• Q 25

List two strategies to reduce the incidence of CMV transmission by blood products. *(p. 681)*

ANSWERS

A1. 10.5 mL/kg body weight is the maximum anyone may donate, but is typically used for donors under the older 110-lb (50-kg) limit. Temperature must be ≤99.5°F or 37.5°C. The blood pressures are ≤180/100. The Hb or Hct must be ≥12.5 g/dL or 38%, respectively.

A2. Isotretinoin carries a 1-month deferral.
Acitretin carries a 3-year deferral.
Etretinate carries an indefinite deferral.

A3. Chagas' disease is an indefinite deferral. Accidental needlestick exposure and syphilis both carry a 1-year deferral. After becoming asymptomatic, a malaria patient must wait 3 years to donate.

A4. With CPDA-1, the storage period is 35 days. Additive solutions (AS-1, AS-3, AS-5) allow for 42 days' storage.

A5. Fibrinogen. DIC is a common clinical setting for use of cryoprecipitate.

A6. The risk of HBV is 1 in 250 000. The risk for HCV is 1 in 2 000 000.

A7. The current risk of HIV is 1 in 2,000,000. Group O viral isolates, such as may be seen in persons from western Africa, are not reliably detected with the EIA platform in current use.

A8. High fever and hypotension shortly after transfusion (or during transfusion) are both key clues to bacterial contamination. Remember that Gram-negative rods (GNR) are often more lethal than Gram-positive cocci (GPC), and that *in general*, GNRs are seen in red cell units, and GPCs in platelets.

A9. This is an acute hemolytic transfusion reaction. In the blood bank, perform a direct antiglobulin test (DAT), both on the pretransfusion and post-transfusion samples from the patient. The pre-DAT should be negative, and the post-DAT positive. Re-type and re-crossmatch the patient and the unit. Spin down the post-sample to look for gross hemolysis. The intern should order a haptoglobin, UA, LDH and indirect bilirubin.

A10. Diphenhydramine (trade name is Benadryl), given orally or i.v. at a dose of 50–100 mg, may prevent allergic reactions.

A11. Deglycerolization requires opening the RBC system in many cases, and an open RBC system has a 24-hour shelf life at 1–6°C. The closed system allows 14 days of shelf life.

A12. Leukocyte-reduced RBCs have less than 5×10^6 WBCs per unit.

A13. FFP is kept at −18°C for 1 year.

A14. They are stored at room temperature (20–24°C) with gentle agitation for 5 days from the date of donation.

A15. Anemia increases cardiac output, increases 2,3-DPG levels in red cells to facilitate the offloading of oxygen, and shift the dissociation curve to the right.

A16. Radiation dosage is recommended as 2500 cGy to the center of the unit bag, with at least 1500 cGy to the outer portions of the bag. This prevents any lymphocytes in the unit from dividing. Lymphocytes are the bad actor in graft-versus-host disease.

A17. Random donor platelets must contain 5.5×10^{10} platelets/unit. Apheresis units must contain 3.0×10^{11}/unit.

A18. $CCI = \dfrac{\text{Post-transfusion platelet increment (per } \mu L) \times \text{Body surface area (m}^2)}{\text{Platelets transfused } (\times 10^{11})}$

If a patient's platelet count rose from 8000/μL to 38 000/μL, the increment would be 30 000. An adequate CCI is ≥ 7500. Average adult body surface area is 1.7 m^2. A standard apheresis dose of platelets has 3×10^{11} platelets, but some platelet units are higher or lower than this, and the dose is indicated on the bag.

A19. Remember this as the 30–30 rule. The goals are a HbS concentration of 30% (or less) and a Hct of 30%.

A20. The 56-year-old woman will get virtually no benefit from 1–2 units of FFP. In the other two scenarios, the benefit will be much greater. FFP is an appropriate therapy to reverse the effects of warfarin, particularly when there is a risk of bleeding. FFP contains the enzyme metalloproteinase, which is deficient in cases of TTP, so FFP would be useful either as the replacement fluid for plasma exchange, or as a simple transfusion.

A21. The commonly accepted definition of massive transfusion is the replacement of one blood volume within 24 hours. For an average adult, this would be 10 units of packed red cells and 10 units of plasma.

A22. If the patient has been pregnant or transfused in the past 3 months, then a sample can be used for just 3 days. Let's remember this as the Rule of 3s. Patients who have been recently transfused may be making antibodies to antigens which they lack, and to which they were exposed in the recent transfusion. By checking a sample for antibodies every 3 days, the blood bank is likely to detect these antibodies early, and be able to provide that patient with antigen-negative units. So if a patient's sample is drawn on Monday and the Type and Screen is negative, the patient can be given group-compatible units through Thursday. If the patient needs blood on Friday, a new sample must be drawn for another Type and Screen.

A23. These febrile reactions have been attributed to the presence of cytokines from donor white blood cells which stimulate a febrile response in the recipient. Pre-storage leukoreduction eliminates most of the WBCs to limit cytokine generation upfront. Leukoreduction will prevent transfusion of most of the donor WBCs, but the cytokines which have already been produced and have leaked out from the WBCs will still be transfused to the recipient.

A24. One mechanism is that donor antibodies to neutrophils or to HLA antigens react with the recipient's WBCs and cause aggregations of WBCs in the pulmonary circulation, with resultant capillary leakage and edema. The second mechanism is the presence of lipid inflammatory mediators in the unit that activate already primed recipient neutrophils to cause capillary leakage and injury.

A25. Leukoreduction clearly helps, as CMV is carried in leukocytes. A second method is to provide seronegative products to recipients. While the term 'CMV-negative' is frequently used, no test for CMV DNA is performed. Rather, these units are from donors who have very low or negative levels of anti-CMV IgG, indicating that they have not been exposed to the virus.

CHAPTER 36

Hemapheresis

QUESTIONS

Q 1

By the AABB *Standards*, what is the maximum amount of blood which can be in the extracorporeal circuit at one time? *(p. 686)*

Q 2

Once random donor platelets are pooled, they have a shelf life of *(p. 687)* _____
_____ .

Q 3

By AABB *Standards*, 90% of apheresis platelets tested must have a count of at least *(p. 687)* _____ .

Q 4

Apheresis platelet donors can donate as often as _____ , but a maximum of _____ times per year. *(p. 687)*

Q 5

If a person donates a unit of whole blood at a blood drive, he must wait _____
_____ before he can donate apheresis platelets again. *(p. 687)*

Q 6

Is there a requirement for a platelet count the first time someone donates apheresis platelets? *(p. 687)*

_____

What about someone who donates every 2 weeks? _____

Q 7

75% granulocyte preparations must have a minimum of _____
_____ granulocytes. *(p. 688)*

Q 8

What are the storage requirements for granulocytes? *(p. 688)*

Q 9

Which of the following are recommended or required for granulocytes donated to another person? *(p. 688)*
ABO or crossmatch compatible: _____
CMV: _____ (if recipient is negative)
HLA match: _____

Q 10

List three advantages of hematopoietic progenitor cell (HPC) harvest and transplant over traditional bone marrow harvest. *(p. 691)*

Q 11

What are two approaches to HPC mobilization, the efforts to maximize the harvest of CD34+ cells? *(p. 692)*

Q 12

True/False. In thrombocytosis, the platelet count does not correlate well with the risk of thrombosis. *(p. 695)*

Q 13

What are the major indications for therapeutic leukapheresis? *(p. 696)*

Q 14

What are the three main categories of transfusions for sickle cell anemia patients? *(p. 696)*

Q 15

Clinical Consultation: A 13-year-old girl with sickle cell anemia presents with acute chest syndrome. Her Hct is 19% and a peripheral blood smear shows almost exclusively sickled cells. The clinician requests 2 units of packed red cells (PRBCs). You reply: *(p. 697)*

Q 16

Photopheresis is a modification of traditional apheresis techniques where T cells are treated with UVA and then returned to the patient. It is used to treat several diseases, but the most complete studies of its efficacy have been on the first disease it was used to treat. This is: *(p. 697)*

Q 17

State the three advantages of red cell exchange (RCE) over simple or chronic transfusion in sickle cell disease patients. *(Table 36–12, p. 697)*

Q 18

What would be the increased benefit of performing a 3 plasma volume (PV) exchange in a therapeutic plasmapheresis versus a 2.0 PV exchange? *(p. 698)*

Q 19

What is the most widely used replacement fluid in therapeutic plasmapheresis? *(p. 699)*

Q 20

Staphylococcal A protein is used to make plasmapheresis a selective procedure, removing unwanted plasma elements. What does the staphylococcal A column selectively remove? *(p. 700)*

Q 21

What two diseases have FDA approval for the staphylococcal A column? *(p. 701)*

Q 22

What methods of low-density lipoprotein (LDL) removal are currently FDA approved in the USA? *(p. 702)*

Q 23

Which diseases are considered Category I for plasmapheresis, meaning that this is the primary or standard form of therapy? *(Table 36–9, pp. 694, 702–704)*

Q 24

Why is FFP the replacement fluid in plasmapheresis for many forms of thrombotic thrombocytopenic purpura? *(p. 703)*

Q 25

What are the first three actions that should be taken for an apheresis patient who complains of perioral tingling and lightheadedness? *(p. 707)*

ANSWERS

A1. The maximum amount of blood that can be extracorporeal is based on the patient's weight. It is 10.5 mL/kg body weight. Note that this is the same volume that can be donated by a blood donor.

A2. Once pooled, platelets have just a 4-hour shelf life. This illustrates an advantage of apheresis platelets over random donor platelets. If an apheresis unit is requested but then not used, it can continue to be available until its expiration date, 5 days from when it was collected.

A3. 90% of apheresis platelet units must contain 3.0×10^{11} platelets.

A4. Platelet donors may donate twice a week and up to 24 times a year.

A5. If a person has donated whole blood, he must wait 8 weeks until he can donate platelets again.

A6. First-time platelet donors need not have a platelet count performed. For those donors who give every 4 weeks or more, they must have a platelet count of at least 150 000/μL.

A7. There is a 75% rule for granulocytes, just as there is a 90% rule for platelets. It is 1.0×10^{10} granulocytes per unit.

A8. Granulocytes are stored at room temperature, 20–24 °C, and have a short 24-hour shelf life.

A9. Because of the high numbers of RBCs in granulocyte units, they must be crossmatch/ABO-compatible. As there are certainly some lymphocytes in the unit, CMV is a concern, and one obviously cannot leukoreduce this type of product. Finally, an HLA match is critical as well.

A10. Donors tolerate a peripheral blood procedure better than they do a marrow harvest, which requires general anesthesia.

    The recipient is restored to hematopoietic and immune function more rapidly in HPC than he is with marrow transplants.

    Patients can donate HPC autologously by peripheral HPC harvest even when there is marrow involvement with tumor. If a marrow harvest were the only option, a tumor-filled marrow would offer little or less in the way of HPCs.

A11. One approach is the postchemotherapy rebound harvest. At about day 14 after chemotherapy has begun, there is a significant increase in the number of peripheral HPCs. The second is treatment of normal (allogeneic) donors with cytokines such as G-CSF and GM-CSF to increase their HPC count prior to donation.

A12. True. However, increasing age, a previous thrombotic event, and a longer duration of thrombocythemia are all risk factors for thrombosis.

A13. The main uses of therapeutic leukapheresis are relieving vascular occlusion symptoms, such as neurologic deficits and pulmonary congestion, and minimizing tumor lysis syndrome.

A14. Patients with sickle cell anemia may receive an acute simple transfusion to improve oxygen-carrying capacity, a chronic simple transfusion to suppress red cell production of cells filled with HbS, or a red cell exchange transfusion (RCE) to treat acute chest syndrome and priapism.

A15. Acute chest syndrome is one of the indications for a RCE instead of an acute simple transfusion. The goals would be to get the Hct to about 30% and the HbS to less than 30%.

A16. Photopheresis was first used to treat cutaneous T cell lymphoma, and we have the most literature on this disease in terms of response to photopheresis.

A17. RCE provides a decreased amount of HbS without increasing the hematocrit/blood viscosity. Fewer units of red cells are needed to achieve the same HbS percentage. Finally, there is a smaller contribution to iron overload, as iron is removed with the patient's own sickled cells in the exchange process.

A18. There is little benefit from exchanging more than 1.5–2.0 plasma volumes.

A19. 5% albumin is the most widely used replacement fluid. It is not indicated for every plasmapheresis situation, as we shall see.

A20. Staphylococcal A protein removes IgG1, 2, and 4, and to a lesser degree IgG3, from plasma.

A21. The FDA has approved the staphylococcal A protein column method for the treatment of immune thrombocytopenic purpura (ITP) and refractory cases of rheumatoid arthritis.

A22. The FDA has approved the dextran sulfate and heparin-induced extracorporeal low-density lipoprotein precipitation (HELP) methods for use.

A23. The key category I diseases are acute inflammatory demyelinating polyneuropathy, anti-basement membrane antibody disease, chronic inflammatory demyelinating polyneuropathy, myasthenia gravis, and thrombotic thrombocytopenic purpura (TTP).

A24. Because many patients with TTP lack the proteinase that cleaves those unusually large vWF multimers, replacing them with normal plasma provides them with at least some level of that proteinase, something they certainly would not get with simple 5% albumin.

A25. In a patient exhibiting symptoms of a low ionized calcium, replenishing with oral calcium (Tums) is a key first step. Also, slowing the reinfusion to allow for greater dilution of the replacement fluid and increasing the blood/citrate ratio will help. Only if these do not alleviate the symptoms does one need to give intravenous calcium.

CHAPTER 37

Tissue banking and progenitor cells

QUESTIONS

Q 1

What two organizations provide standards for tissues banks? *(pp. 716–717)*

Q 2

What is the cryoprotective agent of choice for skin, hematopoietic progenitor cells, and most tissues? *(p. 717)*

Q 3

What layer of skin is provided in a split-thickness skin graft? *(p. 718)* _____
_____
Is this a permanent graft? _____

Q 4

Do bone grafts have ABO antigens? *(p. 718)*

• Q 5

What testing is performed on anonymous sperm donors? *(Table 35–2, pp. 671, 719)*

• Q 6

Do donor pluripotential hematopoietic progenitor cells need to be ABO compatible with the recipient? *(p. 720)*

• Q 7

What is the greatest advantage of using peripheral blood progenitor cells rather than those from the marrow? *(p. 721)*

• Q 8

What flow cytometric cell surface marker is used to identify progenitor cells? *(p. 721)*

• Q 9

Briefly describe the use of immunomagnetic bead technology in processing peripheral blood or marrow for transplant. *(p. 723)*

A1. The American Association of Tissue Banks and the Joint Commission on the Accreditation of Healthcare Organizations.

A2. Dimethyl sulfoxide (DMSO) prevents the formation of ice crystals which would damage the tissues.

A3. Split-thickness skin grafts provide a temporary epidermis to protect a burn victim until he can generate his own autologous graft. The epidermis has no ABO antigens, so an ABO match is not required. The dermis is not engrafted.

A4. No. The marrow and any soft tissue are removed before transplantation, unless large osteoarticular grafts are used. Then, Rh-compatible grafts are provided, if possible.

A5. There is extensive testing of the donor. The sperm is quarantined for 180 days. During this time, the donor is tested monthly for standard serologies that apply to all tissue donors (HIV, HBV, HCV, HTLVI-II, syphilis), as well as for CMV, gonorrhea, and chlamydia. Common genetic diseases such as Tay–Sachs, cystic fibrosis, sickle cell disease, and thalassemia are screened for, and a complete karyotyping is performed.

A6. No. These progenitor cells lack ABO antigens, so this is unnecessary. The HLA match is critical, however.

A7. Peripheral blood progenitors have a much shorter time to engraftment of neutrophils and platelets, 8–12 days on average, compared with 2–4 weeks for marrow progenitors.

A8. CD34.

A9. This technology is applied to both purging, in which tumor cells in autologous grafts and CD3+ T cells in allogeneic grafts are removed, and in positive selection, in which CD34+ cells are selectively removed for transplant. A monoclonal antibody to the cell of interest, tumor, CD3, or CD34, is coupled to an immunomagnetic bead. The antibody–bead complex is incubated with the cell suspension, and after an antibody–bead–cell complex is achieved, the suspension is passed over a magnetic field to remove the cell of interest. In positive selection, the bead is removed from CD34+ cells with a releasing agent.

Part V

Hemostasis and thrombosis

CHAPTER 38

Coagulation and fibrinolysis

QUESTIONS

• Q 1

List the coagulation factors in each of the following pathways. *(Fig. 38–8, p. 735)*

Intrinsic:_____

Extrinsic: _____

Common: _____

• Q 2

Factors Va and VIIIa act as cofactors to mediate the activation of other players in the coagulation cascade. *(Fig. 38–1, p. 730)*

Factor VIIIa acts as a cofactor with factor _____ in the activation of factor _____.

Factor Va acts as a cofactor with _____ in the activation of _____.

• Q 3

Plasmin is the chief biomolecule in fibrinolysis, and it generates fibrinogen degradation products (FDP) and D-dimers. These are not interchangeable terms. Distinguish between the two. *(Fig. 38–5, pp. 732–733)*

FDP:_____

D-dimer: _____

• Q 4

Briefly outline the principle of the prothrombin time test. What coagulation factors are supplied as reagents? *(p. 736)*

Q 5

True/False. The activated partial thromboplastin time (PTT) assesses physiologic hemostasis by evaluating the contact factors in the intrinsic coagulation system. *(p. 735)*

Q 6

Bleeding disorders of platelets typically have a different temporal sequence from disorders of coagulation factors, i.e., early versus late bleeding after a hemostasis challenge. Describe the difference between the two. *(p. 734)*

Q 7

Explain why in a mixing study performed on a patient with a very low factor VIII level and no inhibitor, the PTT corrects to the reference range. If only half of the plasma in a mixing study contains adequate factor VIII, shouldn't the PTT be twice normal? *(p. 737)*

Q 8

If a normal man has 80% clotting factor activity, how many units/mL of a factor does he have? *(p. 738)*

Q 9

The formula for dosing recombinant factor VIII for a hemophilia A patient is:
Dose (IU) = body weight (kg)×0.5 IU/kg×percentage increase required.
A severe hemophilia A patient with <1% activity requires a level of 50% activity for an emergent appendectomy. He weighs 42 kg and has no inhibitor. What is his dose? *(p. 738)*

Q 10

A 45-year-old woman is found to have a markedly prolonged PTT on a routine screening prior to elective surgery. She has had three children and tooth extractions without excess bleeding. A factor level analysis shows one factor to be decreased. What is the most likely diagnosis? *(p. 740)*

Q 11

A 22-year-old male has a mildly prolonged PT and PTT on a routine screen. He reports increased bleeding with wisdom tooth extraction, which resolved in a few hours with extra packing. A fibrinogen antigen assay is within the reference range, but the thrombin time is prolonged. What is your diagnosis? *(p. 740)*

Q 12

What acquired factor deficiency is seen in 8.7% of patients with primary amyloidosis? *(p. 741)*

Q 13

Clinical Consultation: A couple with no clinically apparent bleeding problems have four children. Their son, Andrew, has moderate hemophilia A with usual factor levels of 4–5%. They have three daughters, Anne, Betty, and Cecilia, and would like to know if any are carriers of hemophilia A. What test that does not involve gene analysis is used to predict carrier status? *(p. 738)*

The results of this test are given below. What is the status of each daughter?
Anne 0.45:_____
Betty 0.52: _____
Cecilia 1.09: _____

Q 14

Which routine screening and confirmatory tests are normal, and which are abnormal in factor XIII deficiency? *(p. 741)*

Q 15

A severe hemophilia A patient is known to have developed an inhibitor to factor VIII. Yesterday, his inhibitor was measured at 2 Bethesda units. He is preparing for wisdom tooth extraction and is given a dose of recombinant factor VIII that would raise his level to 100% if he had no inhibitor. His expected factor VIII level will be (p. 739) _____.

• •

ANSWERS

A1. Intrinsic – XII, XI, IX, VIII.
   Extrinsic – III, VII.
   Common – X, V, II, I.

A2. Factor VIIIa helps IXa activate X. Factor Va helps Xa activate II (thrombin).

A3. FDPs may be generated by the degradation of either fibrin or fibrinogen. D-dimers are products of the degradation of fibrin alone and more specifically indicate that clotting has taken place.

A4. In the PT test, reagent tissue thromboplastin (factor III) is mixed with patient plasma. Recall that factor III activates factor VII in the extrinsic pathway in normal clotting. Then, calcium is added as reagent calcium chloride, and the time to clot formation is measured.

A5. False. The contact factors in the intrinsic system are evaluated but the PTT really doesn't assess physiologic hemostasis.

A6. Platelet disorders present with immediate bleeding upon hemostatic challenge but, once controlled, the bleeding remains controlled. These persons have difficulty making that initial platelet plug.
   Coagulation disorders show delayed bleeding after the breakdown of the initial platelet plug. They cannot generate the complete stable clot.

A7. No, it shouldn't. Only 50% levels of any coagulation factor will result in clotting times that fall within the reference range and will ensure adequate hemostasis for routine activities.

A8. 100% activity is equivalent to 1.0unit/mL, so 80% activity is 0.8 units/mL.

A9. He'll need 1050IU. $42\,kg \times 0.5\,IU/kg \times (50-0\%) = 1050\,IU$.

A10. This is most likely to be factor XII deficiency, which is not associated with an increased risk of bleeding.

A11. This is dysfibrinogenemia, a qualitative defect of fibrinogen. These patients may have mild bleeding, as seen here, be asymptomatic, or have thrombotic episodes.

A12. This is factor X deficiency.

A13. The test that will help here is the ratio of factor VIII to vWF. In normal persons, it is 1:1, as vWF is a carrier for VIII. They circulate in pairs. In carriers of hemophilia A, who have factor levels of about 50%, this ratio is roughly 0.5:1.0. Thus, Anne and Betty appear to be carriers, but Cecilia is not.

A14. In factor XIII deficiency, the PT and PTT are normal because the test ends with the formation of the fibrin monomer. Crosslinking need not occur. However, in normal persons, fibrin clots (the crosslinked polymers) are stable in a solution of 5 M urea. In the factor-XIII-deficient person, the clot will dissolve in 5 M urea.

A15. If he has severe hemophilia, consider his starting factor VIII level to be 0–1%. After the dose is given, this boy's factor VIII level will be near 25%. Each Bethesda unit (BU) reduces the amount of factor VIII activity by one half. Here, he went from 100 to 50 and then from 50 to 25 with 2 BU.

CHAPTER 39

Blood platelets and von Willebrand disease

QUESTIONS

Q 1

List six components of the alpha granules of platelets. *(p. 747)*

Q 2

Where are nonmetabolic pools of adenosine diphosphate (ADP), adenosine triphosphate (ATP), and 5-hydroxytryptamine (5-HT) stored? *(p. 747)*

Q 3

Platelet adherence to a site of vascular injury to act as an initial plug is the basis of primary hemostasis. In venules, platelets may bind directly to *(p. 748)* _____ _____, while in arterioles they may bind to von Willebrand factor (vWF) via the platelet glycoprotein _____.

Q 4

Platelets normally rest in a discoid shape. When they are activated during a threat to hemostasis, they change from a discoid to a spherical shape, and this shape change prepares the platelets to release the contents of their alpha and dense core granules. What component of the coagulation cascade is a potent stimulus to platelet activation? *(p. 748)*

Q 5

A stable platelet plug involves binding of the coagulation factor _____ _____ to the platelet glycoprotein _____. *(p. 748)*

Q 6

What is the utility of a bleeding time test as a preoperative screen to predict bleeding in a patient preparing for bypass surgery? *(p. 750)*

Q 7

Platelet aggregation and secretion studies are functional tests used to evaluate abnormal hemostasis. In these tests, which component of dense core granules is measured as an indicator of platelet secretion? *(p. 751)*

Q 8

Which platelet glycoprotein is required for normal clot retraction? *(p. 752)*

Q 9

True/False. The identification of platelet-associated immunoglobulins has a high positive predictive value in the workup of immunologic thrombocytopenic purpura (ITP). *(p. 755)*

Q 10

Clinical Correlation: A 38-year-old woman being treated for a chronic sinus infection with Bactrim presents with petechiae and a platelet count of 12 000/μL. In this case, platelet antibodies may be useful. Should her antibiotic be discontinued? *(Table 39–3, p. 755)* _____ What is the likelihood that she will go into spontaneous remission? _____ Is she more or less likely to have an eventual complete recovery than a child with the same disorder? _____

Q 11

What is the target of antibodies in heparin-induced thrombocytopenia? *(p. 756)*
_____

What is the alternative name of this molecule that indicates its function?
_____

Q 12

Describe the appearance of a blood film made from a fingerstick in a patient with Glanzmann's thrombasthenia? *(p. 758)*

Q 13

In Glanzmann's thrombasthenia, glycoprotein _____
_____ is decreased, absent or functionally abnormal.
How effectively are the person's platelets able to bind fibrinogen? _____
_____

How does this affect clot retraction? _____
(p. 758)

Q 14

In Bernard–Soulier disease, the molecular defect is in platelet glycoprotein _____
_____. Because this glycoprotein binds to VWF, platelet adhesion is typically _____. Also, ristocetin-induced platelet aggregation, which utilizes vWF, is _____. Does ristocetin-induced platelet aggregation correct with the addition of reagent vWF? _____
(p. 758)

Q 15

What is the platelet morphology in Bernard–Soulier disease? *(p. 758)*

Q 16

Platelet aggregation studies on patients with Glanzmann's thrombasthenia and Bernard–Soulier disease show reciprocal patterns. Contrast these patterns, identifying normal vs decreased aggregation in response to the following agents. *(Fig. 39–8, pp. 753, 758)*

	Glanzmann's	Bernard–Soulier
Collagen		
ADP		
Epinephrine		
Ristocetin		

Q 17

True/False. Chediak–Higashi syndrome (CHS), Hermansky–Pudlak syndrome (HPS) and gray platelet syndrome are all platelet storage pool disorders with an autosomal recessive pattern of inheritance and associated oculocutaneous albinism in some of the affected patients. *(p. 759)*

Q 18

What cellular structure is absent in gray platelet syndrome? *(p. 759)*

Q 19

What X-linked disorder is characterized by thrombocytopenia? What are the key clinical manifestations of this disorder? *(p. 760)*

Q 20

What is the duration of the inhibitory effect on platelet function of ibuprofen? *(p. 764)*

Q 21

Briefly describe the dual role of von Willebrand factor (vWF) in hemostasis.
(p. 760)

Primary hemostasis: _____

Secondary hemostasis: _____

Q 22–27

Clinical Consultation: Six patients are seen in one day in a hospital's vWD clinic. Given their histories and laboratory findings, classify their vWD as type 1, 2A, 2B, 3, or platelet-type. *(Fig. 39–11, pp. 761–762)*

Q 22

Susan is a 17-year-old with a 4-year history of heavy menses. Her father had increased bleeding with a tooth extraction as a teenager. Mother and Susan's only sister have no bleeding history. Factor VIII and vWF antigen levels are both decreased at 36% and 25%, respectively. Platelet count is 221 000/μL. A multimer analysis shows absent large and intermediate multimers. Ristocetin cofactor activity is 9%.

Type: _____

Q 23

Karen is a 31-year-old with a history of heavy menses and increased bleeding with her two obstetric deliveries. No family history is available. Factor VIII level is 52%, vWF antigen is 48%, platelet aggregation with ristocetin is increased, and her platelet count is 47 000/μL. Genetic analysis of her vWF gene was normal.

Type: _____

Q 24

Paul is an active 10-year-old boy who develops epistaxis in the waiting room after a minor confrontation with Elaine (see below). His mother has a history of mildly increased bleeding with deliveries. His factor VIII level is 28% and vWF antigen is 30%. His platelet count is 276 000/μL; multimer analysis shows all multimers to be slightly decreased.

Type: _____

Q 25

David is a 35-year-old whose mother was diagnosed with vWD during her pregnancy after a complete blood count showed an abnormality. His factor ristocetin cofactor activity is 28%, vWF antigen is 70%, and he shows an increased response to ristocetin on a platelet aggregation study. The largest multimers of vWF are significantly decreased on his multimer analysis. Platelet count today is 60 000/μL.

Type: _____

Q 26

Elaine is a 12-year-old girl who has demonstrated increased bruising but is otherwise asymptomatic. Her father had significant bleeding with an appendectomy and required cryoprecipitate intraoperatively. Her factor VIII level is 21% and vWF antigen is 26%. Platelet count is 207 000/μL. Multimer analysis shows a mild decrease in low and intermediate-sized forms, but it is difficult to assess if larger multimers are decreased.

Type: _____

Q 27

Amy is a 5-year-old with multiple bruises, purpura, and petechiae sitting quietly in the waiting room. Her factor VIII level is 6%, and vWF antigen level is essentially zero. Her multimer analysis reveal no multimers. Platelet count is 185 000/μL.

Type: _____

Q 28

True/False. Increased bleeding diathesis in myelodysplastic syndromes is due to both quantitative and a myriad of qualitative defects. *(p. 763)*

CHAPTER 39

ANSWERS

A1. Platelet fibrinogen, platelet-derived growth factor, von Willebrand factor, beta-thromboglobulin, heparin neutralizing platelet factor (PF4), P-selectin.

A2. These are the elements of the dense core granules.

A3. In venules, platelets bind to exposed collagen directly. In arterioles, where there is a greater shear force, platelet GP Ib/IX/V binds to vWF.

A4. Thrombin. This factor has many roles in the coagulation cascade.

A5. Fibrinogen binds to platelet GP IIb/IIIa to stabilize the platelet plug.

A6. The bleeding time test is rarely used today. It is not predictive as a preoperative screening test.

A7. ATP is what is measured. It is difficult to measure ADP or 5HT, so ATP is used to assess the dense granules as a whole.

A8. GP IIb/IIIa is required for normal clot retraction. Thus, in Glanzmann thrombasthenia, clot retraction is poor.

A9. False. One may see immunoglobulins to platelets that do not influence platelet function in various clinical settings.

A10. Yes, the antibiotic should be discontinued. Sulfa drugs are well known offenders in ITP. Adults have only a 2% likelihood of spontaneous remission, compared to 83% in children. Complete recovery does occur in 64% of adults and 89% of children.

A11. The target of heparin antibodies is platelet factor 4 (PF4), which we reviewed earlier as heparin-neutralizing factor.

A12. Glanzmann's patients have normal numbers of platelets with a normal morphology. In normal patients, there is some degree of clumping, particularly in fresh blood. This is absent in Glanzmann disease, again because of the inability to bind platelets to fibrinogen.

A13. In Glanzmann disease, GP IIb/IIIa is decreased or defective. The platelets bind fibrinogen poorly, and clot retraction, which depends on fibrinogen binding to the platelets, is decreased.

A14. In Bernard–Soulier disease, the defect is in GP Ib and/or IX. Platelet adhesion, which we discussed as being mediated by platelets binding to vWF via GP Ib, is decreased. Ristocetin assays, which utilize vWF, are abnormal, with low decreased aggregation, and the addition of reagent vWF does not enable the patient's platelets to aggregate any more effectively, because they lack the GP Ib to bind to vWF.

A15. Some platelets are larger than normal.

A16. In Glanzmann's, platelet aggregation is decreased in response to the weak agonists, collagen, ADP, and epinephrine, but normal in response to ristocetin.
In Bernard–Soulier disease, the response to ristocetin is decreased, as the platelets lack GP Ib, but is normal with the weak agonists.

A17. False. Oculocutaneous albinism is not a feature of gray platelet syndrome but is a feature of HPS and CHS. Hermansky–Pudlak syndrome patients may also manifest congenital nystagmus, decreased visual acuity, granulomatous colitis or pulmonary fibrosis. Chediak–Higashi syndrome patients demonstrate immune deficiency (recall that their neutrophils are functionally and structurally abnormal, and their cytotoxic T and NK cells are defective) and neurologic dysfunction.

A18. Alpha granules are deficient in gray platelet syndrome.

A19. This is Wiskott–Aldrich syndrome. These patients usually have eczema and some degree of immunosuppression.

A20. 24 hours after the last dose of ibuprofen, platelet function returns to normal.

A21. In primary hemostasis, vWF binds to GP Ib on the surface of platelets to mediate adhesion, especially in arterioles. In secondary hemostasis, vWF is the protective carrier of factor VIII.

A22. Susan has type 2A.

A23. Karen has platelet type.

A24. Paul has type 1, the most common type.

A25. David has type 2B.

A26. Elaine has type 1.

ANSWERS

A27. Amy has type 3.

A28. True. Patients with myelodysplastic syndromes may have any of a number of structural and/or functional defects, and the impact of these defects may vary in the same patient over time.

CHAPTER 40

Laboratory approach to thrombotic risk

QUESTIONS

• Q 1

List the three major mechanisms that control excess clot formation. *(p. 770)*

• Q 2

Contrast type I and type II mutations of antithrombin. What tests distinguish these two? *(p. 772)*

• Q 3

Heterozygotes for protein C deficiency may be asymptomatic unless other thrombotic risk factors are present, and thus may not be diagnosed until adulthood. At what point will homozygotes for this deficiency manifest symptoms? *(p. 772)*

A6. No. APC, reagent or intrinsic, will inhibit clotting and prolong the PTT, so long as the patient is not resistant to APC. Here, the reagent APC prolonged the PTT; this is a normal result. The PTT without the addition of APC was also within the reference range. A ratio of PTT with APC/PTT without APC that is >2.0 points to the absence of APC-R. This gentleman probably has some clotting disorder, but it's not APC-R.

A7. This is factor VIII.

A8. These antibodies are directed at the β_2-glycoprotein or at another phospholipid binding protein.

A9. The excess phospholipids in this reagent overcome the antibodies in the patient's plasma. Then the time to clot becomes shorter. If the hexagonal phase phospholipids are effective at shortening the time to clot, this is proof of the antiphospholipid antibody.

A10. This is cystathionine-β-synthetase deficiency, the homozygous state.

CHAPTER 41

Antithrombotic therapy

QUESTIONS

• Q 1

Briefly describe the mechanism of action of warfarin. *(p. 778)*

• Q 2

A patient on warfarin has a PT of 30 seconds. The reference range for your laboratory is 11–13 seconds. The international sensitivity index (ISI) is unavailable but review of the package insert for your PT reagent reveals that it is recombinant tissue factor. What is your estimated calculation of the international normalized ratio (INR)? *(p. 779)*

• Q 3

Is the INR calculated in Question 2 appropriate for a patient with atrial fibrillation? *(p. 779)*

Q 4

Briefly describe the mechanisms of action of unfractionated heparin. *(p. 780)*

Q 5

What two assays are recommended to monitor heparin therapy during cardiopulmonary bypass? *(p. 780)*

Q 6

What is the pathophysiology of heparin-associated thrombocytopenia? *(p. 781)*

Q 7

Briefly discuss how heparin-induced thrombocytopenia (HIT) can lead to increased clotting *(Fig. 41–3, pp. 781–782)*.

Q 8

What is the most common laboratory assay used in the diagnosis of HIT? How sensitive and specific is it? *(p. 781)*

Q 9

What is the mechanism of action of the hirudin-derived drugs? *(p. 782)*

Q 10

What factor does the drug fondaparinux indirectly inhibit? *(Fig. 41–5, p. 783)*

Q 11

Briefly describe how aspirin inhibits platelet function. *(p. 783)*

ANSWERS

A1. Warfarin inhibits the enzymes vitamin K reductase to block the regeneration of the active form of vitamin K. The active form of vitamin K performs gamma-carboxylation of specific amino acid residues on factors II, VII, IX, X, protein C, and protein S. If these coagulation factors are not adequately carboxylated, then they cannot bind to complexes in the coagulation cascade and move the cascade toward the generation of fibrin.

A2. The teaching point here is that the recombinant tissue factor has an ISI that is nearly 1.0, so if you do not have it written on the package insert, you can make a fair estimate. The midpoint of the PT for your laboratory is 12 seconds, so 30/12 raised to the first power is 2.5.

A3. An INR of 2.5 is appropriate for a patient with atrial fibrillation.

A4. The key mechanism of action of heparin is that it binds to antithrombin and potentiates this molecule's inhibition of thrombin, so heparin is an indirect inhibitor of thrombin. Its additional effects are that it causes the release of tissue factor pathway inhibitor, increases tissue plasminogen activator and fibrinolysis, and impairs platelet function.

A5. These are the activated clotting time (ACT) and factor Xa inhibition.

A6. Heparin can bind directly to platelets via platelet factor 4 (PF4) and can cause mild and transient thrombocytopenia.

A7. In HIT, the immune system makes IgG antibodies against ultralarge complexes (ULC) of PF4, which are antigenic. IgG bound to these ULC can lead to platelet activation, release of granules and microparticles, and importantly, the generation of thrombin. Thrombin will convert fibrinogen to fibrin to form clots. When HIT is accompanied by thrombus formation, it is referred to as 'heparin-induced thrombocytopenia and thrombosis', or HITT.

A8. This is the PF4-ELISA immunoassay, which is pretty sensitive but not so specific. Functional assays, which offer high sensitivity and specificity, are technically demanding and may not be readily available.

A9. The hirudin-derived drugs form irreversible complexes with thrombin, so they are direct thrombin inhibitors.

A10. This drug is an indirect inhibitor of factor Xa.

A11. Aspirin irreversibly acetylates cyclooxygenase, and it is the cyclooxygenase pathway that generates thromboxane A_2 (TxA_2). TxA_2 activates platelets, so less of this molecule will result in diminished platelet activation, even though the platelets are present in adequate number.

Part VI

Immunology and immunopathology

CHAPTER 42

Overview of the immune system and immunologic disorders

QUESTIONS

Q 1

Which subunits make up the majority of T-cell receptors (TCR), and which subunits are found in a small percentage of TCRs? *(p. 789)*

Q 2

Differentiate between the roles and molecular products of the two classes of helper T cells, Th-1 and Th-2. *(p. 790)*

Q 3

What cell surface markers identify natural killer cells? *(p. 790)*

Q 4

What is the form of IgA found at mucosal surfaces? *(p. 791)*

Q 5

On what chromosome are the genes for the major histocompatibility complex (MHC) antigens? *(p. 791)*

Q 6

Briefly describe the immune reaction in the four types of hypersensitivity. *(pp. 791–792)*

Type I: _____

Type II: _____

Type III: _____

Type IV: _____

ANSWERS

A1. Alpha and beta subunits make up the majority; a few TCRs have delta and gamma subunits.

A2. Th-1 cells facilitate macrophage activity and secrete IL-2 and IFN-γ, the latter being a key activator of macrophages. They aid in synthesis of antibodies with opsonizing action.

   Th-2 cells direct synthesis of other antibodies and secrete IL-4 and IL-5, the former being a major activator of B cells.

A3. These are CD16 and CD56.

A4. Here IgA is in a dimer form.

A5. Chromosome 6.

A6. Type I – anaphylaxis, IgE-mediated release of histamine from basophils and mast cells.

   Type II – antibodies bind to antigens on cell surfaces, activating complement or causing cell-mediated cytotoxicity.

   Type III – immune complexes deposit in tissues causing damage.

   Type IV – delayed-type, cytotoxicity from CD4 and CD8 T cells.

CHAPTER 43

Immunoassays and immunochemistry

QUESTIONS

Q 1

Define the term epitope. *(p. 794)*

Q 2

Avidity is the sum of multiple antigen–antibody interactions that occur when an antibody binds to its corresponding epitope(s) on an antigen. Explain why the avidity of a polyclonal antibody, such as one generated by an immunization, is stronger than that of a monoclonal antibody, for a complex antigen. *(p. 794)*

Q 3

Compare and contrast precipitin reaction and particle agglutination assays. *(p. 794)*

• Q 4

The point at which precipitation in precipitin reactions is maximal is called
(p. 796)

_____ .

• Q 5

Review Figure 43.1 *(Figure 43–4A, p. 798)*. Using the home pregnancy test for hCG
as an example, the hapten-coupled particles are reagent hapten coupled to reagent
hCG. The antibody to hapten is reagent anti-hCG. What is the reaction pattern if
the patient's urine contains hCG? *(Figure 43–4, pp. 797–798)*

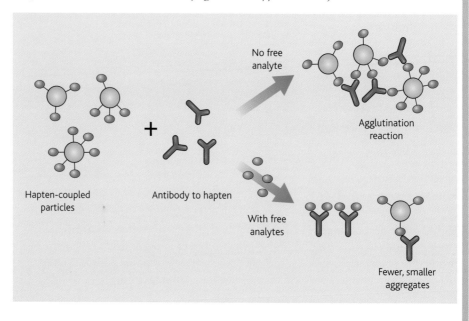

Hapten-coupled particles

Antibody to hapten

No free analyte

Agglutination reaction

With free analytes

Fewer, smaller aggregates

• Q 6

Describe the bivalent mouse monoclonal antibody system of hemagglutination to
test for HIV. *(Fig. 43–7, pp. 797, 800)*

Source of red blood cells (RBC)s: _____ Antibody of interest: _____

_____

Bivalent antibody binds to: _____ and _____
Positive results indicated by: _____

• Q 7

What is a major advantage of the gelatin particle over erythrocytes for agglutination, making this method more sensitive and specific than hemagglutination? *(Fig. 43–8, pp. 797, 801)*

• Q 8

How does the immunoreaction time of latex turbidimetry compare with that of other agglutination methods? *(p. 799)*

• Q 9

In competitive radioimmunoassay (RIA), what is the most common isotope used, and what pattern of decay is measured? *(p. 799)*

• Q 10

What two molecules are competing in competitive RIA methods? *(Fig. 43–10, p. 801)*

• Q 11

In noncompetitive RIA, or immunoradiometric assay (IRMA), how does the level of bound iodine-125 vary with the level of patient antigen? *(Fig. 43–12, pp. 801–802)*

• Q 12

Heterogeneous enzymes immunoassays (EIA), like RIA, may be configured for competitive or noncompetitive (sandwich) interactions. What is the major advantage of EIA over RIA in terms of laboratory safety? *(p. 803)*

• Q 13

Homogeneous EIA eliminates the complicated washing steps of the heterogeneous method, but at present has one key disadvantage compared to heterogeneous EIA. This is: *(p. 805)*

• Q 14

Enzyme-multiplied immunoassay technique (EMIT) is one example of a homogeneous EIA. It is often used to measure drug concentrations. Describe how a drug in patient serum will react with the EMIT reagents to give a positive result. *(Fig. 43–15, pp. 805–806)*

• Q 15

What variation of homogeneous immunoassay is particularly suited to measuring large antigens such as ferritin or α-fetoprotein? *(p. 807)*

• Q 16

Fluorescent immunoassays are often used to detect drugs, hormones, and proteins in patient samples. Describe how polarization is affected by the presence of patient antigen in the fluorescence polarization assay (FPIA). *(Fig. 43–20, p. 809)*

• Q 17

Acridinium esters are molecular labels for what type of assay? *(p. 810)*

• Q 18

Most automated immunoassay systems can treat _____ tests per hour. *(p. 811)*

Q 19

Carryover is when a very high concentration of analyte in one sample is passed on to the next sample, giving a false-positive or falsely elevated result in that following sample. What are some of the strategies to minimize carryover? *(p. 812)*

Q 20

In immunochromatographic devices, the initial reaction between the patient's analyte of interest and the reagent-labeled antigen or antibody takes place at the _____ end of the test strip. What reaction results in the colored line indicating a positive result? *(Fig. 43–24, p. 813)*

ANSWERS

A1. This is the amino acid sequence on an antigen that is recognized by an antibody.

A2. Avidity is the sum of multiple antigen–antibody interactions, a cumulative effect. Polyclonal antibodies recognize multiple epitopes on a single antigen and bind with greater avidity than monoclonal antibodies, which recognize just a single epitope.

A3. The precipitin reaction allows antigens and their corresponding antibodies to react, forming an insoluble lattice that is visible to the naked eye. No additional particle or substrate is required for the reaction to be apparent. This is a qualitative measurement only. The particle agglutination immunoassay introduces a third species, such as erythrocytes or latex beads, which are attached to the reagent antibody (or antigen). This ag–ab-particle complex agglutinates to become visible to the naked eye but, unlike precipitin reactions, may be used for quantitative detection of analytes.

A4. This is the point of equivalence.

A5. Fewer, smaller aggregates. Here hCG binds to the reagent antibody and thus prevents it from agglutinating the reagent hapten–antigen complex. This is an example of reverse agglutination.

A6. RBCs come from the patient/donor. The antibody of interest is anti-HIV.

The bivalent antibody binds to a RBC surface antigen and also to the anti-HIV antibody, if it is present in the patient. Agglutination, from the bivalent antibody binding **both** the RBC surface antigen and the patient's anti-HIV, constitutes a positive result.

A7. The gelatin particle has a very hydrophilic surface that prevents nonspecific binding and has no antigenicity, so it minimizes false-positive reactions from heterophile antibodies, a drawback seen with erythrocyte particles.

A8. Latex agglutination offers shorter incubation time. Some systems can perform 200 tests per hour.

A9. Iodine-125. Gamma radiation is measured.

A10. The patient antigen competes with radiolabeled antigen for binding to a reagent antibody.

A11. Proportionally. The standard curve has a positive slope, in contrast to competitive RIA, in which bound iodine-125 varies **inversely** with the level of patient antigen.

A12. The key advantage is that there is no radioactivity.

A13. Homogeneous systems have decreased sensitivity by one or two orders of magnitude.

A14. The patient drug/analyte/antigen binds to reagent antibody. By complexing with the antibody, the patient's analyte prevents the antibody from binding to the enzyme–reagent analyte complex and inactivating it. Thus, more active enzyme is present and there is a stronger signal indicating that the patient has the drug/analyte onboard.

A15. This is enzyme inhibitory homogeneous immunoassay.

A16. If a patient has no antigen, then a hapten-fluorescent conjugate will bind to a heavy (>160 kDa) reagent antibody, and this will slow rotation of the hapten–fluorescent conjugate, causing a strong polarizing signal.

   If the patient has the antigen of interest, then his antigen will bind to the reagent antibody, and there will still be some hapten–fluorescent conjugate free in the solution. This free conjugate will tumble about in the solution and thereby reduce the polarization.

A17. Chemiluminescence. This method is very similar to heterogeneous and fluorescence immunoassays.

A18. 60–200 tests per hour.

A19. Disposable plastic sample tubes are one method. Another is thorough washing steps, and fixed-probe tips are a third strategy.

A20. This first reaction takes place at the proximal end. The antigen–antibody complex, having migrated by capillary action down the strip, binds to a capture antibody which is immobilized in the detection zone.

CHAPTER 44

Laboratory evaluation of the cellular immune system

QUESTIONS

• Q 1

True/False. Despite the many advances in the field of cellular immunology in the 1980s, there are few tests of this arm of the immune system that are totally and specifically diagnostic, making interpretation of test results challenging. *(p. 820)*

• Q 2

What diseases, besides HIV, would you consider in a child with an inverted CD4$^+$/CD8 ratio? *(p. 820)*

• Q 3

What three tests, measured longitudinally over several months, may predict the severity of DiGeorge syndrome? *(p. 821)*

• Q 4

What mineral is required for the production of functionally mature T cells? *(p. 821)*

• Q 5

There are two classes of helper T cell. Broadly, which arm of the immune system does each help to regulate? *(p. 821)*

• Q 6

What cell surface molecule do lamina propria and intraepithelial T cells use for signal transduction in mucosal immunity? *(p. 822)*

• Q 7

What anticoagulants are appropriate for lymphocyte functional studies? *(p. 822)*

• Q 8

Comment on the utility of the skin test in the assessment of cellular immunity. What are its strengths and weaknesses? *(p. 822)*

• Q 9

Can NK studies be performed on neonates or infants? *(p. 823)*

• Q 10

In the two-signal model of T-cell activation, which T-cell molecules bind to which antigen-presenting cell (APC) molecules? *(p. 824)*

First signal:_____ on T cells bings to _____ on APCs.

Second signal: _____ on T cells bings to _____ on APCs.

• Q 11

T cell responses are divided into type I, a proinflammatory response, and type II, an anti-inflammatory and B-cell-stimulatory response. Which cytokines are involved in each type? *(p. 825)*

Type I: _____

Type II: _____

Q 12

Briefly outline three procedures used by most laboratories to assess T-cell activation and the proliferative capacity of lymphocytes. *(p. 825)*

Q 13

What is the main drawback of the tritiated thymidine incorporation assay and how does flow cytometry address this problem? *(p. 825)*

Q 14

What are two major applications of static image analysis in common use today? *(p. 826)*

Q 15

What is the greatest strength of flow cytometry? *(p. 826)*

Q 16

The two common flow cell systems is use in the clinical laboratory are the flow-in-air flow cell and the quartz tip system. What is the main advantage of the quartz tip system? *(pp. 826–827)*

Q 17

What dye is most commonly used for DNA measurements? *(p. 828)*

• Q 18

Evaluate the flow cytometry panels in *Figure 44–1*. (*p. 827*)
What is the phenotype of the cells in quadrant 4 of panel 2? _____
In quadrant 2 of panel 3? _____

• Q 19

What cell surface marker is typically used as a gate in bone marrow analyses? (*pp. 828–829*)

• Q 20

True/False. The FDA still considers DNA measurements and histogram analysis a research test, probably because of difficulties in standardizing histogram analysis. (*p. 829*)

• Q 21

How is the amount of cell surface antigen per cell quantified in the field of quantitative flow cytometry? (*p. 830*)

. . . .

ANSWERS

A1. True. Flow cytometry is probably the most reliable tool we have currently.

A2. Consider DiGeorge syndrome, Kawasaki disease if the inverted ratio is acute, and possibly protein–calorie malnutrition, although this is rarely seen in the United States except in abuse cases.

A3. The CD4$^+$ T-cell count, the CD4$^+$/CD8$^+$ ratio (as just discussed), and the production of IL-2 are all useful predictors. If all three are low, the prognosis is worse.

A4. This is zinc.

A5. Th-1 regulates the cellular arm, while Th-2 stimulates the humoral arm.

A6. This is CD2.

A7. Sodium heparin without preservative and acid citrate are appropriate.

A8. The skin test correlates well with immune deficiency but does not suggest a reason for the deficiency and is not very quantifiable.

A9. No. This arm of the immune system is not well developed in neonates.

A10. First signal: T-cell antigen receptor – CD4 or CD8 on T cells binds to MHC II or I on APCs. Recall that CD4$^+$ cells bind to MHC II and CD8$^+$ cells bind to MHC I.
Second signal: CD28 on T cells binds to B7 on APCs.

A11. Type I responses – IL-2, IFN-γ, IL-12.
Type II responses – IL-4, IL-5, IL-10, IL-13.

A12. The skin test for delayed-type hypersensitivity is the first test to perform. It is an in vivo test and, although it is not particularly sensitive, it has pretty good specificity with few false positives. Proliferative capacity is assessed in most laboratories by the tritiated thymidine assay. It measures the rate of incorporation of radiolabeled DNA nucleosides over 4–24 hours following incubation of peripheral blood mononuclear cells with mitogens or antigens for several days. Finally, flow cytometry can be used to measure lymphocytes in various phases of the cell cycle by measuring the fluorescence intensity of dyes such as propidium iodide, which intercalate into DNA.

A13. The bulk assays do not tell you which lymphocyte subsets are responding. Flow cytometry can identify cell surface markers to indicate T, B and natural killer cells, and T-cell subsets, using tracking dyes that are incorporated into the lymphocyte membranes.

A14. These are DNA and fluorescence in situ hybridization (FISH).

A15. Flow cytometry can perform multiparameter analysis, simultaneously detecting multiple surface antigens, or cytoplasmic or nuclear constituents.

A16. It is a closed system, which is preferred for biosafety reasons when performing CD4$^+$ counts on HIV-positive patients.

A17. This is propidium iodide.

A18. Quadrant 4 of panel 2 – CD4$^-$, CD8$^+$ cells, cytotoxic or suppressor T cells.
Quadrant 2 of panel 3 – CD3$^+$, CD4$^+$ cells, or helper T cells.

A19. This is CD45.

A20. True.

A21. The antibody-binding capacity of a particular fluorochrome antibody conjugate results in a specific fluorescence intensity, which can be measured.

CHAPTER 45

Laboratory evaluation of immunoglobulin function and humoral immunity

QUESTIONS

Q 1

At which end of the amino acid sequence of an immunoglobulin molecule is the antigen-binding site? *(p. 835)*

Q 2

What is the significance of bivalence of antibodies? *(p. 835)*

Q 3

Describe the cleavage fragments of pepsin and papain. *(Fig. 45–1, p. 836)*
Pepsin:_____
Papain:_____

Q 4

In which domain of the immunoglobulin molecule do the following events occur?
(Table 45–1, pp. 836–837)
Antigen binding: _____
Reactions with macrophages: _____
Binding of complement C1q: _____

Q 5

Define affinity maturation. *(p. 837)*

Q 6

Define somatic hypermutation and give its significance. *(p. 838)*

Q 7

What is the sedimentation rate of normal IgM, and what alternate form is found in many patients with systemic lupus erythematosus (SLE)? *(p. 838)*

Q 8

How does IgG activate complement, and which subclass of IgG is the most effective at this task? *(p. 840)*

Q 9

Briefly outline how IgA dimers are incorporated into epithelial cells in the intestine, bronchi, salivary ducts, etc. *(Fig. 45-4, pp. 840–841)*

Q 10

IgE binds to the Fc receptor on what two related molecules? *(p. 841)*

Q 11

In studies of several communities, black people have been shown to have higher levels than white people of which immunoglobulin? *(p. 842)*

Q 12

Although many disease states are associated with a polyclonal gammopathy involving all classes of immunoglobulin, in some diseases one class predominates in the polyclonal response. Which class of immunoglobulin is typically elevated in these conditions? *(Table 45–6, p. 842)*

Anaphylactoid purpura: _____ Biliary cirrhosis: _____

Narcotic addiction: _____ Chronic active hepatitis: _____

Q 13

Up to 75% of organ transplant patients on immunosuppressive drugs that alter T-lymphocyte functions may have what type of gammopathy? *(p. 843)*

Q 14

What levels of monoclonal IgG and IgA suggest a malignant condition? *(p. 843)*

Q 15

Both immunoelectrophoresis (IEP) and immunofixation (IFE) are sensitive techniques for evaluating gammopathies. What advantages does IFE have over IEP that have led to its replacing IEP in the clinical laboratory? *(p. 845)*

Q 16

Study Figure 45.1 *(pp. 845–846)* and interpret the following serum immunofixation specimens.

Specimen A: _____

Specimen C: _____

Specimen F: _____

ANSWERS

A1. This is the amino-terminal end.

A2. Bivalent antibodies can cross-link multivalent antigen molecules (if the antigens have at least three antigenic determinants) and cross-linking enhances phagocytosis of antigen–antibody complexes.

A3. Pepsin – two identical Fab fragments, one Fc fragment.
Papain – one (Fab')2 fragment, which is bivalent, and smaller fragments with no activity.

A4. Antigen binding – VH, VL.
Reactions with macrophages – CH3.
Binding complement C1q – CH2.

A5. This is an increase in the strength of the bond of an antibody to a single antigenic determinant. It occurs as antibodies are produced after exposure to an antigen. IgM has strong avidity, or cumulative binding power, because it can bind ten sites at once, but lacks affinity. IgG, the secondary response antibody, has stronger affinity.

A6. After exposure to a particular antigen, B cells (not germ cells) can effect mutations in the heavy and light chain variable region genes and in nearby introns to further expand the repertoire of antibody molecules.

A7. Normal is 19S. In SLE patients, there is a monomeric form of IgM that has a rate of 7S.

A8. The Fc portion of IgG binds to the C1 molecule to initiate the classical cascade. IgG3 is most effective at this, although IgG1 and IgG2 can activate complement as well.

A9. Epithelial cells lining these spaces synthesize a receptor for IgA, called secretory component (SC), and then expose SC on the nonluminal surface of the cell. Dimeric IgA binds to this receptor and forms a complex with it. This complex is brought into the cell by receptor-mediated endocytosis. The amino terminus of SC remains attached to IgA and may protect IgA from proteolysis. Thus, secretory IgA is not only a dimer but also has a component that was synthesized apart from the plasma cell.

A10. These are basophils and mast cells.

A11. Black people have higher levels of IgG than white people in studies worldwide.

A12. Anaphylactoid purpura – IgA. (It's IgA, not IgE.)
Biliary cirrhosis and narcotic addiction – IgM.
Chronic active hepatitis – IgG.

A13. Monoclonal gammopathy of undetermined significance (MGUS). It is usually transient.

A14. IgG >2 g/dL, or IgA >1 g/dL suggests a malignancy if monoclonal.

A15. IFE offers speed and ease of interpretation over IEP.

A16. Specimen A – normal.
Specimen C – IgA, λ, monoclonal.
Specimen F – λ light chains, monoclonal.

CHAPTER 46

Mediators of inflammation:

complement, cytokines, and

adhesion molecules

QUESTIONS

• Q 1

List the three general ways in which the complement system destroys foreign cells and microorganisms. *(p. 850)*

• Q 2

C3 is a protein central to all three complement pathways that undergoes multiple degradation steps to yield a variety of bioactive molecules. *(Fig. 46–2, pp. 851–852)*
Does C3 interact with any receptor in its native form? _____
_____

What structure in the α chain is hydrolyzed to yield C3b? _____
_____

What is the end result of C3b bound to a target? _____
_____

What can iC3b promote? _____
What molecule is formed in the alternate pathway from interactions of C3b with factors D, B, and properdin, and what is its purpose? _____
_____

What is the role of properdin in the alternate pathway? _____
_____

Q 3

What molecular interaction usually initiates the classical pathway? *(p. 852)*

Q 4

Which component of the classical pathway is an anaphylatoxin? *(p. 852)*

Q 5

What two alternate pathway components interact to generate the initiation C3 convertase? *(p. 852)*

Q 6

The third pathway of complement involves a series of collectins that are homologous to some of the classical pathway proteins. Mannose-binding lectin (MBL) is structurally related to _____, and MBL-associated serine proteases (MASP)-1 and -2 are related to _____and _____. MASP-2 interacts with the classical pathway by cleaving _____ to generate C3 convertase. *(p. 852)*

Q 7

Which components of the membrane attack complex (MAC) initially insert into the lipid bilayer of cell membranes? *(p. 853)*

Q 8

List some of the biological effects shared by the anaphylatoxins C3a, C4a, and C5a. *(p. 853)*

Q 9

State the fluid-phase or cell-associated regulators of the following complement components, including any required cofactors. *(pp. 853–854)*

C1: _____

C4b: _____

C3b: _____

C5b–7 complex: _____

iC3b: _____

C3 or C5 convertase: _____

Terminal components: _____

Q 10

What is a major physiologic role of complement receptor 1 (CR1)? *(p. 854)*

Q 11

CR2 is the receptor for what complement component and what virus? *(pp. 854–855)*

Q 12

What is the inheritance pattern for most of the complement components? *(p. 855)*

Q 13

Clinical Consultation: A 16-month-old girl has a history of recurrent upper respiratory infections. Her father reports having the same problems as a toddler and still seems to get more colds than others around him. His sister, the girl's aunt, frequently gets colds and was diagnosed with systemic lupus erythematosus (SLE) at age 17. Based on the frequency of complement deficiencies, which one is most likely here? *(Table 46–4, pp. 855–856)*

Q 14

Deficiencies of the components of the membrane attack complex are associated with increased infections with what organism? *(Table 46–4, p. 856)*

• Q 15

Deficiencies in which pathway are well associated with SLE? *(Table 46–4, pp. 855–856)*

• Q 16

Although not true in every case, in some cases of SLE these two complement components are reduced and are useful markers of disease activity. *(p. 856)*

• Q 17

What is the molecular defect causing CD59 and decay-accelerating factor (DAF) deficiencies in paroxysmal nocturnal hemoglobinuria? *(p. 858)*

• Q 18

One of the gold standards in the functional evaluation of the classical pathway is measurement of the total hemolytic activity (CH50). *(p. 860)*
What cells are generally the target of complement-mediated lysis in this system?
_____

What patient specimen is preferred, and which calcium chelators may inhibit complement? _____
Define CH50 units: _____
_____

• Q 19

What technique is commonly used to determine specific complement protein levels by antigenic assays? *(p. 861)*

• Q 20

List the four major proteins of the kinin-generating system. *(p. 861)*

• Q 21

What two cell types are responsible for most cytokine production? *(p. 861)*

• Q 22

Interleukin (IL)-1 is a major cytokine with multiple effects on many aspects of the immune system. Briefly outline its actions in the following areas. *(p. 862)*

Hematopoiesis: _____

Vascular endothelium: _____

_____

Liver: _____

Central nervous system: _____

_____

• Q 23

IL-2 stimulates proliferation of what types of lymphocyte? *(p. 862)* _____

_____

What other cytokine shares some biologic activities with IL-2? _____

_____

• Q 24

Production of which cell lines are increased with high doses of IL-3 in mice? *(p. 862)*

Q 25

IL-4 is another cytokine with several functions. Key among these are its effects on humoral immunity and hematopoiesis. Describe the action of IL-4 in these areas. *(p. 862)*

Q 26

What cell is particularly supported by IL-5? *(p. 863)*

Q 27

IL-6 is an important cytokine in hematopoiesis, and its proinflammatory actions parallel those of IL-1. It is also a growth factor for what neoplastic cell lines? *(p. 863)*

Q 28

IL-7 promotes development of what cell lines? *(p. 863)*

Q 29

What is the chief action of IL-8? *(p. 863)*

Q 30

IL-9 has been shown to have growth factor and antiapoptotic activity in transformed cell lines and is associated with what lymphoid tumors? *(p. 864)*

• Q 31

IL-10 is the major anti-inflammatory cytokine, with several actions. Briefly describe its effects. *(p. 864)*

Inhibits production of what proinflammatory cytokine? _____
_____

Action within macrophages: _____
In allergic conditions: _____
On chemoattractants: _____

• Q 32

IL-11 is another anti-inflammatory cytokine. Additionally it has a role in hematopoiesis. Describe its therapeutic use in this role. *(p. 865)*

• Q 33

IL-12, a major proinflammatory cytokine, stimulates Th1 cells to produce what other proinflammatory cytokine? *(p. 865)*

• Q 34

IL-13 levels are increased in patients with what types of disorder? *(p. 865)*

• Q 35

IL-18 acts with IL-12 to induce the production of what cytokine by Th1 cells? *(p. 866)*

• Q 36

Transforming growth factor (TGF)-β plays what role in wound healing? *(p. 867)*

• Q 37

Tumor necrosis factor (TNF)-α falls into what broad class of cytokines? *(p. 867)*

What is its effect in malignancy and some parasitic infections? *(p. 867)*

• Q 38

Interferon (IFN)-γ chiefly stimulates what cell? *(p. 867)*

• Q 39

What is the role of the integrin LFA-1 (CD11a/CD18)? *(p. 868)*

• Q 40

Margination of leukocytes is facilitated by which endothelial adhesins? *(p. 868)*

• Q 41

Where is P-selectin stored prior to its expression? *(p. 868)*

• Q 42

What additional role do selectins play besides facilitating cell adhesion? *(p. 868)*

A1. Direct lysis, opsonization, and attracting phagocytic cells.

A2. No, C3 can't bind any receptor in its native state.

A thioester in the hydrophobic center of C3 is hydrolyzed to yield C3b.

The end result of C3b bound to cells is continuation of the cascade to the point of lysis.

iC3b can promote phagocytosis but it can't effect lysis.

The alternate pathway forms C3bBb, also known as C3 convertase, which effects further cleavage of C3.

Properdin stabilizes C3 convertase (C3bBb), which would otherwise rapidly decay.

A3. Two IgGs or one IgM binding to an antigen with subsequent binding of C1 by the Fc portion of the antibody start the classical pathway.

A4. This is C4a.

A5. These are factors B and D.

A6. MBL is related to C1q. MASP-1 and 2 are related structurally to C1r and C1s. MASP-2 can act on the classical pathway by cleaving C4 to make C3 convertase.

A7. This is C5b–7. C8 and C9 bind once this complex is already in the lipid bilayer.

A8. The anaphylatoxins all effect vasodilation via histamine release from basophils, smooth muscle contraction, polymorphonuclear lymphocyte (PMN) aggregation, enhanced vascular permeability, and stimulation of mucus secretion from goblet cells. C5a has some unique actions as well.

A9. C1 – C1 inhibitor.

C4b – factor I. Cofactor – C4-binding protein.

C3b – factor I. Cofactor – factor H, CR1.

C5b-7 – S-protein (vitronectin), clusterin.

iC3b – factor I. Cofactor – CR1 or CR2.

C3 or C5 convertase – decay-accelerating factor (DAF).

Terminal components – homologous restriction factor or CD59.

A10. CR1 facilitates opsonization.

A11. C3d and Epstein–Barr virus.

A12. Most are inherited in an autosomal co-dominant fashion.

A13. 5% of individuals have some mutation in the mannose-binding lectin leading to a deficiency. This is inherited as an autosomal dominant trait and may be associated with SLE.

A14. This is *Neisseria meningitidis*.

A15. This is the classical pathway.

A16. C3 and C4 are often useful markers of disease activity.

A17. These patients lack the cell membrane anchor for CD59 and DAF, the glycosyl phosphatidylinositol-linked proteins. This is due to a mutation in the gene for phosphatidylinositol glycan A. Without the membrane anchor for CD59 and DAF, these proteins are essentially absent. The red cells have little defense against complement-mediated lysis (the alternate name for Cd50 is membrane inhibitor of reactive lysis, or MIRL). After the red cells lyse, hemoglobin is passed out in the urine.

A18. Sheep red blood cells (RBCs) are the target of lysis.

Serum is the preferred sample. Ethylenediaminetetraacetic acid (EDTA) and heparin may be anticomplementary.

CH50 units are the reciprocal of the dilution of complement that lyses 50% of the sensitized (by rabbit antibody) sheep RBCs.

A19. This is single radial immunodiffusion, using the Fahey or Mancini method.

A20. These are Hageman factor, clotting factor XI, prekallikrein, and high-molecular-weight kininogen.

A21. T cells and macrophages generate most of the cytokines.

A22. IL-1 stimulates progenitor cell proliferation along with the colony-stimulating factors.

It upregulates adhesion molecules at sites of inflammation to promote accumulation of white blood cells, and also induces nitric oxide production to cause hypotension.

In the liver, it promotes synthesis of acute phase reactants.

In the central nervous system, it promotes fever, anorexia, slow-wave sleep, and lethargy.

A23. CD4$^+$, CD8$^+$, NK and B cells are all favored by IL-2 although IL-2's effects are thought of as primarily targeting the T-lymphocyte populations. IL-15 shares some activities with IL-2. If you can remember the actions of IL-2, then just try to link IL-15 along with IL-2.

A24. IL-3 stimulates all three cells lines – red cells, white cells, and platelets.

A25. IL-4 activates and promotes differentiation of B cells and regulates B-cell apoptosis and isotype switching. It also stimulates colony formation for RBCs, platelets, granulocytes, and monocytes.

A26. Eosinophils. Virtually every aspect of their existence is promoted by IL-5. E (for eosinophils) is the fifth letter of the alphabet; this is a helpful way to remember the target of IL-5.

A27. Human myeloma and plasmacytoma.

A28. T cells, B cells, and myeloid precursors are all favored by IL-7.

A29. IL-8 is a chemokine. Its main action is the accumulation of neutrophils at sites of inflammation, facilitated by the activation of CD11b/CD18 on PMNs.

A30. These are Hodgkin, anaplastic and lymphoblastic lymphomas.

A31. IL-10 inhibits production of IL-1, IL-3, IL-6, IL-8, TNF-α, G-CSF, GM-CSF, and MIP-1α.

It suppresses release of free radicals and inhibits nitric-oxide-dependent killing in macrophages.

It prevents IL-5 production in T cells to slow the allergic response.

It inhibits production of chemoattractants at sites of chronic inflammation.

A32. IL-11 has been used in chemotherapy patients to improve hematopoiesis and thus reduce the morbidity of bone-marrow suppressive agents.

A33. Interferon (IFN)-γ.

A34. IL-13 is associated with allergic disorders. It seems to have both pro- and anti-allergic effects.

A35. IFN-γ.

A36. TGF-β promotes fibroblast proliferation and collagen synthesis. Excess TGF-β can lead to fibrosis and scarring, and researchers are studying the use of an anti-TGF-β antibody to prevent this in scleroderma patients.

A37. TNF-α is another major proinflammatory cytokine. It causes wasting syndrome in cancer patients and in some patients with severe parasite infections.

A38. The macrophage is the key recipient of the effects of IFN-γ.

A39. LFA-1 on leukocytes mediates adhesion to the vascular endothelium during migration.

A40. These are E-selectin and P-selectin.

A41. P-selectin is stored in the Weibel–Palade bodies of platelets and in endothelial cells.

A42. The selectins also play a role in signal transduction.

CHAPTER 47

Human leukocyte antigen:
the major histocompatibility complex
of man

QUESTIONS

Q 1

On which chromosome is the major histocompatibility complex (MHC) located? *(p. 878)*

Q 2

Define linkage disequilibrium, a key feature of the MHC system. *(p. 878)*

Q 3

Describe the basic structure of the HLA Class I molecule, including which domains give rise to polymorphism and which is/are conserved. *(Fig. 47–3, pp. 878–879)*

Q 4

What two cytokines can up-regulate expression of HLA-I molecules? *(p. 880)*

Q 5

In adaptive immunity, what cell recognizes processed peptide/antigen in conjunction with HLA-I molecules? *(p. 880)*

Q 6

The absence or down-regulation of HLA-I molecules may lead to direct cell lysis by which immune cells? *(p. 880)*

Q 7

How do HLA-E, F, and G molecules compare with HLA-A, B, and C in terms of polymorphism and cell surface expression? *(p. 881)*

_____

What is the putative role of HLA-G? _____

_____

Q 8

Describe the basic structure of HLA-II molecules. *(Fig. 47–3, pp. 879–881)*

Q 9

Which is the predominant subregion in class II molecules? *(p. 882)*

Q 10

Which lymphocyte subset recognizes HLA-II and processed antigen? *(p. 882)*

• Q 11

Describe which type of peptide is bound by each class of MHC molecule. *(p. 883)*

Class I: _____

Class II: _____

• Q 12

What are the two HLA-B public epitopes, such that all HLA-B molecules carry one of these epitopes? *(p. 884)*

• Q 13

Class I and II antigens are now typed using DNA-based methods. Briefly state how DNA-based typing is advantageous. *(p. 884)*

Specific: _____

Flexible: _____

Robust: _____

Large-scale: _____

Discriminating: _____

• Q 14

The older microcytotoxicity assay is still sometimes used with which HLA molecules? *(p. 886)*

• Q 15

In tissue and organ transplants, which three HLA loci are matched (each with two alleles) as closely as possible? *(p. 887)*

• Q 16

What is tested in the panel reactive antibody (PRA) and donor-specific crossmatch tests? *(pp. 888–889)*

• Q 17

Are HLA matching and donor-specific crossmatch testing performed on heart, liver, lung, and pancreas transplant organs? *(p. 890)*

• Q 18

What level of resolution of HLA typing is needed for hematopoietic progenitor cell transplants compared to that needed for renal transplants? *(p. 890)*

ANSWERS

A1. MHC is encoded on the short arm of chromosome 6, at 6p21.

A2. Linkage disequilibrium is when alleles at different loci occur more frequently on the same haplotype in a population than would be expected by chance alone.

A3. HLA-I consists of a heavy chain, a transmembrane glycosylated peptide, with three extracellular domains: α_1, α_2, and α_3. α_1 and α_2 are polymorphic, while α_3 is conserved. The heavy chain is noncovalently associated with β_2-microglobulin. α_3 and β_2-microglobulin have similar tertiary structures, as do α_1 and α_2. Antigenic peptide fragments fit in a groove made by α_1 and α_2.

A4. IFN-γ and TNF.

A5. This is the $CD8^+$ cytotoxic T lymphocyte.

A6. These are the natural killer (NK) cells. Elegant intermolecular signaling regulates this process.

A7. These other class I molecules are less polymorphic and have lower expression than do the main players. HLA-G contributes to maternofetal tolerance by acting as a ligand for NK inhibitory receptors to protect placental tissue from NK cells.

A8. Class II molecules consist of two noncovalently associated transmembrane glycoproteins, an α and a β chain. The α_1 and β_1 regions are polymorphic, while the α_2 and β_2 regions are conserved. The α_2 and β_2 regions are homologous to the constant region of the immunoglobulin molecule.

A9. This is DR, which accounts for over half the HLA-II molecules on the cell surface. DR is the key MHC class II molecule in transplant medicine.

A10. These are the CD4⁺ T cells.

A11. Class I – binds peptides synthesized de novo from endogenous antigens.
Class II – binds peptides from soluble or particulate antigens (exogenous).

A12. These are HLA-Bw4 and Bw6.

A13. Specific – synthetic oligonucleotide probes are generated from known nucleotide sequences; they bind base to base precisely.
Flexible – as new alleles are discovered, new oligonucleotide probes can be made.
Robust – viable lymphocytes are not required, as in serologic methods. DNA methods are also reproducible.
Large-scale – automated instruments allow batching so that many potential donors can be screened quickly, to find a match in a short time (hopefully).
Discriminating – older serologic methods could not always discriminate between two similar alleles, but DNA methods can. This is what we mean by specificity.

A14. HLA-A and B.

A15. HLA-A, B and DR. Thus, there are six alleles that may be matched. 6/6 is a perfect match.

A16. In PRA, recipient serum is tested against a panel of HLA antigens to determine if the recipient has any preformed antibodies that would rule out donors with those specific HLA antigens. This sounds analogous to the antibody screen done in the blood bank.
    The donor-specific crossmatch incubates recipient serum with a specific donor's lymphocytes to check for antibodies to the donor's cells. Donor lymphocytes are rich in HLA antigens, so they would readily elicit an antibody response by the recipient, and are thus chosen for this test.

A17. No, not routinely. An HLA match has no effect on the survival of liver transplants in one study, though the same study found a significant impact of HLA matching on first heart transplants.

A18. Higher resolution is required for progenitor cell transplants because the entire immune system is being transferred from the donor to the recipient.

CHAPTER 48

The major histocompatibility complex and disease

QUESTIONS

Q 1

The class III molecules are encoded by genes located between those for class I and class II molecules and are a varied group, in contrast to HLA-I and II proteins. *(p. 895)*

Which complement proteins are encoded here? _____

_____

Which cytokines? _____

Which steroid biosynthetic enzyme? _____

Q 2

Both C2 and factor B are serine proteases, and they show considerable homology. It is not surprising, then, that they have a common function in their respective complement pathways. This is: *(p. 896)*

Q 3

C4 variants carry the antigenic determinants of what blood groups? *(pp. 896–897)*

Q 4

C2, C4, and factor B all show some polymorphism among races. This is most pronounced in _____, where most white people have a slowly migrating variant, and most black people have a fast variant. *(p. 897)*

Q 5

What four regions of the HLA genes make up the extended haplotype? *(p. 898)*

Q 6

What are the two main methods used for complement typing, and what unique method can be used for C4 typing? *(p. 896)*

Q 7

What is the most common complement protein deficiency state in Caucasians, and what is the implication of this deficiency for most patients? *(p. 897)*

Q 8

Most patients with 21-hydroxylase deficiency do not have an extended haplotype, but 20% of patients with severe disease/salt-wasting do have a rare extended haplotype. What two genes are deleted in these cases? *(p. 900)*

Q 9

In addition to *HLA-DR3* and *DR4*, this gene is now considered a major marker for type 1 diabetes susceptibility. *(p. 900)*

Q 10

What are the most common rheumatoid arthritis (RA) associated *HLA-D4* alleles in Caucasians? *(p. 900)*

• Q 11

What HLA antigens are found mostly in Caucasians and are associated with rapid progression in HIV disease? *(p. 901)*

• Q 12

A recent study has suggested that the *DQB1*0003* allele is associated with susceptibility to progressive clinical tuberculosis. Briefly describe the molecular structural abnormality in the gene product and how it contributes to a blunted response. *(p. 901)*

• Q 13

Give the formula for calculating relative risk (RR), and state what the RR estimates. *(p. 901)*

RR =

RR calculates _____

_____

• Q 14

What are the two common missense mutations seen in hereditary hemochromatosis? *(p. 899)*

ANSWERS

A1. The complement proteins C2, C4, and factor B are coded for in the MHC III region.

The cytokines TNF and lymphotoxins (LT) α and β are encoded here. 21-hydroxylase is also in the MHC III region.

A2. C2 and factor B both mediate cleavage of C3.

A3. C4A carries the Rodgers blood group antigen, while Chido is on the C4B variant.

A4. Factor B has the most marked racial variation.

A5. These are HLA-B, complotype (C2, BF, C4A, and C4B), HLA-DR, and the most recent addition, HLA-Cw.

A6. Electrophoresis and isoelectric focusing are the two main methods. Serum containing antibodies to the Chido (C4B) or Rodgers (C4A) blood groups can also be used for C4 typing.

A7. The deficiency of C2 is the most common. Fortunately, most patients are asymptomatic. However, up to 25% of homozygotes have an increased susceptibility to bacterial infections, and 20–40% have a systemic-lupus-like disease.

A8. Both *C4B* and *CYP21B* are deleted in 20% of severe cases.

A9. *DQB1*0002* in linkage disequilibrium with *HLA-DR4* is the major marker for type 1 DM.

A10. In RA, *DR4* associated with *DRB1*0001* and *0004* are common findings.

A11. These are HLA-B35 and Cw4.

A12. Researchers believe they have identified the peptide binding pocket of the DQ molecule. Patients with the DQB1*0503 gene product may not be able to bind the peptide derived from the tuberculosis bacterium when it is presented by macrophages, and thus they have a diminished immune response.

A13. $RR = \dfrac{a \times d}{b \times c}$

Where 'a' individuals are patients with the character, 'b' individuals are patients lacking the character, 'c' persons are controls with the character, and 'd' persons are controls lacking the character.

RR calculates the risk of carrying a marker in a population of persons with the disease of interest compared to the control population.

A14. These are C282Y and H63D.

CHAPTER 49

Immunodeficiency disorders

QUESTIONS

• Q 1

What aspect of the immune system is affected in approximately half of reported immune defects? *(p. 906)*

• Q 2

A patient with a phagocytic defect will probably have a history of infections with this genus of bacteria *(p. 908)* _____

A patient with a complement deficiency will have recurrent infections with these genera _____

• Q 3

Clinical Consultation: A 5-year-old boy develops a *Haemophilus influenzae* type B infection despite having received the full vaccine series. His platelet count is 48 000/μL, and mean platelet volume is 6.5 fL. A skin rash is noted. *(pp. 908–909)*
What is your leading diagnosis? _____

How might immunoglobulin levels support this diagnosis? _____

• Q 4

A chest X-ray demonstrates splaying of the ends of the ribs, squaring off of the scapulae, and unusual articulations of the transverse rib processes. In a patient with multiple types of recurrent infection, what is the likely biochemical defect and clinical syndrome? *(p. 910)*

• Q 5

Both chronic granulomatous disease and hyper-IgE syndrome may present with recurrent skin and pulmonary abscesses. What clinical features will help distinguish hyper-IgE syndrome from chronic granulomatous disease? *(p. 911)*

• Q 6

Which four vaccines are most useful in assessing post-booster antibody titers? *(p. 910)*

• Q 7

Functional assessment of T cells in young children is hampered by the fact that skin tests cannot be used until the child has been exposed to the antigen in the skin test (usually occurs by 3–5 years), and also by the fact that response to mitogen stimulation may not equate with effective in vivo T-cell immunity. Which test can be used in infants and demonstrates a severe T-cell defect when negative? *(pp. 910–911)*

• Q 8

What is the classic laboratory method for diagnosing chronic granulomatous disease? *(p. 911)*

• Q 9

What cell type(s) is/are affected by a deficiency of purine nucleoside phosphorylase (PNP)? *(p. 911)*

• Q 10

A complete deficiency of natural killer (NK) cells is characterized by recurrent infections with what organisms? *(p. 911)*

• Q 11

Which integrin is defective in leukocyte adhesion defect (LAD)-1? *(p. 912)*

LAD-2 is associated with what unusual blood group?

• Q 12

Briefly describe the molecular defect in human X-linked severe combined immunodeficiency syndrome (SCID). *(p. 912)*

ANSWERS

A1. Defects in antibody production are particularly common.

A2. The patients with phagocytic defects have trouble handling *Staphylococcus* species, while those with complement deficiencies struggle with *Streptococcus* and *Neisseria*.

A3. In Wiskott–Aldrich syndrome, IgA, and often IgE levels are typically elevated, while IgM levels are decreased.

A4. This is adenosine deaminase deficiency in severe combined immunodeficiency (SCID).

A5. Patients with hyper-IgE syndrome present with bony abnormalities, unusual facies and cutaneous candidiasis.

A6. The four vaccines are tetanus, diphtheria, haemophilus, and pneumococcus.

A7. Mitogenic concentrations of monoclonal anti-CD3 are incubated with the patient's peripheral blood mononuclear cells. An absence of proliferation of all CD3 demonstrates a severe defect. This is another mitogenic reaction, but is presented in Henry as being more useful than other mitogenic studies.

A8. This is the nitroblue tetrazolium test. It has largely been replaced by flow cytometry. Either method will assess for the presence or absence of intracellular killing by respiratory burst.

A9. PNP deficiency results in T-cell deficiency but has no effect on B cells.

A10. Although rare, complete NK cell deficiency has been described and is associated with recurrent herpes infections.

A11. LAD-1 is a defect in CD18, the common β chain of LFA-1, Mac-1, and p150,90. White blood cells lacking CD18 cannot adhere to the walls of blood vessels to prepare for migration to a site of injury.
    LAD-2 individuals have the Bombay phenotype.

A12. In X-linked SCID, there is a defect in the interleukin receptor gene (*IL2RG*). This gene codes for the shared component, the γ-chain, for the receptor for the cytokines IL-4F, IL-7R, IL-9r and IL-15. If the lymphocytes cannot receive the signal from these cytokines, then they cannot effect an optimal immune response. IL-4 activates B cells, IL-7 is necessary for T-cell development in the thymus, and IL-15 works in concert with IL-2, a key player in T-cell activity.

CHAPTER 50

Clinical and laboratory evaluation of systemic rheumatic diseases

QUESTIONS

• Q 1

Which autoantibody class is the hallmark of the systemic rheumatic diseases? *(p. 916)*

• Q 2

What is the greatest risk factor for systemic lupus erythematosus (SLE)? *(p. 917)*

• Q 3

The average number of autoantibodies in SLE patients is *(p. 917)*:

• Q 4

Which four autoantibodies are part of the criteria for a diagnosis of SLE? *(Table 50–2, p. 917)*

• Q 5

Which four antibodies are considered the most specific for SLE? *(p. 918)*

• Q 6

Immune complexes of DNA–anti-DNA have a tropism for what tissue structure? *(p. 918)*

• Q 7

What are the components of the Sm antigen? *(p. 919)*

• Q 8

What two test methodologies are widely used to detect and discriminate between anti-Sm and antinuclear ribonucleoprotein (nRNP) antibodies (not epitopes)? *(p. 919)*

• Q 9

What are the likely demographics and HLA profile of a person with anti-SS-A/Ro but not anti-SS-B/La who has SLE? *(p. 919)*

How about a person with both Ro and La?

• Q 10

What complement deficiencies are associated with anti-SS-A/Ro? *(p. 919)*

• Q 11

An SLE patient with antiribosomal ribonucleoproteins (rRNPs) may have what specific symptoms? *(p. 919)*

• Q 12

Describe the mechanism by which SLE patients test falsely positive for the Venereal Disease Research Laboratory (VDRL) test. *(pp. 919–920)*

What is the specific epitope on phospholipids to which the antibodies are directed?

• Q 13

Which specific autoantibody is characteristic of systemic drug-induced lupus? *(p. 920)*

• Q 14

What type of Sjögren syndrome is indicated by the presence of both anti-SS-A/Ro and anti-SS-B/La? *(p. 920)*

• Q 15

What is the major antibody in diffuse scleroderma and in CREST? *(Table 50–5, p. 921)*

Diffuse: _____   CREST: _____

• Q 16

Describe the rheumatoid factor (RF) antibody, including its usual immunoglobulin class and its target. *(p. 922)*

QUESTIONS

• Q 17

What enzyme class is the target of several key autoantibodies in polymyositis? *(p. 923)*

• Q 18

Patients with mixed connective tissue disease (MCTD) typically have a high titer of this autoantibody. *(p. 923)*

• Q 19

Comment on the sensitivity of the immunofluorescence method, using Hep-2 cells, to detect antinuclear antibodies. *(p. 924)*

• Q 20

Study the figure below *(Fig. 50–8, p. 929)* and interpret this immunoblot analysis for autoantibodies. Lane 1 is the negative control.

What is the most likely diagnosis for lane 2? _____

CENP-A and B bands indicate anticentromere antibodies. What disease is likely in the patient in lane 4? _____

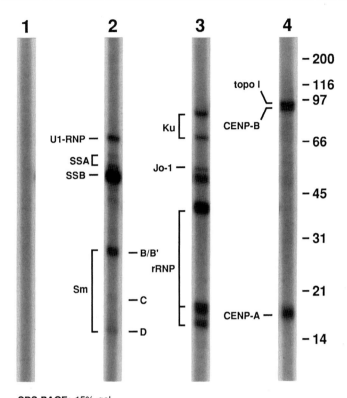

SDS-PAGE: 15% gel
Antigen extract: MOLT-4 whole cell
Detection system: ^{125}I-protein A

ANSWERS

A1. These are the antinuclear antibodies (ANAs).

A2. Female gender is the biggest risk factor.

A3. Three. The antibodies are heterogeneous and polyclonal.

A4. Anti-native/ds DNA, anti-Sm, antiphospholipid, and ANA.

A5. Anti-native DNA and anti-Sm are the two key players for specificity.
Additionally, antiribosomal and PCNA antibodies are fairly specific for lupus.

A6. Basement membranes. This is the mechanism by which renal damage is inflicted in SLE.

A7. Sm, as well as nuclear ribonucleoproteins (nRNPs), are small nuclear RNAs complexed with proteins.

A8. Immunodiffusion and enzyme-linked immunosorbent assay (ELISA).

A9. Anti-SS-A/Ro – This person is probably young and positive for HLA-DR2. He or she may have more serious renal disease than other SLE patients.
Ro and La – This person is probably older and positive for HLA-DR3.

A10. A homozygous deficiency of complement factor C2 and C4 is associated with anti-SS-A/Ro. Patients with this profile often go on to have a lupus-like syndrome.

A11. Psychosis.

A12. The VDRL test uses carbon particles coated with several phospholipids, among them cardiolipin, to elicit flocculation (a positive result). The SLE patient often has antibodies to cardiolipin and thus shows a positive reaction.
The specific epitope is β_2 glycoprotein.

A13. Patients who have systemic disease often have anti-IgG to the H2A–H2B dimer complex of histones. Asymptomatic patients often have IgM with a broad reactivity to all the histones.

A14. This is primary Sjögren syndrome, usually with no other autoimmune disorder but occasionally coexisting with SLE.

A15. Diffuse – anti-Scl-70.
CREST – anticentromere.

A16. RF is usually IgM against the Fc portion of IgG. It may also be of the IgG or IgA class, the latter being associated with more severe disease.

A17. Several different transfer RNA synthetases are the target in polymyositis.

A18. MCTD patients are often restricted to antiribonucleoproteins, either U1-RNP or nRNP.

A19. This is a very sensitive test, with 98% sensitivity. Recall that screening tests should have a high sensitivity, even at the expense of specificity.

A20. Lane 2 – SLE. This patient is positive for Sm and SS-B. SS-A is poorly detected by the immunoblot method. U1-RNP is also positive.
Lane 4 – Scleroderma. This patient has both the anti-Scl-70 and anticentromere antibodies.

CHAPTER 51
Vasculitis

QUESTIONS

Q 1

List the three mechanisms of immune-mediated vascular injury. *(pp. 933–934)*

Q 2

Leukopenia and thrombocytopenia are rare in the idiopathic vasculitides. A patient with the histology of polyarteritis nodosa (PAN) and pancytopenia may have what lymphoid malignancy? *(p. 935)*

Q 3

What is the most sensitive and, along with ELISA, the most common method of detecting antineutrophil cytoplasmic antibody (ANCA)? *(p. 935)*

Q 4

Clinical Consultation: A 40-year-old female with allergic rhinitis is being worked up for Churg–Strauss syndrome. A peripheral blood sample from a normal person is processed for removal of the neutrophils, which are fixed in formalin. Staining with fluorescein-labeled polyspecific antihuman immunoglobulin conjugate after these neutrophils are incubated with the woman's serum reveals a cytoplasmic pattern. You thought she would be positive for p-ANCA, and an ELISA is positive for p-ANCA. Explain this discordant result. *(pp. 935–936)*

Q 5

What are the antigenic specificities of c-ANCA and p-ANCA? *(p. 936)*

c-ANCA:_____ p-ANCA: _____

Q 6

Is a positive indirect fluorescence microscopy (IFM) sufficient by itself for the diagnosis of p-ANCA positivity? *(p. 936)*

Q 7

Describe the hallmark microscopic lesion of active polyarteritis nodosa (PAN). *(p. 938)*

Q 8

What is the prognosis for untreated PAN? *(p. 938)*

Q 9

What laboratory finding is the hallmark of Churg–Stauss syndrome? *(p. 938)*

Q 10

Review the typical laboratory features of Wegener's granulomatosis. *(p. 939)*

WBC: _____ Eosinophils: _____

Autoantibodies: _____ ESR: _____

BUN, creatinine: _____

Q 11

Clinical Consultation: A 7-year-old boy develops palpable purpura in May, a couple of weeks after having a cold. He complains of abdominal pain and has passed bloody, mucoid stools. Renal function is only mildly impaired, with a creatinine of 1.3 mg/dL, 1+ proteinuria and 5–7 RBCs/hpf in the urine sediment. The pediatrician feels confident making a clinical diagnosis but asks if there are any laboratory tests that would be useful. What is the diagnosis, and what test might be helpful for future reference? *(pp. 940–941)*

Q 12

What rheumatic disease is associated with giant cell arteritis? *(p. 942)*

Q 13

What vessels are particularly targeted in Takayasu arteritis? *(p. 942)*

Q 14

Primary angiitis of the central nervous system is a rare disorder with no specific laboratory findings to assist one in the diagnostic process. What is the most consistent laboratory finding, although it is not specific? *(p. 943)*

_____

What is the prognosis? _____

ANSWERS

A1. Vascular injury may occur by immune complex deposition, direct autoantibody binding to vessels walls or to PMNs, or T-cell-mediated effects.

A2. This combination suggests hairy cell leukemia.

A3. Indirect fluorescence microscopy (IFM).

A4. When neutrophils are fixed in formalin, the target antigen, myeloperoxidase (MPO), is immobilized in the cytoplasm. The characteristic perinuclear staining is actually an artefact of fixation with alcohol; the MPO redistributes to the perinuclear area. Another sample of normal polymorphonuclear leukocytes (PMNs), this time fixed in 99% ethanol, should clarify her pattern.

A5. c-ANCA – proteinase 3 (PR-3) in the primary granules of PMNs.
p-ANCA – myeloperoxidase, or sometimes other PMN enzymes.

A6. No, p-ANCA should be confirmed by ELISA. Nonspecific staining can occur with other antibodies, such as antinuclear antibodies (ANA), granulocyte-specific ANA and antineutrophil elastase.

A7. A circumferential or segmental lesion of the vessel wall consisting of a mixed cell inflammatory infiltrate with fibrinoid necrosis is typical of PAN.

A8. Poor. The 5-year survival rate is only 13%. Glucocorticoids have improved survival rates to 50–60%.

A9. Peripheral blood eosinophilia, at least 1000/μL in the majority of patients.

A10. In Wegener's granulomatosis, the WBC is elevated without eosinophilia. c-ANCA is the characteristic autoantibody, but rheumatoid factor is seen in more than 50% of patients. c-ANCA is not specific but, in conjunction with clinical findings, it is sufficient for many clinicians for a diagnosis. ESR is elevated. BUN and creatinine are often elevated with glomerular involvement, which does occur in the majority of patients at some point in their disease course.

A11. This is Henoch–Schönlein purpura. A C2 level might be a good idea here. It is associated with Henoch–Schönlein purpura and may portend a lupus-like illness for this boy at some point in his life.

A12. This is polymyalgia rheumatica.

A13. The aortic arch and pulmonary arteries are particularly affected. ESR is a helpful marker to monitor disease.

A14. An elevated ESR is usually present, and many other markers are negative. This disease carries a poor prognosis, with 60–70% of patients succumbing within 1 year of diagnosis.

CHAPTER 52

Organ-specific autoimmune diseases

QUESTIONS

• Q 1

What is the most common method of detecting circulating autoantibodies to specific target organs or tissues? *(p. 945)*

• Q 2

What are the three main tissue targets in autoimmune diseases of the skin? *(p. 947)*

• Q 3

While indirect immunofluorescence microscopy (IIFM) detects circulating autoantibodies in patient serum, direct immunofluorescence microscopy (DIFM) identifies: *(p. 947)*

• Q 4

In the pemphigus disorders, the inciting antigen is a desmosomal adhesion molecule, so it is not surprising that DIFM will show intercellular space (ICS) staining. *(p. 947)*

What is the major antigen in pemphigus vulgaris?_____

What is the major antigen in pemphigus foliaceus? _____

What is the main class of immunoglobulins produced? _____

• Q 5

Bullous pemphigoid (BP) is a subepidermal bullous disease, so it is not surprising that antibodies are directed at the basement membrane zone (BMZ), the junction between the epidermis and the dermis. State the type of proteins which are the targets in BP and the predominant immunoreactants (Ig type, C') *(p. 948)*

• Q 6

Clinical Consultation: A 43-year-old male presents to a dermatologist with blisters and erosions on his knees, elbows, and the dorsa of both hands. A biopsy demonstrates a subepidermal blister but a routine IIFM to normal human skin is negative. What disease do you suspect, and what technique might be more sensitive for any autoantibody that may be present? *(p. 949)*

• Q 7

What is the characteristic DIFM pattern in dermatitis herpetiformis (DH)? *(p. 949)*

These patients often have another autoantibody associated with another autoimmune disease. What is this?

• Q 8

Describe how the pattern of IgA staining will help distinguish DH from linear IgA dermatosis. *(p. 949)*

• Q 9

Explain how multiple skin biopsies can be used to distinguish SLE from discoid lupus (DLE). *(p. 950)*

• Q 10

Which two mitochondrial antigens are the most important diagnostic markers of primary biliary cirrhosis? *(p. 950)*

• Q 11

What are the predominant antibodies in the following subclasses of autoimmune hepatitis? *(Table 52–3, pp. 951–952)*

Type 1: _____

Type 2: _____

Type 3: _____

• Q 12

What are the two key autoantibodies in primary sclerosing cholangitis (PSC)? *(pp. 952–953)*

What disease is seen in 50% of patients with PSC?

• Q 13

Which autoantibody clearly plays a causal role in autoimmune thyroid disease? *(p. 953)*

• Q 14

Which autoimmune thyroid disease(s) is/are characterized by anti-thyroid peroxidase antibodies? *(p. 953)*

• Q 15

How do anti-thyroid-stimulating hormone receptor antibodies cause both hyper- and hypothyroidism? *(p. 955)*

• Q 16

What is the Goodpasture's antigen? *(p. 955)*

• Q 17

Which autoantibody is detected in most newly diagnosed type 1A diabetes patients and prediabetic first-degree relatives of patients, and is also associated with stiff-man syndrome? *(p. 956)*

• Q 18

Describe the two types of antibody to intrinsic factor (IF) seen in pernicious anemia. *(p. 957)*

Contrast antiparietal cell (APC) and anti-IF autoantibodies in terms of sensitivity and specificity in the diagnosis of pernicious anemia.

• Q 19

Which two IgA autoantibodies may be used to monitor a celiac sprue patient's adherence to a gluten-free diet? *(p. 957)*

• Q 20

Briefly outline the competitive radioimmunoassay used to test patients for myasthenia gravis. *(p. 958)*

A1. This is indirect immunofluorescence microscopy (IIFM).

A2. These are the basement membrane zone (BMZ), epidermal intercellular spaces (ICS), and dermal blood vessels.

A3. DIFM uses a biopsy from the patient to identify tissue-bound autoantibodies and complement.

A4. Pemphigus vulgaris – desmoglein 3.
Pemphigus foliaceus – desmoglein 1.
IgG is the predominant immunoglobulin, but some pemphigus vulgaris patients have IgA or IgM.

A5. The major antigens are two keratinocytic hemidesmosome proteins called bullous pemphigoid antigens 1 and 2 (BP 1 and BP 2). C3 and IgG or C3 alone are most often seen in DIFM.

A6. This sounds clinically like epidermolysis bullosa acquisita (EBA). Roughly 40% of patients have a positive IIFM with the routine skin technique. A salt-split-skin technique will increase sensitivity to 50–85%. In EBA, autoantibodies are on the dermal, or floor, side of the split.

A7. DH shows granular IgA at the tips of dermal papillae. 80% of DH patients have antiendomysial antibodies, reflecting the association with celiac sprue.

A8. DH – staining at the tips of the dermal papillae, but not the BMZ.
IgA dermatosis – linear staining along the BMZ, but not in the dermal papillae.

A9. In SLE, uninvolved skin will show characteristic coarse granular deposits of Ig or C3, about 40% of the time (not always). In DLE, deposits are confined to involved, or lesional, skin. They are not seen in uninvolved skin.

A10. M2 and M9 of the nine identified antigens.

A11. Type 1 – ANA, smooth muscle antibody (SMA).
Type 2 – Liver-kidney microsomal antibody (LKMA)-1.
Type 3 – Anti-soluble liver autoantibody.

A12. ANA and p-ANCA. There is a strong correlation between PSC and ulcerative colitis.

A13. Anti-thyroid stimulating hormone receptor antibody (anti-TSHR).

A14. This is seen in both Graves disease and Hashimoto thyroiditis.

A15. There are two types of anti-TSHR: stimulating and blocking types. The stimulating variant is called thyroid-stimulating immunoglobulin (TSI) and is a confirmatory finding for Graves disease.

A16. This is the NC1 domain of type IV collagen, located in the basement membrane of the glomerulus.

A17. This is anti-glutamic acid decarboxylase (GAD). The GAD65 isoform is found in the pancreas.

A18. Type 1 is a blocking autoantibody that prevents IF from binding to vitamin B_{12} in the stomach. Type 2 is a binding autoantibody that reacts with the B_{12} complexed to IF.

APC is sensitive, seen in 90% of PA patients.

Anti-IF is more specific. Type 1 anti-IF is presented as more diagnostically sensitive, but I think that Henry means when compared to type 2 anti-IF.

A19. Either IgA antiendomysial or antigliadin may be used as a monitor.

A20. Acetylcholine receptors (AChR) are obtained from denervated muscle, such as from amputees or from tissue cultures, and incubated with the snake venom protein α-bungarotoxin (α-BTx). This toxin binds irreversibly to AChR, but at a different site than where the autoantibody binds. Patient serum is then added. If antibodies to AChR are present, they will also bind to AChR. This three-part complex is precipitated with polyvalent anti-human immunoglobulin, and the radioactivity is measured. This radioactivity correlates directly with the amount of anti-AChR in the patient's serum.

CHAPTER 53

Allergic diseases

QUESTIONS

• Q 1

List the cytokines encoded on chromosome 5q that influence IgE production. *(p. 962)*

• Q 2

Which subset of lymphocytes produces IL-3, IL-4, IL-5, and IL-13 to promote IgE synthesis by B cells? *(p. 962)*

• Q 3

Does IgE cross the placenta? *(p. 963)*

• Q 4

What is the initial signal for histamine release by mast cells and basophils, and what is the role of IgE in the signaling process? *(p. 964)*

• Q 5

What are the two main in vivo tests of immediate hypersensitivity? *(p. 965)*

Q 6

A variety of immunodeficiency disorders are associated with either increased or decreased levels of serum IgE. State whether IgE is high or low in the following disorders. *(p. 966)*

Ataxia telangiectasia: _____ SCID: _____

Partial deficiency of cellular immunity: _____

Q 7

Comment on the diagnostic sensitivity of an elevated serum IgE level in a symptomatic child with a strong family history of atopy. *(p. 966)*

Q 8

Briefly describe the principle underlying the radioallergosorbent test (RAST), a first generation immunometric assay. *(p. 966)*

Q 9

Comment on the utility of the IgE antibody test along the following parameters and in the following situations. *(pp. 967–970)*

Risk to the patient: _____

Cost with wide battery of tests: _____

Foods causing anaphylaxis (fish, nuts): _____

Foods not associated with clinical signs: _____

Confirming skin test for *Hymenoptera*: _____

Confirming penicillin anaphylaxis: _____

Q 10

What protein is released from mast cells and basophils and remains in the blood for up to 12 hours after anaphylaxis? *(p. 970)*

A1. Interleukin (IL)-4, IL-5, and IL-13.

A2. These are the Th2 helper T cells.

A3. No, IgE does not cross the placenta in any significant amount.

A4. Crosslinking of FCεRI molecules by a multivalent allergen is the initial signal. IgE binds to the FCεRI molecule and serves as a bridge to the crosslinking event.

A5. The two key in vivo tests are the skin test and the end-organ challenge.

A6. In ataxia telangiectasia and SCID, diseases of humoral immunity, IgE is low. In incomplete diseases of cellular immunity, such as Wiskott–Aldrich syndrome and Nezelof syndrome (thymic alymphoplasia), IgE is usually elevated.

A7. Serum IgE adds little to the diagnosis in this situation. It may be more useful when the clinician suspects a nonallergic disease process but cannot rule out allergic disease. Even then, a normal serum IgE does not exclude the possibility of allergy later in life.

A8. Patient serum containing specific IgE antibodies (if the test is positive) is reacted with the allergen of interest coupled to a solid-phase support. After a wash step to remove nonspecific antibodies, a second, anti-IgE, antibody is added to demonstrate the patient immunoglobulin.

A9. The IgE antibody test presents no risk to the patient, as skin tests do. If used as a broad screening tool, however, it can be costly. This test is particularly useful for identifying persons who will have anaphylactic reactions to certain foods, such as fish or nuts, but is beset by false positives when applied to foods rarely associated with clinical signs, particularly in children. It is well suited to confirm positive skin test in venomous animals and to confirm a recent reaction to penicillin.

A10. This is tryptase, a serum protease in mast cells and basophils. Histamine has a very short half-life, just minutes long, and tryptase may be a more useful marker of immediate hypersensitivity.

Part VII

Medical microbiology

CHAPTER 54
Viral infections

QUESTIONS

Q 1

What are the seasonal peaks for enteroviruses and rotavirus? *(Fig. 54–1, p. 976)*

Enteroviruses: _____

Rotaviruses: _____

Q 2

From the selection in *Figure 54–3 (pp. 977–979)*, which two cell lines would you select to culture influenza virus?

Q 3

Which two cell lines would you select to culture herpes simplex virus (HSV)? *(Fig. 54–3, p. 978)*

Q 4

What are the two advantages of enzyme immunoassay (EIA) over direct fluorescent antibody (DFA)? *(p. 978)*

Q 5

What is the transport temperature for viral transport media, for all samples except blood? *(p. 979)*

Q 6

Cell culture isolation is still the gold standard for diagnosis of HSV. Cytopathic effect (CPE) by standard culture methods is usually evident in _____ days. Describe the characteristic CPE. *(p. 981)*

Q 7

What is the role of DFA in both standard and centrifugation-enhanced cultures for HSV? *(p. 981)*

Q 8

Which of the influenza viruses is more common and produces more serious illness? *(p. 981)*

Q 9

What two laboratory methods are useful for rapid diagnosis of influenza and utilize a nasopharyngeal swab? *(p. 982)*

Q 10

What are the two rapid diagnostic methods for respiratory syncytial virus? *(p. 983)*

Q 11

What two cell types does Epstein–Barr virus (EBV) infect in humans? *(p. 984)*

• Q 12

To what EBV antigen are the heterophile antibodies directed? *(p. 984)*

• Q 13

What four other primary infections might be demonstrated in a mononucleosis-like illness that is EBV-negative? *(p. 986)*

• Q 14

What is the most common intrauterine infection and infects 1% of liveborn infants in the USA? *(p. 987)*

• Q 15

What test performed on amniotic fluid is reliable in the diagnosis of CMV? *(p. 987)*

• Q 16

What is the first test to perform if one suspects acute rubella in a woman who is 10 weeks pregnant? *(p. 987)*

• Q 17

What test can be performed to diagnose human immunodeficiency virus (HIV) in an infant, and what is the earliest age this test can be performed? *(p. 989)*

• Q 18

What subfamily of viruses accounts for nearly 75% of cases of viral meningitis in the USA? *(p. 990)*

• Q 19

To diagnose varicella zoster virus in a patient, what specimen should be taken for culture? _____

_____

What tissue culture cells work well, and what method of culture is preferred?

_____

A DFA conjugate stain is applied to confirm positives in _____ days. *(pp. 991–992)*

• Q 20

Two viral exanthems with similar sounding names are erythema infectiosum, which is due to _____,
and exanthem subitum, due to _____

_____. *(p. 992)*

• Q 21

Rotavirus is a major cause of diarrhea in the pediatric population. What are three other viruses that cause diarrhea in this age group? *(p. 992)*

• Q 22

In a community hospital setting, what are the two main methods of diagnosing rotavirus? *(p. 992)*

• Q 23

Can any of the hepatitis viruses be grown in standard tissue culture cell lines? *(p. 993)*

• Q 24

Which is the most common genotype of hepatitis C virus (HCV) in the US? *(p. 993)*

How effective is treatment with α-interferon in patients with this genotype?

• Q 25

A 28-year-old male with HIV has a viral load of 10 000 copies/mL prior to starting antiretroviral therapy. 2 months after initiating therapy and maintaining good compliance, his viral load has fallen by 1.0 log copies/mL. How many copies are present by the polymerase chain reaction (PCR) assay? *(p. 993)*

• Q 26

What technique is used to determine the viral load in hepatitis C? *(p. 993)*

• Q 27

What type of culture has shortened the incubation time for cytomegalovirus (CMV) to 1–2 days? *(p. 995)*

What is the main cell line for culturing CMV?

ANSWERS

A1. Enteroviruses peak in late summer and early fall. Rotavirus is a wintertime disease.

A2. Rhesus monkey kidney and the R-Mix hybrid of mink lung/A549 are the most sensitive for influenza.

A3. For HSV, choose human diploid fibroblast (HDF), Hep-2, or rabbit kidney.

A4. EIA is more easily automated and is less subjective in the interpretation of positive vs negative than DFA.

A5. 4°C is the transport temperature for viral culture specimens.

A6. The standard cell culture for HSV shows syncytial formation in 2–3 days. For most cell cultures, the centrifugation method speeds up growth, and for HSV, cultures may show CPE after only 1 day.

A7. DFA is used to confirm positive CPE in cultures.

A8. This is influenza A.

A9. One is the DFA stain. If you aspirate several columnar epithelial cells where the virus is lurking, you can pick them up right away with DFA. EIA is rapid and easy to perform; sensitivity is better with nasopharyngeal aspirates than with throat swabs with this method.

A10. DFA and EIA. These are much faster methods than the 3–10 days needed to culture this virus. Respiratory syncytial virus (RSV) is a serious illness in infants, and prompt diagnosis is critical to the initiation of therapy.

A11. Recall that EBV infects pharyngeal epithelial cells (infectious mononucleosis starts with a sore throat) as well as the B lymphocytes.

A12. None. That is why we use the complicated tests with cells from other species to sort out nonspecific antibodies from those that are associated with EBV. The antibodies that bind to EBV antigens are those binding to the early antigen (EA) and to the viral capsid antigen (VCA).

A13. *Toxoplasma gondii*, CMV, human herpes virus 6 (HHV 6), and HIV all may cause a mononucleosis-like illness.

A14. CMV. Thankfully, 90% are asymptomatic.

A15. PCR, along with culture.

A16. Serology is the mainstay to begin the diagnostic process. Start with an antirubella IgM for an acute infection.

A17. Maternal antibodies to HIV transmitted transplacentally can persist for up to 15 months, so this is not a useful method for detecting vertical HIV infection. The PCR assay for transcribed DNA in lymphoid cells can be performed at 1 month of age, and RT-PCR can be performed at birth if the neonate was infected transplacentally.

A18. Enteroviruses are the main player here. The gold standard is RT-PCR of the cerebrospinal fluid.

A19. Vesicle fluid (a new lesion) is cultured on human diploid fibroblasts (HDF) in a shell vial. At 3–5 days, one may perform a DFA conjugate stain to look for positivity.

A20. Erythema infectiosum is due to parvovirus B19. This illness is commonly called 'slapped cheek' in children because of their facial erythema. Exanthem subitum is due to HHV 6.

A21. Other pediatric gastroenteritis viruses include adenovirus serotypes 40 and 41, astroviruses, and caliciviruses.

A22. These are latex agglutination or EIA. Electron microscopy is quite specific, but it cannot easily be performed in hospital settings.

A23. No. Diagnosis of the hepatitides rests on serology and PCR.

A24. Genotype 1 is found in 75% of US HCV patients, but it is not very responsive to therapy with α-IFN.

A25. 1000 copies/mL will be present after a 1.0 log reduction. Do not forget your basic math skills when taking an examination. Some questions are as simple as this one. This reduction in viral load (at least 0.5–1.0 log copies/mL) correlates with slowed disease progression in HIV, so this patient is doing OK.

A26. Viral load is determined by RT-PCR. HCV is an RNA virus and the nucleic acid must be converted to DNA. The same is true for HIV.

A27. The centrifugation-enhanced shell vial shortens the incubation time. CMV strongly prefers HDF as its cell line for culture.

CHAPTER 55

Chlamydial, rickettsial, and mycoplasmal infections

QUESTIONS

• Q 1

There are two distinct forms in the life cycle of chlamydias. Which is the infectious form? *(p. 1000)* _____
DNA, RNA and protein synthesis and replication occur in the _____
_____

• Q 2

Review the names of the diseases caused by *Chlamydia trachomatis*. *(p. 1001)*
Children and adults – ocular: _____
Adults – STD: _____
Neonates – ocular: _____
Neonates – pulmonary: _____

• Q 3

Compare and contrast *C. psittaci* and *C. pneumoniae*. *(pp. 1002–1003)*

	C. psittaci	*C. pneumoniae*
Avian reservoir		
Human–human transmission		
Laboratory diagnosis		
Severity of illness		

• Q 4

The DFA test for *C. trachomatis* has the advantage over other nonculture methods of the ability to assess for specimen adequacy. Define specimen adequacy for *C. trachomatis*. *(p. 1003)*

• Q 5

Complete the following chart on these rickettsial infections. The first infection is completed as an example. *(pp. 1004–1009)*

Type of illness	Etiologic agent	Disease name	Transmission/Vector
Bartonellosis	*Bartonella henselae*	Cat scratch fever	Cat bite, scratch
	Rickettsia rickettsiae		
			Louse feces
		Monocytic ehrlichiosis	
		Q fever	
	Anaplasma phagocytophila		

• Q 6

What cell is the target of infection by *R. rickettsiae*? *(p. 1004)*

• Q 7

Laboratory diagnostics play a relatively small role in the rickettsial illnesses, most being diagnosed by clinicoepidemiologic suspicion. Nevertheless, a fourfold rise in titer may be very useful in the proper setting. What methodology is used for performing titers? *(p. 1006)*

• Q 8

The older method for diagnosing rickettsioses, no longer recommended in the USA, is the Weil–Felix test. What is the principle of this test? *(p. 1006)*

Q 9

What three ticks can transmit *Ehrlichia chaffeensis*? *(p. 1007)*

Q 10

What genus of tick can transit *Anaplasma phagocytophila*? *(p. 1007)*

Q 11

True/False. Empiric treatment should be initiated in suspected cases of ehrlichiosis because serologic titers, the mainstay of diagnosis in most hospitals, may not become diagnostic for 2–4 weeks. *(p. 1008)*

Q 12

Chronic Q fever is associated with what cardiac illness? *(p. 1008)*

Q 13

Because traditional microbiological culture methods, including biochemical tests, are not very specific, these two serologic methods are often used to diagnose *Bartonella henselae* and *B. quintana*. *(p. 1009)*

Q 14

What red cell antigen does *Mycoplasma pneumoniae* alter, resulting in the production of cold agglutinins? *(p. 1010)*

• Q 15

True/False. Colonies of M. pneumoniae grow rapidly and show the characteristic 'fried egg' appearance in about 48 hours. *(p. 1011)*

ANSWERS

A1. The elementary body is infectious. The reticulate body replicates.

A2. Ocular disease in children and adults is chronic follicular keratoconjunctivitis. The STDs in adults are lymphogranuloma venereum, urethritis and cervicitis. Neonates may get inclusion conjunctivitis from the birth canal. Neonates may also get interstitial pneumonitis.

A3. *C. psittaci* has several bird reservoirs, is not transmitted from human to human, is diagnosed chiefly by serology, and can be serious, even fatal.

C. pneumoniae only infects humans and is thus transmitted from person to person. It is also diagnosed by serologic titers and is usually mild and self-limiting.

A4. The presence of columnar and/or metaplastic squamous cells equates with adequacy.

A5. One of the spotted fevers is due to *R. rickettsiae*, is called Rocky Mountain spotted fever, and is transmitted by ticks.

One of the typhus fevers is due to *R. prowazekii*; this is epidemic typhus and is spread by louse feces. It is associated with wartime, overcrowding, and filth.

One ehrlichiosis is due to *E. chaffeensis*. This is human monocytic ehrlichiosis and is transmitted by tick bite.

One coxiellosis is due to *C. burnetii* and is called Q fever. It is most often acquired from inhalation of the rickettsia, but can also be from handling animals.

The other important ehrlichiosis is due to *E. phagocytophila*. This is human granulocytic ehrlichiosis and is also spread by ticks.

A6. The vascular endothelium is the target of this organism.

A7. The primary method is indirect fluorescent antibody (IFA).

A8. The Weil–Felix test measures agglutination of *Proteus vulgaris* strains. It is still performed in some developing countries.

A9. *E. chaffeensis* causes human monocytic ehrlichiosis and may be transmitted by the Lone Star tick (*Amblyomma americanum*), *Dermacentor variabilis*, or *Ixodes pacificus*.

A10. Three species of *Ixodes* can transmit the agent of human granulocytic ehrlichiosis.

A11. True.

A12. Chronic Q fever causes an endocarditis.

A13. EIA and indirect immunofluorescence are used with the species of *Bartonella*. Of course, if a lymph node is aspirated from cat scratch fever, then a Warthin–Starry stain might be very helpful.

A14. This is the I antigen.

A15. False. *M. pneumoniae* is a slow-grower and is given 3 weeks to grow. A much more rapid diagnostic method is specific IgM. By contrast, *M. hominis* usually grows in 5 days or less.

CHAPTER 56

Medical bacteriology

QUESTIONS

• Q 1

What two preparatory procedures are performed on a slide prior to Gram staining? *(p. 1016)*

• Q 2

What two media are commonly used to inhibit the growth of Gram-negative bacilli while allowing Gram-positive bacteria to grow? *(p. 1017)*

• Q 3

What chemical is used as a catalyst to achieve anaerobic conditions for culturing bacteria? *(p. 1017)*

• Q 4

Review the key biochemical features of the genus *Staphylococcus*. *(Table 56–2, pp. 1017–1018)*

Catalase: _____

Bacitracin: _____

Coagulase: _____

Growth in NaCl: _____

• Q 5

Briefly describe the traditional antimicrobial resistance testing procedure for the penicillinase-resistant penicillins, using disk diffusion. *(p. 1019)*

• Q 6

Clinical Consultation: A 25-year-old male has a necrotizing fasciitis. The blood agar plate (BAP) shows small white colonies with β-hemolysis. To confirm a suspicion of group A *Streptococcus*, which three biochemical tests would you perform, beginning with one to rule out *Staphylococcus*? *(Fig. 56–4, p. 1021)*

• Q 7

What two tests offer presumptive identification of group B *Streptococcus*, if positive? *(Fig. 56–4, p. 1021)*

• Q 8

What is the first test to perform to presumptively identify *S. pneumoniae* in a mucoid α-hemolytic isolate? *(Fig. 56–5, p. 1022)*

• Q 9

Clinical Consultation: A blood culture on a 67-year-old female has grown out Gram-positive cocci in chains that are γ-hemolytic. Describe how L-pyrrolidonyl-β-naphthylamide (PYR) hydrolysis, growth in 6.5% NaCl and esculin hydrolysis will help you distinguish between *Enterococcus* and *viridans*. *(Fig. 56–5, p. 1022)*

• Q 10

Does S. pneumoniae require penicillin sensitivity testing? *(p. 1022)*

• Q 11

Name the immunodiffusion test that discriminates between oral and skin diphtheroids or corynebacteria, and the more pathogenic *Clostridium diphtheriae*. *(p. 1023)*

• Q 12

Clinical Consultation: A 3-day-old female has meningitis. Small colonies with a narrow zone of β-hemolysis are isolated. What three tests, including growth patterns and motility characteristics, will distinguish this as *Listeria monocytogenes* and rule out group B *Streptococcus*? *(Table 56–6, pp. 1024–1025)*

• Q 13

Clinical Consultation: A 31-year-old fisherman develops an elevated cutaneous eruption with a violaceous zone around the site of inoculum, which was a cut he sustained on the back of his hand. After 5 days, a BAP reveals some growth. What will be the result of these tests if your suspicion of *Erysipelothrix rhusiopathiae* is correct? *(Table 56–6, p. 1025)*
Oxidase: _____
Catalase: _____
Motility: _____
H$_2$S in TSI: _____

• Q 14

What are the three components of the complex anthrax toxin? *(p. 1025)*

• Q 15

True/False. The 'Medusa head' colony morphology in a Gram-positive, spore-forming rod that is catalase-positive is diagnostic of *Bacillus anthracis*. *(p. 1026)*

• Q 16

Both *Nocardia* spp. and *Actinomyces* have a similar Gram stain morphology. Describe this morphology and state which stain is used to differentiate between the two. *(p. 1026)*

• Q 17

Which *Nocardia* species are most likely in these patients? *(p. 1026)*

22-year-old Venezuelan male with leg ulcer: _____

_____

60-year-old US female with multiple central nervous system (CNS) abscesses:

_____

• Q 18

List three selective and differential media that would be useful in the workup of a *Salmonella* outbreak. *(p. 1031)*

• Q 19

All members of the Enterobacteriaceae family are oxidase _____
_____ and nitrate _____. *(p. 1030)*

• Q 20

How are *Escherichia coli*, *Klebsiella* spp. and many of the *Enterobacter* spp. differentiated from other members of the Enterobacteriaceae family on MacConkey agar (MAC)? *(Table 56–9, p. 1031)*

• Q 21

Clinical Consultation: A 36-year-old oyster fisherman was hospitalized for gastroenteritis and became septic over a 24-hour period. Your differential diagnosis includes members of the *Vibrio* genus, including *V. vulnificus* because he is septicemic, *V. cholerae*, and *V. parahaemolyticus*. Isolates from blood cultures are motile, curved, Gram-negative rods (GNRs). How will the following tests support a general diagnosis of *Vibrio* spp.? *(Table 56–12, pp. 1034–1035)*

Nitrate: _____

Oxidase: _____

Growth at 42°C: _____

Growth in 3% NaCl: _____

Which *Vibrio* species is supported by positive salicin and cellobiose tests?

• Q 22

Two genera of GNR that are implicated in gastroenteritis are *Aeromonas* and *Plesiomonas*. A common biochemical test that suggests these two genera, rather than one of the Enterobacteriaceae, is _____,

which is positive in *Aeromonas* and *Plesiomonas*. *(pp. 1032, 1035)*

• Q 23

Campylobacter jejuni is the most common cause of bacterial enteritis in the USA. Review its characteristic features. *(p. 1036)*

Growth temperatures: _____, and selective for *C. jejuni*,

particularly _____

Oxygen concentration for growth: _____ CO_2: _____

Fecal leukocytes: _____ Motility: _____

Gram morphology: _____ Oxidase: _____

• Q 24

Clinical Consultation: An 8-year-old girl with cystic fibrosis is hospitalized with pneumonia. The differential diagnosis includes *Pseudomonas aeruginosa* and *Burkholderia cepacia*. Are there media that will select for *B. cepacia*? *(p. 1034)* _____

_____

Review Table 56–11 *(p. 1034)* and note that fluorescein and pyocyanin are positive in *P. aeruginosa* but negative in *B. cepacia*. If your laboratory did not offer these tests, which three biochemical tests would clearly differentiate between the two? *(Table 56–11, p. 1034)*

• Q 25

The HACEK organisms are well-known agents of endocarditis. They may be distinguished by their biochemical characteristics. Except for *Kingella kingae*, they each have a particular test, which is positive in just one of the organisms and negative in all of the others, including *Kingella*. Review which HACEK organism is uniquely positive for the following tests. *(Table 56–14, p. 1038)*

Lactose: _____

Indole: _____

Lysine decarboxylase: _____

Catalase: _____

• Q 26

What culture medium is used to isolate *Legionella* spp.? *(p. 1039)*

• Q 27

What is the principal virulence factor of *Neisseria meningitidis*? *(p. 1028)*

• Q 28

What are the incubation parameters for *Neisseria* spp? *(p. 1028)*

• Q 29

Because *Moraxella* spp. will occasionally yield positive carbohydrate reactions, what two biochemical tests distinguish them from Neisseria spp? *(Table 56–8, p. 1029)*

• Q 30

The tetravalent polysaccharide vaccine for *N. meningitidis* protects against what four serogroups? *(p. 1029)*

• Q 31

Review the differential characteristics of the *Haemophilus* species by identifying which bacteria require which supplemental factors. *(Table 56–13, pp. 1037–1038)*

Requires X and V: _____

Requires X only: _____

Requires V only: _____

Requires neither: _____

• Q 32

Haemophilus aphrophilus is the H in the HACEK organisms. In question 25, we identified _____ as a characteristic test in differentiating *Haemophilus* among the HACEKs. *(Table 56–14, p. 1038)*

• Q 33

What is the action of the pertussis toxin of *Bordetella pertussis*? *(p. 1040)*

• Q 34

B. pertussis is a slow-grower but, after 4 days, one may look for this characteristic colony morphology. *(p. 1041)*

• Q 35

What are the typical biochemical reactions of *Brucella* spp.? *(p. 1041)*

Catalase: _____

Oxidase: _____

Urease: _____

• Q 36

How well do *Pasteurella* spp. grow on the following media? *(p. 1041)*

BAP: _____

EMB: _____

MAC: _____

• Q 37

What nutrient is necessary for the growth of *Francisella*? *(p. 1041)*

• Q 38

What is the etiologic agent of Haverhill disease? *(p. 1043)*

• Q 39

Which toxin is predominantly responsible for the enterotoxicity of *Clostridium difficile*? *(p. 1044)*

• Q 40

A double zone of hemolysis on BAP and boxcar-shaped, large, Gram-positive rods are presumptively diagnostic for what anaerobe in a case of massive tissue necrosis? *(p. 1044)*

ANSWERS

A1. Air drying and fixation with methanol or gentle heat.

A2. Colistin–nalidixic acid (CNA) and phenylethyl agar (PEA) are two common media that select for Gram-positives.

A3. This is palladium.

A4. Staphylococci are catalase-positive, bacitracin-resistant, coagulase-positive (*S. aureus*) or -negative (*S. epidermidis* and *S. saprophyticus*), and grow in NaCl.

A5. A 1 μg oxacillin disk is placed on Mueller–Hinton agar and incubated 24 hours at 35°C.

A6. Start with catalase (negative). Then perform PYR hydrolysis (positive). Finally, test for bacitracin (S).

A7. Hippurate hydrolysis and cAMP test are both positive in group B *Streptococcus*.

A8. Optochin (P) is the first test to do. It is an old standard, and *S. pneumoniae* is positive.

A9. Enterococci are PYR-positive, grow in 6.5% NaCl, and are esculin-positive. Viridans is negative for all three, except that about 10% of viridans will test esculin-positive.

A10. Yes. Use the 1 μg oxacillin disk.

A11. The Elek test is an immunodiffusion test, rarely performed in routine laboratories now that diphtheria is so uncommon. A paper impregnated with a strip of diphtheria antitoxin is incubated with a streak of culture laid out at a 90° angle to the strip. A precipitin line at 45° between the two lines indicates toxin production and thus *C. diphtheriae*.

A12. *L. monocytogenes* is catalase-positive, grows at 4°C and displays tumbling motility at room temperature. In this age group, group B *Streptococcus* must be considered.

A13. *E. rhusiopathiae* is oxidase-, catalase- and motility-negative. It is H_2S-positive in TSI.

A14. The three toxins are edema factor, contributing to pulmonary edema; protective antigen; and lethal factor.

A15. False. This pattern can also be seen in the other major pathogen in this genus, *B. cereus*.

A16. Both are Gram-positive, long, beaded, branching bacilli. *Nocardia* spp. are partially acid-fast, while *Actinomyces* spp. are not.

A17. The leg ulcer is due to *N. brasiliensis*. The systemic illness with CNS abscesses is due to *N. asteroides*.

A18. Three good media are xylose–lysine deoxycholate (XLD), Hektoen enteric (HE), and bismuth sulfite (BS). *Salmonella* colonies will have black centers, in contrast to *Shigella*.

A19. Enterobacteriaceae are all oxidase-negative and nitrate-positive (reducers).

A20. All are lactose fermenters that will manifest as pink colonies on MAC.

A21. Vibrios are nitrate-, oxidase- and NaCl-positive. They do not grow at 42°C, but *C. jejuni* does, and should be ruled out in a case of gastroenteritis. *V. vulnificus* is positive for salicin and cellobiose.

A22. *Aeromonas* and *Plesiomonas* are both oxidase-positive, but Enterobacteriaceae are negative.

A23. *Campylobacter* species grow at 37°C and *C. jejuni* grows at 37°C as well as 42°C, requiring reduced oxygen (5–10%) and increased CO_2 (10%). Fecal leukocytes are seen in only 25% of cases, so this is not helpful in the diagnosis. It is motile, is an S-shaped small GNR, and is oxidase positive.

A24. As *B. cepacia* portends a worse prognosis for cystic fibrosis patients, distinguishing it from *P. aeruginosa* is important. Three media, *Pseudomonas cepacia* (PC), oxidative fermentative base, polymyxin B, bacitracin lactose (OFBL), and *B. cepacia*-selective agar (BCSA) are all helpful, as are the following biochemical characteristics:
Lysine decarboxylase is negative in *P. aeruginosa* and positive in *B. cepacia*.
Arginine dihydrolase is positive in *P. aeruginosa* and negative in *B. cepacia*.
Maltose oxidation is negative in *P. aeruginosa* and positive in *B. cepacia*.

A25. Lactose – *Haemophilus aphrophilus*.
Indole – *Cardiobacterium hominis*.
Lysine decarboxylase – *Eikenella corrodens*.
Catalase – *Actinobacillus actinomycetemcomitans*.

A26. Buffered charcoal yeast extract (BCYE) is used to grow *Legionella spp.*

A27. This is the lipopolysaccharide–endotoxin complex, which activates the clotting cascade.

A28. 2–8% CO_2 at 35°C.

A29. DNase and nitrate reduction are both positive in *Moraxella* spp. but negative in *Neisseria* spp.

A30. The vaccine protects against serogroups A, C, Y, and W135. It does not protect against serogroup B.

A31. X and V are required by *H. influenzae* and *H. hemolyticus*.
X only is required by *H. ducreyi*. Chancroid, the disease caused by *H. ducreyi*, is sexually transmitted. One may think of the 'X-rated' disease agent as requiring only the X factor.
V only is required by *H. parainfluenzae* and *H. paraphrophilus*. The two 'paras' go together.
H. aphrophilus requires neither.

A32. Lactose fermentation.

A33. The pertussis toxin inhibits intracellular signal transduction factors.

A34. *B. pertussis* colonies are described as 'a drop of mercury.' They are small and shiny.

A35. *Brucella* is positive for catalase, oxidase, and urease.

A36. *Pasteurella* grows well on BAP but poorly on EMB and MAC. This growth pattern is a key aid to diagnosis of *P. multocida*.

A37. *Francisella* requires cystine or cysteine for growth.

A38. *Streptobacillus moniliformis* is the agent of Haverhill disease. In this section of the text, this disease is also called rat bite fever. However, in Chapter 58, the spirochete *Spirillum minus* is identified as the agent of rat bite fever.

A39. Toxin A. There is also a toxin B, which plays a minor role in human disease.

A40. *Clostridium perfringens*. It is important to identify patients with gas gangrene as opposed to those with an anaerobic cellulitis, as the former disease may require amputation while the latter generally does not.

CHAPTER 57

In vitro testing of antimicrobial agents

QUESTIONS

Q 1

In what circumstances can an antibiotic falling in the 'intermediate' category of antimicrobial resistance be used to treat an infection due to a specific isolate? *(pp. 1048–1049)*

Q 2

What organization establishes recommendations for antimicrobial testing? *(p. 1048)*

Q 3

The CLSI provides a list of antimicrobial agents that should be considered for testing against commonly-isolated bacteria. State the antibiotic to be tested against the following β-lactam bacteria. *(p. 1053)*

Staphylococcus and *Streptococcus* _____

Enterococci and Enterobacteriaceae _____

Staphylococcus _____

Enterococci (some institutions) _____

Q 4

Define minimum inhibitory concentration (MIC). *(p. 1049)*

Q 5

What three methods are used to determine MIC? *(p. 1049)*

Q 6

What culture medium is recommended for antimicrobial testing of aerobic and facultative anaerobic bacteria? *(p. 1050)*

Q 7

What is the concentration of McFarland suspension used for agar disk diffusion? *(p. 1051)*

Q 8

The original VITEK automated antimicrobial susceptibility system measured only turbidity to assess resistance. What parameters does the Vitek II analyze? *(p. 1051)*

Q 9

Define minimum bactericidal concentration (MBC). *(p. 1056)*

Q 10

How well does the serum bactericidal test correlate with the outcome of antimicrobial therapy? *(p. 1057)*

A1. Such an antibiotic can be used if the patient can tolerate high doses, or if the infection is in an anatomic site where the antibiotic is concentrated, such as a β-lactam in the urine.

A2. The Clinical and Laboratory Standards Institute (CLSI). Previously, this organization was known as the National Committee for Clinical Laboratory Standards (NCCLS).

A3. Test penicillin for *Staphylococcus* and *Streptococcus*.
Test ampicillin for Enterococci and Enterobacteriaceae.
Test oxacillin against *Staphylococcus*.
Test vancomycin against enterococci at institutions where resistance is suspected or has occurred.

A4. MIC is the lowest concentration of an antimicrobial that will inhibit visible growth.

A5. The three main methods of determining MIC are the dilution test, the disk diffusion test, and the Etest. Although microdilution systems now provide more rapid results and are more efficient, Henry stresses the continued utility of the disk diffusion test.

A6. The Mueller–Hinton medium is the CLSI recommendation.

A7. CLSI recommends a 0.5 McFarland suspension for disk diffusion.

A8. The Vitek II still measures turbidity, but also uses a multichannel fluorometer and photometer to record fluorescence and colorimetric data every 15 minutes.

A9. The minimum bactericidal concentration (MBC) is defined as the lowest concentration of antimicrobial agent that is bactericidal or lethal to at least 99.9% of the original inoculum.

A10. It does not correlate well with outcome, and its utility has been questioned.

• Q 4

Proper preparation of a slide is critical to the diagnosis of T. pallidum. When should a slide with tissue fluid be allowed to air dry, and when should it not? *(p. 1061)*

• Q 5

Briefly describe the principle of the microhemagglutination–*Treponema pallidum* test (MHA-TP). *(p. 1062)*

• Q 6

What is the etiologic agent of Weil's disease? *(p. 1063)*

• Q 7

The eastern, midwest and southern tick carrier of the etiologic agent of Lyme disease has undergone a species name change (genus is the same). *(p. 1064)*
The older name is:_____ The new name is: _____

• Q 8

According to the CDC, Lyme Disease may be diagnosed by clinical findings and physical examination, with laboratory confirmation required only for more subjective signs that occur later in the disease course. CDC has proposed that if laboratory testing is undertaken, then ELISA or IFA results are followed up with a second method. What is this method? *(p. 1066)*

• Q 9

True/False. Serologic tests for Lyme disease are very specific, with few false positives clouding the diagnostic picture. *(p. 1066)*

Q 10

What is the etiologic agent of louse-borne relapsing fever, and what is the genus and species of the louse carrier? *(p. 1068)*

ANSWERS

A1. Pinta – *Treponema carateum*.
Venereal syphilis – *T. pallidum pallidum*.
Endemic syphilis – *T. pallidum endemicum*.
Yaws – *T. pallidum pertenue*.

A2. To counter humoral immunity, the spirochete has few exposed antigens. The important antigens are its proteolipids, and they are beneath the surface. It also coats itself with host proteins to look less foreign.
T. pallidum downregulates cellular immunity in animal models.

A3. Interstitial keratitis, Hutchinson's teeth, and eighth nerve deafness are the classic triad.

A4. In darkfield microscopy, you want to examine a coverslipped slide immediately in order to visualize the motility, a key to diagnosis. Do not let the treponemes dry out and die.
In the direct fluorescent antibody (DFA) test, the slide must air-dry and be fixed prior to staining with the monoclonal antibody.

A5. Patient serum is mixed in a microtiter tray with sheep red blood cells that have been sensitized with *T. pallidum*. If the patient's serum contains antibody to *T. pallidum*, agglutination will occur.

A6. This is another name for icteric leptospirosis, the more severe form of leptospirosis. It is caused by *Leptospira interrogans*.

A7. The old name is *Ixodes dammini*. The new name is *Ixodes scapularis*.

A8. Western blot is used to supplement enzyme-linked immunosorbent assay (ELISA) and the indirect fluorescent antigen test (IFA).

A9. False. Lack of specificity is a major problem in Lyme serology.

A10. *Borrelia recurrentis* is carried by *Pediculus humanus*.

CHAPTER 59

Mycobacteria

QUESTIONS

• Q 1

Name the four members of the *Mycobacterium tuberculosis* complex. *(p. 1074)*

• Q 2

Define rapid growth for the nontubercular mycobacteria. *(Table 59–1, p. 1075)*

• Q 3

Can *Mycobacterium bovis* be transmitted from human to human? *(p. 1075)*

• Q 4

What is the most common clinical manifestation of *Mycobacterium kansasii*? *(p. 1076)*

Q 5

What is the usual history in a person with a cutaneous lesion due to *Mycobacterium fortuitum* or *M. chelonae*? *(p. 1077)*

Q 6

List four of the more common nontuberculous mycobacteria for which skin and subcutaneous lesions are the chief manifestation. *(p. 1077)*

Q 7

What type of leprosy develops in persons lacking specific cell-mediated immunity? *(p. 1078)*

Q 8

What are the three categories of persons for whom a 5 mm induration indicates a positive Mantoux test? *(p. 1078)*

Q 9

What two chemicals are used to liquify and decontaminate specimens being evaluated for mycobacteria? *(Fig. 59–1, pp. 1078–1079)*

• Q 10

Clinical Consultation: A 5-year-old boy develops a cellulitis with focal abscess formation in his left upper arm 1 month after receiving a dose of diphtheria–pertussis–tetanus (DTP) vaccine. A fluorochrome stain for mycobacteria is negative. What do you recommend to the laboratory technician to further pursue a diagnosis? What organism should be ruled out in this case? *(pp. 1077–1081)*

• Q 11

Name the three commonly encountered species of *Mycobacterium* that are notable for their rapid growth, with colonies evident in less than 1 week. *(p. 1077)*

• Q 12

Which *Mycobacterium* species are photochromogens? *(Table 59–6, p. 1081)*

• Q 13

What is currently the most rapid method for diagnosis of pulmonary tuberculosis? *(p. 1081)*

• Q 14

Briefly outline the four strategies for controlling tuberculosis as described by the Centers for Disease Control (CDC). *(p. 1082)*

• Q 15

What is the risk posed to immunosuppressed persons receiving the bacillus Calmette–Guérin (BCG) vaccine? *(p. 1083)*

ANSWERS

A1. These are *Mycobacterium tuberculosis*, *M. bovis*, *M. africanum* and *M. canettii*. The last is seen in West Africa, and possibly elsewhere in the world, but it is not well identified in laboratories.

A2. Rapid growth means less than or equal to 7 days. This growth rate does not apply to liquid media, only to solid media.

A3. Yes. This mycobacterium can be transmitted in many ways, and human to human is one of them.

A4. The most common manifestation is chronic cavitary pulmonary disease in the upper lobes.

A5. Most people report a penetrating injury/trauma with soil and/or water contamination.

A6. The skin-lesion-associated mycobacteria are *Mycobacterium fortuitum–chelonae* complex, *M. marinum*, *M. haemophilum*, and *M. ulcerans*. Not all of these are rapid-growers. *M. mucogenicum* and *M. immunogenum* are not listed as they are uncommon.

A7. Lepromatous leprosy is markedly disfiguring and due to a defect in cell-mediated immunity. Recall that tuberculoid leprosy is associated with anesthetic skin lesions and is seen in persons with a normal immune system.

A8. Persons who are human immunodeficiency virus (HIV)-positive, have had recent close contact with someone with infectious tuberculosis, or who have a characteristic X-ray for old tuberculosis fall under the 5 mm rule.

A9. *N*-acetyl-L-cysteine is the liquefying agent, and 2% sodium hydroxide is the decontaminant.

A10. *Mycobacterium chelonae* is associated with the DPT vaccine but does not always stain well with fluorochromes. The technician should restain the slide with carbol fuscin, which has better sensitivity for *M. chelonae*.

A11. The rapid growers are *Mycobacterium fortuitum*, *M. chelonae*, and *M. abscessus*.

A12. The photochromogens are *Mycobacterium kansasii*, *M. simiae*, *M. marinum*, and *M. szulgai*.

A13. This is nucleic acid amplification of *MTBC* from a clinical specimen.

A14. The first strategy is early identification and treatment of infectious persons. The second is identification and treatment of persons with noncontagious tuberculosis. The third is creation of a safe environment to limit spread of the disease. The fourth is vaccination with the BCG vaccine, a strategy not currently practiced in the USA.

A15. There is a risk of disseminated *Mycobacterium bovis*, as this is a live-attenuated vaccine.

CHAPTER 60
Mycotic diseases

QUESTIONS

● Q 1

Most fungi may reproduce by sexual and asexual means. The terms to describe the spores of each are: *(Table 61–1, p. 1087)*
Asexual spore: _____
Sexual spore: _____

● Q 2

The structure of yeast and hyphal forms may offer useful clues to the organism present. While a definitive speciation cannot always be made, reasonable assertions can. For the morphology below, give the classically associated genus or group. *(pp. 1088–1089)*
Acute angle branching: _____
Right angle branching: _____
Pseudohyphae: _____

● Q 3

A fungal colony is noted to be darkly pigmented on the obverse (front) of the plate. How will you determine if this is truly a dematiaceous colony? *(p. 1089)*

● Q 4

What is a cleistothecium, and what fairly common fungal organism reproduces via this structure? *(p. 1091)*

• Q 5

Define thallic conidiogenesis and describe how this process results in the high degree of infectivity seen with *Coccidioides immitis*. *(p. 1090)*

• Q 6

A respiratory specimen demonstrating only yeast forms that is positive for urease and is inhibited by cycloheximide is likely: *(p. 1096)*

• Q 7

What molecular technique may be used to diagnose the three major dimorphs as well as *Cryptococcus neoformans*, and may be a more efficient alternative to phase conversion? *(p. 1091)*

• Q 8

How does immunologic detection of cryptococcal antigen compare with the India ink test in terms of sensitivity in the diagnosis of *C. neoformans* in cerebrospinal fluid (CSF) specimens? *(p. 1092)*

• Q 9

Clinical Consultation: An ulcerated skin lesion in a 27-year-old male from Arkansas demonstrates budding yeast on a wet preparation. Select or describe three tandem media on which to culture this contaminated specimen and give your reasons for each. *(pp. 1092–1094)*

• Q 10

What simple technique can sterilize a plate culture suspected to be *Coccidioides immitis* before the plate is opened up for microscopic examination? *(p. 1092)*

• Q 11

True/False. The serum germ tube test is typically set up at the end of the workday, incubated overnight at 37°C, and is read the following morning. *(Table 60–8, p. 1095)*

• Q 12

Diagnosis of *Candida albicans* can be made, often within 48 hours, by two morphologic findings. If these are both absent, then one relies on pseudohyphae. Name the two characteristic microscopic findings. *(Table 60–10, p. 1095)*

• Q 13

What is the role of mucicarmine or Alcian blue stains in the workup of *Cryptococcus neoformans*? *(p. 1092)*

• Q 14

What supplement should be added to an agar medium when one suspects *Malassezia furfur*? *(p. 1100)*

• Q 15

True/False. Serology unfortunately aids little in the diagnosis of *Histoplasma capsulatum*, but the combination of typical morphology in a Giemsa-stained tissue specimen, characteristic tuberculated macroconidia in mould colonies, and a positive nucleic acid hybridization are sufficient for diagnosis. *(p. 1102)*

Q 16

What morphologic feature helps distinguish *Blastomyces dermatitidis* from *Histoplasma capsulatum* in microscopic preparation of the mould form? *(p. 1103)*

Q 17

What three organ systems are most commonly affected in disseminated coccidioidomycosis? *(p. 1103)*

Q 18

A nucleic acid hybridization, as well as an alternating pattern of cells, would confirm the diagnosis of *Coccidioides immitis* over two other fairly common isolates with arthroconidia. These two mimickers are from the genera: *(p. 1104)*

_____ and _____

Q 19

An alcoholic rose gardener is at risk for demonstrating the Splendore–Hoeppli phenomenon. Describe the morphology of this tissue reaction, as well as its sensitivity and specificity for sporotrichosis. *(pp. 1104–1105)*

Q 20

Describe the characteristic macroconidia of *Microsporum* spp. *(Figures 60–32, 60-33, p. 1106)*

Q 21

Describe three nonmorphologic tests which differentiate *Trichophyton mentagrophytes* from *T. rubrum*. *(p. 1107)*

Q 22

Muriform bodies are diagnostic of what disease? *(p. 1108)*

Q 23

Madurella mycetomatis and *Pseudallescheria boydii* are both etiologic agents of what indolent skin and soft tissue infection? *(p. 1107)*

Q 24

What genus is most commonly isolated from patients with zygomycosis? *(p. 1109)*

Q 25

Review the features of the zygomycete *Rhizopus*. *(pp. 1109–1110)*
Growth rate in vitro: _____
Presence of hyphae: _____
Presence of rhizoids: _____
Branching angle of hyphae: _____

Q 26

A 68-year-old male with chronic obstructive pulmonary disease develops a fungal infection in his right lung. A mass of infected tissue is removed and a sample of it grows within 1 week on an agar plate, manifesting as blue-green fluffy colonies. A second plate, treated with cycloheximide, shows no growth. What is the organism? Are you surprised that it did not grow in the presence of cycloheximide? *(p. 1111)*

Q 27

A rapidly growing, fluffy, salmon-colored colony that demonstrates crescent-shaped macroconidia in a patient with a history of ocular trauma is likely to be: *(Fig. 60–46, p. 1112)*

Q 28

The 5 μm cysts of *Pneumocystis carinii* must be differentiated from what other fungal pathogen of a similar size? *(pp. 1102, 1113)*

· ·

ANSWERS

A1. Asexual – sporangiospore.
   Sexual – ascospore.

A2. Acute angle – *Aspergillus* sp.
   Right angle – *Zygomycetes* sp.
   Pseudohyphae – *Candida albicans*, occasionally *C. tropicalis*.

A3. Turn the plate over. Dematiaceous colonies are dark on both sides of the plate, while nondematiaceous fungi have a light-colored reverse.

A4. A cleistothecium is a sexual fruiting body in which the ascospores are entirely enclosed and are released only by rupture of the cleistothecial wall. *Pseudallescheria boydii* reproduces via this structure.

A5. Thallic conidiogenesis is a form of reproduction where the conidium does not form until a septum has formed between the conidium and the parent cell. In *C. immitis*, the characteristic barrel-shaped conidia develop as part of conidiogenesis, and these conidia fragment easily, and disseminate in the air (such as the dry air of the south-west) to flow into the respiratory tracts of humans.

A6. Although nucleic acid tests have largely replaced these older biochemical tests, urease and phenol oxidase positivity still point toward *C. neoformans*.

A7. Nucleic acid hybridization, as mentioned in the answer to question 6.

A8. The immunologic tests, such as latex agglutination or enzyme immunoassay, have 90–100% sensitivity, whereas India ink offers only about 50% sensitivity.

A9. This is probably *B. dermatitidis*. Start with a general purpose medium, such as Sabouraud dextrose. A second choice might be a cycloheximide + antibacterial plate, which would inhibit saprophytic fungi and contaminating bacteria. Finally, brain–heart infusion agar with blood selects for dimorphs in tissue and would support *Blastomyces*.

A10. *C. immitis* is very dangerous to laboratory workers. Flood the plate with 10% formalin and incubate for several hours or overnight at room temperature.

A11. False. Other species begin to form germ tubes after 4 hours. *Candida albicans* produces germ tubes at just 2–4 hours, so the specificity of this test depends on reading it at the correct time.

A12. Germ tubes and chlamydospores are characteristic of *C. albicans*.

A13. These stain the mucopolysaccharide capsule and may be helpful with strains with little capsular material.

A14. A source of long-chain fatty acids, such as olive oil or peanut oil.

A15. True. Serologic tests for *H. capsulatum* show crossreactions with *B. dermatitidis*.

A16. *B. dermatitidis* has only microconidia. *H. capsulatum* has both micro- and macroconidia.

A17. The skin, skeletal system, and meninges are the most commonly affected systems.

A18. *C. immitis* may be confused with *Trichosporon* and *Geotrichum* spp.

A19. This appears as radiating eosinophilic material up to 10 μm in thickness around the yeast cell. It is not seen very often in sporotrichosis (poor sensitivity) and is also seen in other fungal infections (poor specificity).

A20. *Microsporum* macroconidia are thick-walled, roughened, tapered, and spindle-shaped.

A21. *T. rubrum* is appropriately named. Potato flake or cornmeal agar with 1% dextrose encourages a deep red pigment in *T. rubrum*, which is much more striking than the red pigment of *T. mentagrophytes*.

   At 3–5 days, *T. mentagrophytes* produces urease, while *T. rubrum* does not.

   The hair penetration test demonstrates the defects which *T. mentagrophytes* produces in hair in vitro, which is not seen with *T. rubrum*.

A22. This is chromoblastomycosis.

A23. This is mycetoma.

A24. *Rhizopus* spp. are the most common. *Mucor* was thought to be the second most common genus, but some members of the genus have been reclassified into other genera.

A25. *Rhizopus* is a rapid grower, filling the Petri dish in just 48–72 hours. It does have rhizoids, or roots, hence the name. Henry does not mention it, but *Mucor* lacks these root-like structures, and this is a helpful discriminating feature microscopically. As a zygomycete, *Rhizopus* is completely inhibited by cycloheximide. It has characteristic 90° angles between hyphae.

A26. This is *Aspergillus fumigatus* manifesting as a fungus ball. Most members of the *Aspergillus* genus are at least partially inhibited by cycloheximide. If the colonies had been yellow–tan, this would have *Aspergillus flavus*.

A27. A crescent or canoe shape along with a salmon- or pink-colored colony should immediately suggest *Fusarium*.

A28. Patients at risk for *Pneumocystis* are also at risk for *H. capsulatum*, and these two can look similar. Direct fluorescent antibody (DFA) may be helpful here.

CHAPTER 61
Medical parasitology

QUESTIONS

• Q 1

The optimal blood specimen is not often provided for malaria smears. State what this specimen is and also what the second choice is in terms of anticoagulant. *(p. 1121)*

• Q 2

What is the only stain that allows visualization of erythrocyte stippling in malaria smears? *(p. 1121)*

• Q 3

Which two fecal matter fixatives contain mercury and are thus difficult to dispose of safely in the laboratory? *(p. 1122)*

• Q 4

What are the three types of microscopic examination routinely performed on stool specimens? *(p. 1123)*

• Q 5

What three organisms may be better visualized with either a modified iron hematoxylin or modified acid-fast stain? Discuss the sensitivity and specificity of the acid-fast stain for these organisms. *(p. 1123)*

• Q 6

Several human cells and types of organic material resemble parasites and can make diagnosis challenging. What do *Entamoeba histolytica* trophozoites look like? *(Table 61–4, p. 1124)*

• Q 7

Review the lifecycle of Plasmodium species by stating whether the following events or parasite forms are found in the mosquito or in humans. *(Fig. 61–1, pp. 1128–1130)*

Fertilization of macrogamete: _____

Immature schizont: _____

Release of merezoites: _____

Liberation of sporozoites: _____

Mature schizont: _____

• Q 8

Differentiate between true disease relapse and recrudescence in malaria and state which Plasmodium species exhibit each. *(pp. 1128–1129)*

Q 9

Clinical Consultation: A 23-year-old female returned from a 1-week trip to West Africa 3 months ago and has complained of fevers and chills for the past week. She is now hospitalized and is noted to have fevers to 102.5°F every other day at about 2:00pm. The clinician suspects malaria. Based on her history and fever curve, what two species are now unlikely or at least less likely? *(Table 61–8, pp. 1130–1133)*

_____   _____

Using what you learned from question 1 in this chapter and the guidance on *page 1121*, what do you recommend for collection of a blood sample?

_____

What age of red blood cells (RBCs) will you pay particular attention to in your microscopic examination?

_____

You find several intracellular parasites on the thick smear, and note ameboid forms, Shüffner's dots, and 13–16 merozoites in the few mature schizonts you find. You diagnose:

_____

The woman then reveals to the clinician that her brother had an episode of hemolytic anemia when he was treated for vivax malaria last year. She wonders if she is at risk for hemolysis. Is she? Explain your answer.

_____
_____

Q 10

Are both trophozoites and gametocytes seen in humans with babesiosis? *(p. 1134)*

Q 11

Review the morphologic forms of the two important genera of hemoflagellates, stating which form is found in which vector or host. *(pp. 1134–1135)*
Leishmania spp. in humans: _____
Trypanosoma cruzi tissue in humans: _____
Leishmania spp. in insect vector: _____
Trypanosoma in insect vector: _____
Trypanosoma in bloodstream in humans: _____

Q 12

Compare and contrast the trypanosomiases. *(p. 1135)*

	East African	West African	American
Hemoflagellate			
Vector			
Illness severity (describe)			
Length of parasite (blood)			

Q 13

Review the major hemoflagellates causing the various forms of leishmaniasis.
(pp. 1135–1136)
L. donovani causes _____
L. braziliensis causes the aggressive _____
L. mexicana and *L. braziliensis* cause the less severe New World _____
L. tropica and *L. major* cause Old World _____

Q 14

How will you distinguish *Leishmania* spp. from *Histoplasma capsulatum* in a tissue biopsy? *(p. 1136)*

Q 15

What three types of serologic tests are employed to diagnose toxoplasmosis?
(p. 1137)

Q 16

What is the etiologic agent of primary amebic meningoencephalitis? *(p. 1137)*

• Q 17

What genus causes granulomatous amebic meningoencephalitis, and keratitis in contact lens wearers? *(p. 1138)*

• Q 18

List the three genera of ameba that inhabit the intestinal tract of humans. *(p. 1138)*

• Q 19

The only amebic species that is invasive and causes disease in humans is *Entamoeba histolytica*. What nonpathogenic species looks identical to *E. histolytica* in stool specimens? *(p. 1139)*

What commercially available test will discriminate between the two?

• Q 20

How useful is the serologic test for diagnosing amebic liver abscess if stool samples are negative? *(p. 1139)*

• Q 21

Differentiating between Entamoeba histolytica and the nonpathogenic Entamoeba coli is challenging. Erythrophagocytosis by a trophozoite, if present, is diagnostic for E. histolytica. Otherwise, cyst forms may be compared and contrasted. Review these. *(Table 61–10, p. 1142)*

	E. histolytica	*E. coli*
Usual size		
No. of nuclei (mature cyst)		
Appearance of chromatid bodies		

• Q 22

Dientamoeba fragilis is an ameboid flagellate which causes diarrhea, often in young children. Trophozoites are roughly 10 μm, with binucleation being the predominant form. A positive specimen should raise suspicion for what other intestinal parasite? *(p. 1142)*

• Q 23

Describe in the box below how you can differentiate between *Giardia lamblia* and *Chilomastix mesnili*. *(Figs. 61–13 and 61–14, pp. 1143–1144)*

	G. lamblia	*C. mesnili*
Nuclei in trophs		
Nuclei in cysts		
Patient symptoms		

• Q 24

Clinical Consultation: A 48-year-old male pig farmer has had diarrhea for 1 week. Colonoscopy showed ulcerations, and a biopsy was performed. List some of the morphologic features that will help you diagnose *Balantidium coli*. *(p. 1144)*

• Q 25

List the four coccidian parasite genera that infect humans. *(p. 1144)*

• Q 26

State how the size of the organism will distinguish oocysts of *Cryptosporidium parvum* from those of *Cyclospora cayetanensis* on an acid-fast preparation of a stool specimen. *(pp. 1145–1146)*

• Q 27

Describe the appearance of microsporidia on a modified trichrome stain. *(p. 1146)*
Color: _____
Size: _____
Shape: _____

• Q 28

The Cellophane test is the method of choice for diagnosing *Enterobius vermicularis*. Adult females measuring up to _____ in length and colorless ovoid eggs _____ long are easily identified. *(Fig. 61–16, p. 1147)*

• Q 29

How does pneumonitis occur in ascariasis if ova are ingested orally, and the adults live in the duodenum and jejunum? *(p. 1148)*

• Q 30

Describe how the buccal chamber morphology can be used to distinguish between rhabditoid larvae of hookworms and *Strongyloides stercoralis*. *(Fig. 61–19, pp. 1149–1150)*

• Q 31

Like *Ascaris lumbricoides*, *Strongyloides stercoralis* adults live in the duodenum and may cause Löffler syndrome/pneumonitis in the migration stage. They differ from *A. lumbricoides* in several ways. Outline these by reviewing the life cycle of *S. stercoralis*. *(pp. 1149–1150)*
How parasite enters host (human): _____
Form found in stool specimens: _____
Variant of life cycle in immunosuppressed host: _____

• Q 32

How may the number of lateral branches of a gravid uterus differentiate between *Taenia saginata* and *T. solium*? *(Fig. 61–21, p. 1150)*

• Q 33

Infection with the pork tapeworm and cysticercosis are not acquired in the same way and are not interchangeable terms. Distinguish between the two. *(pp. 1150–1151, 1157)*

• Q 34

The common first intermediate host of all trematodes is: *(p. 1152)*

• Q 35

Differentiation between the ova of *Fasciolopsis buski* and those of *Fasciola hepatica* is not usually possible. What clinical symptoms or laboratory tests would suggest one fluke over the other? *(pp. 1152–1153)*

• Q 36

Longstanding infection with *Clonorchis sinensis* is linked to what malignancy? *(p. 1153)*

• Q 37

Both *Fasciola hepatica* and the lung fluke *Paragonimus westermani* have unembryonated, operculated ova. Describe the size difference that distinguishes the two. *(Fig. 61–16, pp. 1147, 1153)*

• Q 38

What form/stage of the schistosome penetrates the skin of humans? *(p. 1154)*

• Q 39

Which two species of *Schistosoma* have a lateral spine? *(p. 1154)*

• Q 40

Review the periodicity of the common filarial worms by stating the optimal time to draw blood for examination. *(p. 1155)*

Wuchereria bancrofti: _____

Brugia malayi: _____

Loa loa: _____

Mansonella spp: _____

• Q 41

Differentiation of the filarial worm is based on morphology, but there may be other clues to their identity on an exam question, such as the insect vector. Review both of these features. *(Figure 61 –25, pp. 1155–1156)*

	Sheath	Nuclei in tail tip	Vector(s)
Wuchereria bancrofti			
Brugia malayi			
Loa loa			
Onchocerca volvulus			
Mansonella spp.			

• Q 42

Clinical Consultation: A 10-year-old boy whose parents are sheep farmers develops abdominal pain and is found to have a single, unilocular, 9 cm cyst filled with clear fluid in his liver. His primary chore at home is to clean up after the family's Australian shepherd dog. Give three species of cestode, from two genera, that are diagnostic possibilities. *(pp. 1158–1159)*

ANSWERS

A1. A drop of fresh blood, directly from a finger stick or syringe, is preferred because it does not distort the parasite. If anticoagulant must be used, then ethylenediaminetetraacetic acid (EDTA) is preferred.

A2. Giemsa stain will allow for visualization of the Shüffner's dots.

A3. Schaudinn's and polyvinyl alcohol (PVA) both contain mercury. The modified PVA fixatives replace mercury with either zinc sulfate or copper sulfate.

A4. The three basic examinations are the direct wet mount with a drop of saline or iodine, the wet mount of a concentrate, and the permanent stain. The direct mount is best for identifying motility, the concentration method is more sensitive if few organisms are present, and the stains can bring out small organisms such as amebae.

A5. The oocysts of *Cryptosporidium*, *Cyclospora*, and *Isospora* are better visualized with these stains than with Wheatley's trichrome, so this is a more sensitive method. It is not, however, specific, and careful attention must be paid to size and comparison with positive controls.

A6. *E. histolytica* trophozoites resemble macrophages, which are likely to be present in the specimen along with parasites.

A7. Fertilization of the macrogamete and liberation of sporozoites occur in the mosquito. Both schizont forms and the release of merozoites occur in humans.

A8. True disease relapse occurs when there is a renewal of exoerythrocytic schizony by latent hepatic sporozoites, called hypnozoites. This occurs with *P. vivax* and *P. ovale*.

Recrudescence does not involve the liver. It is a rise in parasitemia from undetectable to clinically detectable levels. It occurs with *P. falciparum* and *P. malariae*.

A9. *P. falciparum* usually presents within 1 month, and *P. malariae* has quartan periodicity, so these are less likely.

Collect blood by syringe or fingerstick near 2:00 pm on a 'febrile' day.
Examine the smear for younger red blood cells (reticulocytes).
Diagnosis: *P. vivax*.

If this woman is a heterozygote with a dual population of red blood cells, she may experience some degree of hemolysis, but not as severe as her brother's.

A10. No, just trophozoites. As *P. falciparum* often shows only the ring forms, distinguishing between the two with no travel history can be tough.

A11. *Leishmania* and *T. cruzi* in humans are in the amastigote form.
The promastigote is found in the insect vector for *Leishmania*.
The epimastigote form is in the insect vector for *Trypanosoma*.
The trypomastigote is found in the bloodstream of humans.

A12. East African trypanosomiasis is caused by *Trypanosoma brucei rhodesiense*, 30 μm long, carried by the tsetse fly, *Glossina* spp. It is rapidly fatal.

West African trypanosomiasis is caused by *T. brucei gambiense*, 30 μm long, also carried by *Glossina* spp. flies. It is more chronic, but can be fatal.

American trypanosomiasis (Chagas disease) is caused by *Trypanosoma cruzi*, 20 μm long, carried by the reduviid bug. It may have an acute or chronic course.

A13. *L. donovani* – visceral form.
L. braziliensis – mucocutaneous.
L. mexicana and *L. braziliensis* – New World cutaneous.
L. tropica and *L. major* – Old World cutaneous.

A14. *Leishmania* have a kinetoplast but lack a cell wall. *H. capsulatum* lacks the kinetoplast but its cell wall may stain with Gomori's methenamine silver or periodic-acid–Schiff.

A15. Sabin–Feldman (an antibody titer), indirect fluorescent antibody (IFA), and enzyme immunoassay (EIA).

A16. *Naegleria fowleri*. This is nearly always fatal.

A17. *Acanthamoeba* spp. are classically associated with keratitis in contact lens wearers.

A18. These are *Entamoeba*, *Endolimax*, and *Iodamoeba*.

A19. *E. dispar* is the nonpathogen. EIA antigen detection can help distinguish the two.

A20. Very useful. It has a 95% sensitivity if one has a liver abscess. By contrast, serologies are much less often positive (10%) in asymptomatic carriers.

A21. *E. histolytica* and *E. coli* cysts are nearly the same size, with *E. coli* a little larger (15–25 μm vs 12–15 μm). *E. histolytica* cysts have four nuclei and blunt or rounded chromatoidal bodies. E. coli cysts have eight nuclei and splintered or pointed chromatoidal bodies.

A22. *Enterobius vermicularis*, the agent of pinworms.

A23. *G. lamblia* has two nuclei in the trophozoite and four in the cyst stage. It also causes diarrhea. *C. mesnili*, in contrast, has just one nucleus in either stage and is nonpathogenic. If a person is symptomatic, and one finds only *C. mesnili*, one must continue to search for a cause.

A24. *B. coli* is the largest parasite one will see under the microscope. The trophozoite is 50–100 μm, and the cyst is 50–70 μm. It is ciliated, another feature that makes it unique among pathogens. It has a large macronucleus and many cytoplasmic food vacuoles.

A25. *Isospora*, *Sarcocystis*, *Cryptosporidium*, and *Cyclospora* are the four coccidians that infect humans.

A26. *C. parvum* is just 4–6 μm in diameter, while *C. cayetanensis* is 8–10 μm.

A27. Microsporidia are extremely small, but the modified trichrome stain helps bring them out. They are elliptical in shape, just 1.5–3 μm in size, and red with this stain.

A28. Adults are up to 13 μmm long, and ova are 50–60 μm in length.

A29. Ingested eggs hatch in the intestine and migrate through the wall of the bowel as larvae to enter the bloodstream. They travel to the lungs and mature briefly in the alveolar capillaries before being coughed up, swallowed, and returning to the intestines, where they mature into adults. A large load of larvae in a person previously sensitized to *Ascaris lumbricoides* can lead to an allergic reaction.

A30. *Strongyloides* has a short buccal cavity, about as long as the (narrowed) anterior tip is wide. Hookworms have a longer buccal cavity, about as long as the body is wide.

A31. Humans are infected by penetration of the skin by infective (third-stage) larvae. They pass first-stage larvae in their stool, and rarely pass ova. Autoinfection can occur in the debilitated host.

A32. *T. saginata* has 15–20 branches, while *T. solium* has 7–13.

A33. Ingestion of undercooked pork containing cysticerci results in the tapeworm developing in the gut and passage of *T. solium* ova in the feces. This is mildly debilitating. Ingestion of *T. solium* eggs, from one's own tapeworm or from poor hygiene, with spreading of the ova to others, causes cysticercosis. This is a serious, often fatal illness.

A34. The snail is the common intermediate host. Many trematodes have a second intermediate host, such as a fish or crab.

A35. *F. buski* causes diarrhea and nausea. The geographic range is south-east Asia, China, and India and is found in people who eat water chestnuts (and possibly have contact with pigs). Peripheral blood eosinophilia may be seen even in asymptomatic persons. *F. hepatica*, with a wider geographic distribution and acquired by ingestion of watercress, causes biliary colic and obstructive jaundice, so an elevated direct bilirubin or alkaline phosphatase might be helpful. Eosinophilia would be seen with *F. hepatica* as well, so this would not be a useful discriminator.

A36. Cholangiocarcinoma is an adverse outcome associated with chronic *Clonorchis* infestations.

A37. *F. hepatica* is about 140 μm long, while *P. westermani* is about 90 μm.

A38. The cercaria stage penetrates the intact skin of humans.

A39. Both *S. mansoni* and *S. japonicum* have lateral spines, but they are often poorly visible in *S. japonicum*.

A40. Both *W. bancrofti* and *B. malayi* are nocturnal, so 10:00 pm to 2:00 am is the recommended time to draw blood. *L. loa* is best harvested at noon. *Mansonella* spp. lack periodicity and can be found any time.

A41. *W. bancrofti* have a sheath, have no nuclei in the tail, and are transmitted by several mosquito vectors – *Culex*, *Aedes*, and *Anopheles*.

 B. malayi have a sheath, have two nuclei in the tail, and are transmitted by *Aedes*, *Anopheles*, and *Mansoni* spp. mosquitos.

 L. loa has a sheath, has some nuclei in the tail, and is transmitted by the *Chrysops* deer fly.

O. volvulus lacks a sheath, has no nuclei in the tail, and is transmitted by the *Simulium* black fly.

Mansonella spp. lack a sheath, have nuclei in the tail, and are transmitted by *Culicoides* gnats.

A42. *Echinococcus granulosus* is associated with sheep and is probably the first choice. Also consider the dog or cat tapeworms *Taenia multiceps* or *Taenia serialis* in this case.

CHAPTER 62

Molecular pathology of infectious diseases

. . . .

QUESTIONS

• Q 1

Direct DNA probe detection methods are chiefly used in the diagnosis of diseases in what two organ systems? *(p. 1170)*

• Q 2

What is the dual role of *Thermus thermophilus* in the molecular detection of hepatitis C virus (HCV)? *(p. 1174)*

• Q 3

Your laboratory has been using reverse-transcriptase polymerase chain reaction (RT-PCR) to monitor human immunodeficiency virus (HIV) RNA levels for the hospital's large HIV-positive population. A representative for a company using a different technology for HIV RNA quantification presents a slightly more cost-effective arrangement for this assay. What reason can you give for staying with your current RT-PCR technology? *(p. 1174)*

Q 4

Discuss how molecular techniques may be used in the case of a 55-year-old male housepainter with a cough and an acid-fast bacilli (AFB)-positive sputum specimen. *(p. 1175)*

Q 5

What is the utility in performing molecular typing of HCV? *(p. 1180)*

ANSWERS

A1. The infectious agents of the genitourinary (sexually transmitted diseases) and respiratory systems are the target of the commonly used direct DNA probes.

A2. The enzyme derived from this bacteria can perform both reverse transcription and amplification. Usually, two separate enzymes are needed for these two tasks.

A3. HIV RNA measurements varied from patient to patient among three methods used to quantify this virus in a recent study. The authors of the study recommended that the methods should not be used interchangeably. The teaching point is that there may be variation in results between different methods, or different manufacturers' platforms, for *any* assay. If you change your method, you must carefully review and compare your results between the old method and the new, and inform clinicians of any significant changes in interpreting the results.

A4. A nucleic acid amplification method would allow the more rapid discrimination of *Mycobacterium tuberculosis* and *M. kansasii* so that appropriate therapy could be started promptly, as well as isolation, if indicated. In real practice, however, false positives of *M. tuberculosis* occur, limiting the utility of this method.

A5. There are different strains of HCV, and some respond better to interferon-α than others. Typing allows one to predict the response to treatment.

CHAPTER 63

Specimen collection and handling for diagnosis of infectious diseases

QUESTIONS

Q 1

For most specimens, a polyester-tipped swab, such as Dacron, is appropriate for collection. For several sexually transmitted diseases, a particular swab is inappropriate. State which swab should not be used to collect for recovery of: *(p. 1188)*

Herpes simplex virus (HSV): _____

Neisseria gonorrhoeae: _____

Chlamydia trachomatis: _____

Q 2

What are the four functions of sodium polyethanol sulfonate in blood culture bottles? *(p. 1190)*

Q 3

What white blood cell types are collected for culture of cytomegalovirus? *(p. 1191)*

Q 4

What serologic test is used to diagnose neurosyphilis from a cerebrospinal fluid specimen? *(p. 1192)*

Q 5

Give three methods of diagnosing *Chlamydia trachomatis* from conjunctival scrapings? *(pp. 1193–1194)*

Q 6

Clinical Consultation: A 4-year-old girl is hospitalized with what is suspected to be whooping cough. The clinician wants to perform a nasopharyngeal culture. You ask him to stop by the laboratory before going to her bedside. What do you give him and why? *(p. 1194)*

Q 7

Is a sputum sample with eight epithelial cells and 30 polymorphonuclear leukocytes (PMNs) acceptable for further processing? *(p. 1195)*

Q 8

Compare the utility of sputum vs bronchoalveolar lavage (BAL) to recover *Legionella* spp. *(p. 1196)*

Q 9

Clinical Consultation: A 43-year-old nun has mild urinary frequency and provides a midstream clean-catch urine specimen. A standard loop is used to inoculate sheep's blood agar and MacConkey's agar (MAC) plates. After 48 hours of incubation, 125 bright pink colonies are counted on the MAC plate. What is the most likely agent? Is this a significant number of bacteria, indicating infection? *(pp. 1196–1197)*

Q 10

What culture media are used for recovery of *Leptospira interrogans* in urine specimens? *(p. 1197)*

Q 11

What transport temperature and culture medium are used to recover *Neisseria gonorrhoeae* from an endocervical specimen? *(p. 1198)*

Q 12

What medium is used to recover shiga-toxin-producing enterohemorrhagic *Escherichia coli* (STEC), and how does culture compare with toxin detection in terms of sensitivity? *(p. 1199)*

Q 13

Outline collection and processing of stool for *Clostridium difficile* toxin evaluation by the cell culture method. *(p. 1200)*

Q 14

Compare and contrast the advantages of the saline and iodine methods in wet preps of stool examined for parasites. *(p. 1200)*

· ·

ANSWERS

A1. Calcium alginate can inactivate HSV.
Cotton can be toxic to *N. gonorrhoeae*.
Wood can be toxic to *C. trachomatis*.

A2. Sodium polyanethanol sulfonate inhibits coagulation, phagocytosis, complement activation, and the aminoglycoside antibiotics.

A3. Neutrophils are the main cell type that cytomegalovirus infects, but it is also seen in mononuclear cells, so both should be harvested.

A4. The Venereal Disease Research Laboratory (VDRL) test is the only one that can detect antibodies. Recall that this is one of the nonspecific tests.

A5. A Giemsa stain directly from the conjunctival swab, a direct fluorescent antibody test (DFA), and a culture are all methods for detecting *C. trachomatis*.

A6. The clinician should pick up a Regan–Lowe plate and inoculate it right at the bedside for optimal recovery. Regan–Lowe is recommended currently over the older Bordet–Gengou potato agar.

A7. Yes. There are a few different criteria for acceptability of sputum samples, all based on the number of squamous cells from the oral cavity and PMNs from the pulmonary system. A good rule of thumb is the more PMNs, the better, and a greater number of PMNs than epithelial cells is satisfactory.

A8. Sputum for DFA and culture is preferred for recovery of Legionella. Culture takes up to 1 week. BAL may be too diluted to be fruitful, and the anesthetic can inhibit *Legionella* organisms.

A9. This is classic for *Escherichia coli*. Greater than 1×10^5 organisms is significant. A standard loop contains 0.001 mL of urine. 125 colonies $\times 1000 = 125\,000$ CFU/mL, so this is a real infection. Do you remember that the three major lactose-fermenting organisms are *E. coli*, *Klebsiella*, and *Enterobacter*?

A10. *L. interrogans* should be cultured on Fletcher's or Ellinghausen–McCullough–Johnson–Harris medium.

A11. The important fact to remember for *N. gonorrhoeae* is to maintain it at room temperature. Do not refrigerate. There are a few media for this organism; one is the modified Thayer–Martin with added CO_2.

A12. STEC should be plated on, among other standard media such as sheep blood agar, MAC, and sorbitol MAC. STEC does not ferment sorbitol but almost all other *E. coli* do. The toxin detection method is actually more sensitive.

A13. This is a cell culture assay. Collect 25–50 mL of liquid stool in a clean container and process within 2 hours of collection. Extracting the toxin involves centrifugation, either at 2000 g for 20 minutes, or 10 000 g for 10 minutes. The stool is then filtered through a 0.45 µm membrane filter. Serial dilutions are prepared on cell monolayers and incubated for 24–48 hours. The enzyme-linked immunosorbent assay (ELISA) method of toxin detection is simpler and faster but may not be as sensitive.

A14. Saline shows movement of trophozoites, its greatest advantage over other techniques, but will also show cysts and ova fairly well. Iodine destroys trophozoites unless the sample was previously fixed. It neatly highlights the features of cyst forms, though. Usually, a wet preparation is performed with side by side saline and iodine mounts.

CHAPTER 64

Bioterrorism:
microbiology

QUESTIONS

Q 1

The Laboratory Response Network (LRN) is a consortium of laboratories that provide testing and communication in support of public health emergencies, particularly bioterrorist attacks. LRN has classified laboratories into three levels according to their capabilities and roles in an emergency. To familiarize yourself with this classification, complete the following table. *(p. 1208)*

Type of lab	Biosafety level guidelines	Primary responsibility	Type of facility/location
Sentinel			
Reference			
National			

Q 2

Would you expect to see spores from an impression smear from a clinical specimen from the gastrointestinal tract in a case of anthrax?

How about from a sheep's blood agar plate after incubation for 18 h? *(p. 1209)*

Q 3

Contrast the growth rate of *Brucella* spp. with that of *Bacillus anthracis*. *(p. 1209)*

Q 4

What is the etiologic agent of melioidosis? *(p. 1211)*

Q 5

Clinical Consultation: A 23-year-old man presents to your community hospital with fever, headache, cough with a vague pulmonary infiltrate, and elevated liver enzymes. Two weeks ago, he was in a small town where there is a suspected outbreak of Q fever. As medical director of your facility's sentinel laboratory, what should you do in the work-up of his blood and sputum samples? The clinician understands the risk of Q-fever samples but states that an adenovirus is in her differential diagnosis and asks if you could set up a cell culture in your laboratory to explore this. What's your next step? *(Table 64–11, p. 1214)*

Q 6

Francisella tularensis infection may present with nonspecific symptoms such as cough, chest pain, weakness and chills. If a blood culture is positive for a small, Gram-negative coccobacillus, what test can you perform to distinguish this organism from *Haemophilus influenzae*, another agent of a respiratory system illness? *(Fig. 64–6, p. 1216)*

• Q 7

Smallpox is a serious bioterrorism threat as it is very contagious and immunity from those vaccinated a generation ago may be lost. Chickenpox on the other hand, is a fairly benign illness that is still common, despite vaccination of children. Contrast the clinical presentation of the lesions of these two diseases. *(p. 1216)*

Characteristic	Smallpox	Chickenpox
Temporal development of lesions		
Distribution/dispersion		
Key locations of lesions on bod		
Constitutional, associated symptoms		

• Q 8

At your sentinel laboratory, should you inoculate a cell culture with clinical material from a suspected smallpox case, contacting your local public health official only if growth in cell culture occurs? *(p. 1217)*

• Q 9

Can plague be transmitted from human to human? *(p. 1220)*

ANSWERS

A1.

Type of lab	Biosafety level guidelines	Primary responsibility	Type of facility/ location
Sentinel	BSL-2	Rule out and refer suspicious agents to the appropriate reference laboratory	Clinical laboratories, as found in local hospitals
Reference	BSL-3	Definitive confirmation of organisms, including toxin testing, sent by the sentinel labs	Local and state public health labs, some academic or university-based labs, designated specialty labs
National	BSL-4	Isolation of BSL-4 agents, genetic characterization and archiving of bioterrorism agents	CDC, USAMRID

A2. Spores will not be present from the clinical specimen, but central to subterminal spores are visible from culture plates such as SBA.

A3. *Brucella* spp. are fairly slow-growers, with peak isolation occurring at 3–4 days. *B. anthracis* is a rapid grower, with growth visible in just 6–8 hours and individual colonies present in 12–15 hours.

A4. This is *Burkholderia mallei*. It is the human equivalent of glanders, and typically presents as an acute pneumonia.

A5. The role of the sentinel laboratory in cases of suspected Q fever is *not* to attempt to culture this highly infectious organism but to refer all specimens to the appropriate reference laboratory. Your first phone call should be to your hospital's infection control officer, who will then contact the state or local public health department and coordinate transportation of specimens. You should also NOT set up a cell culture, as *Coxiella burnetii* is an obligate intracellular organism which can be cultured in all fibroblast cell lines.

A6. Recall that *H. influenza* requires both hemin and NAD for growth, so it will have a positive XV test. *F. tularensis* will be negative for this test.

A7.

Characteristic	Smallpox	Chickenpox
Temporal development of lesions	Simultaneous, with uniform maturation	Progressive, with lesions at different stages at different body sites
Distribution/dispersion	Uniform	Crops of lesions clustered together
Key locations of lesions on body	Face, forearms, lower legs	Trunk, head
Constitutional, associated symptoms	Fever, severe myalgia	Fever, myalgia, but also coryza

A8. No. *Do not* inoculate specimens from suspected smallpox cases. While the patient is present in the hospital, contact your infection control officer so that s/he can evaluate the patient and contact local public health authorities for specimen handling and transport.

A9. Yes, primary pneumonic plague can be transmitted from human to human.

Part VIII

Molecular pathology

CHAPTER 65

Introduction to molecular pathology

QUESTIONS

• Q 1

What common autosomal recessive disease may manifest in a mild form with such findings as bilateral absence of vas deferens or sinopulmonary complaints? *(p. 1226)*

• Q 2

On average, 1 in _____ base pairs differs between any two individuals as a result of polymorphisms in coding and noncoding regions of the genome. *(p. 1226)*

• Q 3

What agency publishes guidelines for the standardization of methods in molecular pathology? *(p. 1226)*

ANSWERS

A1. Cystic fibrosis. Some persons have a mild form of the disease but have the mutation in the cystic fibrosis transporter protein.

A2. 1 per 1000 base pairs differs as a result of polymorphisms.

A3. This is the Clinical Laboratory Standards Institute (CLSI), previously known as the National Committee for Clinical Laboratory Standards.

CHAPTER 66

Molecular diagnostics:
basic principles and techniques

QUESTIONS

• Q 1

What pH will disrupt helical DNA? *(p. 1229)*
Below _____ and above _____

• Q 2

Which DNA purine–pyrimidine base pair requires more energy to disrupt the hydrogen bonds? (circle correct choice) *(p. 1229)*
G–C   A–T

• Q 3

Why is RNA inherently less stable than DNA? *(p. 1229)*

• Q 4

What is the role of the spliceosome in transcription–translation? *(p. 1231)*

Q 5

Promoters are regions of DNA that help regulate gene transcription and protein translation. The most common promoter sequence is _____ _____. Two others are the _____ box and the _____ motif. *(p. 1231)*

Q 6

State the type of repair pathway that would be used to correct the following errors. *(Table 66–3, p. 1232)*
Small adducts: _____
Mispaired base: _____
Error due to radiation: _____
Alkylation lesion: _____
Large adducts: _____

Q 7

Which DNA repair pathway is nonfunctional in xeroderma pigmentosum? *(p. 1232)*

Q 8

A fundamental principle in nucleic acid analysis is nucleic acid hybridization. Compare and contrast the terms hybridization and annealing, two events in the analysis process. *(p. 1234)*

Q 9

A hybridization cocktail is a mixture of reagents that favors the interaction of nucleic acids – it facilitates hybridization. It has several components. What is the role of formamide in the cocktail? *(p. 1235)*

Q 10

Many hospital laboratories now employ hybridization assays, which allow detection of the hybridization process to give a clinically meaningful result. One such commercial assay is the Hybrid-Capture system. Detection of the hybrids utilizing the hybrid capture technique involves DNA, RNA, and an antibody. What is the role of each? *(p. 1236)*

_____ is the target. _____ is the probe. _____ binds to the RNA–DNA hybrid.

Q 11

Both dot/blot assays and Southern and Northern blots utilize solid-support media to detect hybridization. What additional information do Southern and Northern blots provide and what technique provides this data? *(p. 1236)*

Q 12

True/False. Positional cloning uses restriction fragment length polymorphism (RFLP) analysis to identify abnormal protein products of mutated genes. *(p. 1238)*

. . . .

ANSWERS

A1. A pH below 4 or above 9 will disrupt the DNA molecule.

A2. G–C has three hydrogen bonds, compared to just two for A–T, so G–C requires more energy to disrupt. If a DNA strand is rich in G–C pairs, then overall, more energy is required to unravel the helix.

A3. RNA is naturally a single-stranded molecule, so it lacks the stabilizing forces of those hydrogen bonds we just reviewed in question 2. It also has the hydroxyl group at the 2′ position on its sugar, and this moiety is vulnerable to attack by alkaline hydrolysis. Finally, ubiquitous RNA-specific enzymes may rapidly degrade the RNA molecule.

A4. The spliceosome excises introns, or noncoding regions, from messenger RNA (mRNA), leaving only the exons to be translated. Exons are expressed.

A5. The TATA box is the most common promoter region. Also known are the GC box and the CAA motif.

A6. Small adducts – base excision repair.
Mispaired base – mismatch repair.
Error due to radiation – double-strand break repair.
Alkylation lesion – direct repair.
Large adducts – nucleotide excision repair.

A7. The nucleotide excision repair activity is lost. Damage from ultraviolet radiation cannot be repaired and these children are prone to skin cancers at an early age.

A8. Hybridization refers to the binding of unlabeled DNA to a labeled probe. The new double strand is a hybrid of labeled and unlabeled strands.

Annealing is simply two unlabeled strands of DNA joining together to form a double strand.

RNA can also participate in the hybridization process.

A9. Formamide denatures the sample DNA to expose its base pairs.

A10. DNA is the target, as human papilloma virus (HPV) is a DNA virus. An RNA probe is employed, and the RNA–DNA hybrid is bound by an antibody for detection.

A11. Southern and Northern blots use electrophoretic separation of the test nucleic acid, which permits determination of the molecular weight of the species.

A12. False. Positional cloning works without the knowledge of the protein product in a given disease. It uses family analysis to locate the gene first.

CHAPTER 67

Polymerase chain reaction and other nucleic acid amplification technology

QUESTIONS

• Q 1

Polymerase chain reaction (PCR) is an enzyme-mediated process that amplifies a target nucleic acid from one copy to millions of copies. What enzyme is used to amplify the nucleic acid? *(p. 1239)*

• Q 2

Two enzymes are used in conventional reverse transcriptase PCR (RT-PCR). First, _____ produces copy DNA (cDNA) from an RNA target. Then, _____ amplifies cDNA by the PCR methodology. What is the key advantage of the enzyme derived from *Thermus thermophilus*? *(p. 1239)*

• Q 3

What is the chief advantage of multiplex PCR? *(p. 1240)*

● Q 4

Quantitative PCR assays, such as those for CMV, human immunodeficiency virus (HIV)-1, and hepatitis C virus (HCV), make use of the competitive PCR (cPCR) approach. In cPCR, two templates are amplified at once. What parameters are the same between the two templates? (circle correct choices) *(p. 1241)*

Template base sequence   Primer   Thermodynamics   Amplification efficiency

● Q 5

Fluorescent dyes are the foundation of this type of PCR. *(p. 1241)*

● Q 6

Transcription-mediated amplification and nucleic-acid-sequence-based amplification are techniques used to amplify RNA that involve isothermal rather than thermal cycling. Give three advantages of the isothermal technique? *(pp. 1243–1244)*

● Q 7

True/False. One disadvantage of strand-displacement amplification (SDA) is that it has relatively poor sensitivity compared to its specificity, requiring more than 1000 copies of the target molecule for detection. *(p. 1245)*

● Q 8

The invader probe amplification assay can be adapted to detect _____ ____ mutations, such as those in the genes for Apo E and factor V Leiden. *(p. 1247)*

● Q 9

How do signal amplification assays reduce the number of false positives (increase specificity) compared to target amplification assays? *(p. 1247)*

ANSWERS

A1. This is DNA polymerase.

A2. Reverse transcriptase makes cDNA from RNA. Then DNA polymerase continues, as in regular PCR, to amplify the cDNA. *T. thermophilus* has provided a thermostable DNA polymerase that functions as both reverse transcriptase and DNA polymerase.

A3. More than one target sequence can be used in a single tube.

A4. The primer, thermodynamics, and amplification efficiency are all the same. The templates are of a similar length but are not the same. The principle is that if you know the quantity, before and after, of your second template, you can calculate the quantity of your patient template to make PCR a quantitative process.

A5. This is real-time PCR.

A6. DNA is never denatured by heat in these isothermal systems. Thus, DNA cannot bind to primers. You don't want DNA getting in the way when you are amplifying RNA, and dsDNA cannot bind to primers in its double-stranded state.

They don't require sophisticated thermal cyclers. These are closed tube system techniques, which further reduce contamination by DNA.

A7. False. SDA is very sensitive, requiring only 10–50 copies of the target molecule, except when there is excess background DNA. This can overwhelm the system, and sensitivity falls as a result.

A8. Point mutations.

A9. In this method, the signal is directly proportional to the amount of target sequence present. When the target sequence is amplified, there is risk of crosscontamination with background DNA. When the signal is the component that is amplified, you eliminate the risk.

CHAPTER 68

Hybridization array technologies

QUESTIONS

• Q 1

Define hybridization array technology (HAT). What is the fundamental principle of HAT? *(p. 1250)*

• Q 2

There are two types of hybridization array – macroarrays and microarrays. Which one is the diagnostic platform of choice in most commercial labs? *(p. 1251)*

• Q 3

Microarray technology is still on the horizon, but the FDA recently granted clearance to Roche Molecular Systems to market a testing platform. What does the platform test for? *(p. 1256)*

ANSWERS

A1. HAT is a method in molecular pathology that enables the base pairing of two strands of nucleic acid (hybridization) to occur in a solid substrate, in order to perform thousands of hybridization reactions simultaneously in a single procedure. Thus, the fundamental principle is the detection of specific hybridization between complementary strands of nucleic acid. Prior to arrays, hybridization evaluated one DNA sample with one probe at a time.

A2. Microarrays save time and money and are the platform of choice.

A3. Roche has produced a genotyping test for the cytochrome P450 206 and 2C19 genotypes, which code for enzymes involved in the metabolism of drugs. Their goal is to aid clinicians in identifying patients for whom a particular drug may or may not be appropriate.

CHAPTER 69

Applications of cytogenetics in modern pathology

QUESTIONS

Q 1

In what phase of mitosis are chromosomes usually observed in cytogenetics?
(p. 1261)

Q 2

What is the preferred specimen for routine cytogenetic studies, and what is the appropriate preservative? *(p. 1262)*

Q 3

What is the purpose of phytohemagglutinin (PHA) in cell cultures? *(p. 1262)*

Q 4

An infant is born with ambiguous genitalia. While endocrine studies are being initiated, the genotypic sex of the infant must also be determined. What stain will mark the Y chromosome, if present? *(p. 1263)*

Q 5

State three advantages of fluorescence in situ hybridization (FISH) over older autoradiography techniques. *(p. 1264)*

Q 6

True/False. A partial mole is classified as euploid. *(p. 1267)*

Q 7

A child is homozygous for the F508 mutation and has cystic fibrosis. However, studies on both parents reveal that only the mother carries for the mutation. She is heterozygous. Explain how this has occurred. *(pp. 1267–1268)*

Q 8

Uniparental disomy is defined as (circle correct choices):
one copy   two copies   of a chromosome from   one parent   each parent.
(p. 1268)

Q 9

Nondisjunction in meiosis I results in (circle correct choices):
one   two   normal   abnormal   gametes.
In this same case, after meiosis II, there are two gametes with
isodisomy   heterodisomy   and two gametes that lack a chromosome.
(Fig. 69–11, pp. 1267–1268)

Q 10

Reviewing Figure 69.1 *(Fig. 69–13, pp. 1268–1269)*, assume that the pink chromosome represents a point mutation in the β-globin gene of 6 Glu ⟶ Lys in the mother. The blue maternal chromosome and both paternal chromosomes (green, purple) are normal. What would be the hemoglobin genotype of each of the three 'children' shown in the figure?

Uniparental isodisomy child: _____

Uniparental heterodisomy child: _____

Biparental heterodisomy child: _____

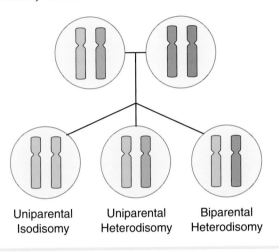

Uniparental Isodisomy   Uniparental Heterodisomy   Biparental Heterodisomy

Q 11

A ring chromosome has lost (circle correct choices)   one   both
telomere(s)   centromere(s). *(p. 1272)*

Q 12

A 15-year-old girl was born to a father with Becker muscular dystrophy (BMD) and a normal mother. One of the girl's X chromosomes had undergone midivision of the centromere, generating isochromosome X (iXq) and resulting in Turner's syndrome. It is unknown whether the isochromosome is of maternal or paternal origin. Now the child is demonstrating vague muscle weakness. Is BMD a consideration? Why? *(Fig. 69–14, pp. 1271–1272)*

Q 13

The most common trisomy seen in abortus material is: *(p. 1273)*

Q 14

What percentage of newborns have a chromosomal abnormality? *(p. 1273)*

Q 15–20

For the following common cytogenetic rearrangements in leukemias and lymphomas, name the type of leukemia or lymphoma. *(Table 69–3, p. 1275)*

Q 15

t(8;21)(q22;q22): _____

Q 16

inv(16)(p12q22): _____

Q 17

t(1;19)(q23;p13.3): _____

Q 18

t(8;22)(q24;q11): _____

Q 19

14q11.2 rearrangements: _____

Q 20

5q–, del(5)(q13q33): _____

Q 21

What region of chromosome 21 is critical to the manifestation of the Down syndrome phenotype? *(p. 1277)*

Q 22

True/False. Both Turner and Klinefelter syndromes may present as a mosaic *(p. 1278)*

Q 23

State the two causes of a phenotypic male with a 46, XX genotype. *(p. 1278)*

Q 24

State the more common cause of a phenotypic female with a 46, XY genotype *(p. 1278)*

Q 25

What deletion is present in Wolf–Hirschorn syndrome? *(p. 1279)*

Q 26

Both Angelman and Prader–Willi syndromes have deletions at chromosome _____. Which is the more sensitive diagnostic tool for these syndromes, FISH or high-resolution cytogenetic analysis? *(p. 1279)*

Q 27

DiGeorge syndrome and _____ _____ share an abnormality at chromosome _____. *(Table 69–5, p. 1279)*

Q 28

Williams syndrome involves a deletion of the gene for which protein? _____

This gene is located at chromosome _____. *(p. 1280)*

Q 29

True/False. Fragile X syndrome is due to a trinucleotide repeat on the short arm of the X chromosome. *(Fig. 69–24, p. 1280)*

Q 30

Ataxia telangiectasia has been localized to chromosome _____, and is associated with translocations involving chromosomes _____ and _____. *(Table 69–6, p. 1281)*

ANSWERS

A1. Metaphase is the common phase of mitosis for chromosome analysis.

A2. Peripheral blood in a heparin (green top) tube is preferred.

A3. PHA stimulates lymphocytes, which are naturally in a nondividing state, into mitosis, so they may be observed in metaphase.

A4. This is quinacrine, or Q-stain. This is a fluorescent stain but it is not used for routine analysis because it is transient. It marks the distal end of the Y chromosome very brightly, though, so it is still used for this purpose.

A5. FISH is faster, more specific, and allows the use of multiple probes in a single hybridization procedure.

A6. True. Euploid is defined as any exact multiple of haploid, so 23, 46, 69 are all euploid.

A7. This is a complex sequence of events. This child began embryonic life with monosomy for chromosome 7; he only got a 7 from his mother, and he got the 7 with the *CF* mutation. The paternal 7 was never transmitted as a result of meiotic nondisjunction. Monosomy of any autosomal chromosome is lethal in utero but in this case the child was rescued by duplication of the existing maternal 7. Unfortunately, the *CF* mutation was duplicated along with the rest of the genetic material on 7, and the child was homozygous for the *CF* mutation. This is called uniparental (both copies of a chromosome from one parent) disomy (two copies of the chromosome).

A8. Reinforce what we have just reviewed in question 7. Uniparental disomy is two chromosomes (both copies) from one parent.

A9. When nondisjunction occurs in meiosis I, both gametes produced at that division are abnormal. One has both chromosome pairs, and one has none. After meiosis II, in which a 'normal' disjunction occurs, two gametes have one copy of each of the persons' parental genes, say a paternal chromosome 5 and the maternal 5 heterodisomy. The other two gametes lack chromosome 5 altogether.

A10. Uniparental isodisomy – Hb CC, or Hb C disease.
Uniparental heterodisomy – Hb AC, or Hb C trait.
Biparental heterodisomy – Hb AC, or Hb C trait.

A11. Ring chromosomes have lost both telomeres.

A12. You need to know that BMD is an abnormality on the short arm of the X chromosome. This girl has two long arms in her isochromosome, so she has only one short arm. If her isochromosome came from her mother, then her only X with a short arm came from her father, who has the BMD deletion/insertion. So, yes, BMD is a possibility.

A13. This is trisomy 16.

A14. 0.6% of live newborns have a chromosomal abnormality.

A15. Acute myeloid leukemia (AML) M2 in the old FAB classification.

A16. AML M4 in FAB.

A17. Pre-B acute lymphoblastic leukemia (ALL).

A18. Burkitt lymphoma. The World Health Organization no longer classifies the ALLs as L1, L2, L3.

A19. Pre-T-cell ALL.

A20. Myelodysplastic syndromes.

A21. This is 21q22.12 to 21q22.3. Some Down syndrome individuals have just a partial trisomy but, if it is in this region of chromosome 21, then it is enough to confer the phenotype.

A22. True. Some of the mosaics of both sexes are able to reproduce.

A23. Congenital adrenal hyperplasia (CAH) is the common cause, due to a lack of 21-hydroxylase enzyme and a subsequent in utero accumulation of androgens. Less commonly, recombination, which occurs with the sex chromosomes during meiosis, moves the sex-determining region of the Y chromosome (SRY) over to the tip of the X. The genotypic female has the genetic material to develop the male phenotype.

A24. This is testicular feminization or androgen insensitivity syndrome. Here, the Y chromosome is intact, and the testes-determining factor is located in the SRY region. Yet the fetus lacks the androgen receptor gene on the long arm of X (Xq21), testosterone cannot be complexed to dihydrotestosterone, and male genital development does not take place.

A25. This is 4p– syndrome. It is a terminal deletion – del(4)(p16).

A26. These classic imprinting syndromes are at 15q11.2. FISH is more sensitive, picking up 80–85% of cases.

A27. Both DiGeorge and velocardiofacial syndrome are at 22q11.2.

A28. Williams syndrome involves a defect in elastin on chromosome 7q11.23. Abnormalities in elastin account for most of the phenotype but do not account for the observed behavioral problems.

A29. False. It's the long arm, at Xq27.3.

A30. This disorder has been localized to 11q22.3. Its breakage manifests in several ways, one of which is translocations involving 7 and 14.

CHAPTER 70

Establishing a molecular diagnostics laboratory

QUESTIONS

• Q 1

The overriding consideration in the design of a molecular diagnostics laboratory is minimizing *(p. 1284)*

• Q 2

Ultraviolet radiation, deoxyuridine triphosphate, and uracil-*N*-glycosylase are all aspects of preventing contamination of the: *(p. 1285)*

• Q 3

What act specifies the educational and training requirements of laboratory personnel in molecular diagnostics laboratories? *(p. 1285)*

• Q 4

Which step in molecular diagnostic testing is particularly labor-intensive and has been the focus of development of customized platforms using technologies such as magnetic bead isolation? *(p. 1287)*

Q 5

You are establishing a new molecular diagnostics laboratory. Where do you turn for guidance in writing your quality control procedure plan? *(p. 1293)*

Q 6

What agency has been granted the status of an enforcement agency by the Department of Health and Human Services (HHS enforces CLIA '88) to accredit laboratories performing molecular diagnostics? *(p. 1294)*

ANSWERS

A1. This is contamination.

A2. Amplicon. The amplicon is what you are trying to amplify via polymerase chain reaction (PCR).

A3. The Clinical Laboratory Improvement Amendment 1988 (CLIA '88).

A4. This is nucleic acid extraction. Newer devices such as those described in *Table 70–2* have increased throughput, precision, and personnel savings.

A5. The Clinical and Laboratory Standards Institute (CLSI, formerly NCCLS) addresses both of these issues.

A6. This is the College of American Pathologists (CAP).

CHAPTER 71

Molecular diagnosis of hematopoietic neoplasms

QUESTIONS

• Q 1

The leukemias are typically characterized by variability in the intronic breakpoint and fusion sites of transcribed genes. Despite this variability, diagnosis of these translocations is still achieved. State the invariant species that can be detected and the technology used in its detection. *(pp. 1296–1297)*

• Q 2

What is the translocation of chronic myelogenous leukemia (CML)? Include specific sites on chromosomes. *(p. 1297)*

• Q 3

t(9;22) is seen in de novo acute lymphoblastic leukemia (ALL) as well as CML. How can reverse-transcriptase polymerase chain reaction (RT-PCR) distinguish these two disorders in many cases? *(Fig. 71–1, pp. 1297–1298)*

• Q 4

The *BCR–ABL* fusion protein in CML is a constitutive tyrosine kinase. Which chromosome and which gene code for normal tyrosine kinase? *(Fig. 71–1, pp. 1297–1298)*

• Q 5

A subset of acute myeloid leukemias (AMLs) is characterized by extensive karyotypic abnormalities and an aggressive course. These acute leukemias sometimes evolve out of myelodysplasia. Which two chromosomes are usually involved in this subset of AMLs? *(p. 1299)*

• Q 6

The most common translocation in all of childhood ALL cases is _____ _____ and carries a _____ prognosis. *(p. 1302)*

• Q 7

Clinical Consultation: A clinician is treating a 3-year-old girl for ALL. She has been identified by RT-PCR as having the t(1;19)(q23;p13.3) translocation. Your reference laboratory performs only qualitative PCR. The clinician wants to repeat the RT-PCR at the end of consolidation chemotherapy to evaluate for minimal residual disease (MRD). Is RT-PCR sensitive enough for MRD, or should another methodology be used? *(p. 1314)*

• Q 8

How useful is RT-PCR for the *PML–RARα* fusion protein in predicting relapse in acute myeloid leukemia (AML) M3? *(p. 1313)*

• Q 9

A patient treated for AML M2 2 years ago has had normal blood counts and has felt clinically well since completing chemotherapy. She now has a bone marrow examination, and for the first time, RT-PCR is applied for t(8;21). It is positive. Is relapse imminent? *(p. 1313)*

• Q 10

Where is the immunoglobulin heavy chain gene located? *(p. 1305)*

• Q 11

True/False. In light chain production, the B cell first attempts to generate the κ light chain. If unsuccessful, the cell then generates the λ light chain. *(p. 1305)*

• Q 12

Study Figure 71.1B and C *(Fig. 71–1, p. 1298)* and interpret this PCR by classifying the type of leukemia demonstrated.

Lane E1: (e1–a2 product) _____
Lane B2: (b2–a2 product) _____
What is lane M? _____
What is lane N? _____

• Q 13

Compare and contrast the two main techniques for determining lymphoid clonality, PCR, and Southern blot hybridization (SBH). *(pp. 1307–1308)*

PCR advantages: _____
_____
PCR disadvantages: _____
_____
SBH advantages: _____
_____
SBH disadvantages: _____
_____

• Q 14

Which of these two methods, PCR or SBH, should be the first or front-line choice for determining lymphoid clonality? *(p. 1308)*

• Q 15

What is the normal function of the *BCL2* gene product? *(p. 1309)*

• Q 16

What is the location of the *BCL2* gene? *(p. 1309)*

• Q 17

Overexpression of cyclin D1 is strongly correlated with _____ _____ lymphoma. *(p. 1310)*

• Q 18

Why is FISH a better methodology for diagnosing the t(11;14)(q13;q32) translocation than SBH or PCR? *(p. 1310)*

• Q 19

What is the role of normal BCL6 protein? *(p. 1311)*

Q 20

Why is there no t(3; —)(q27; —) established translocation for the *BCL6* gene? *(p. 1311)*

Q 21

The *c-myc* locus at 8q24, associated with Burkitt and some other high-grade lymphomas, is translocated to one of three different loci to generate a fusion product. List these three loci and their genes. *(p. 1311)*

Q 22

What is the role of the normal c-Myc gene product? *(p. 1311)*

Q 23

Why is RT-PCR a sensitive and specific methodology for diagnosis of the t(2;5)(p23;q35) translocation? *(p. 1312)*

Q 24

ALK protein expression can help distinguish what two CD30 positive lymphomas? *(p. 1312)*

• Q 25

TaqMan and LightCycler are two examples of what type of PCR? What is their key application in the management of hematolymphoid malignancies? *(p. 1312)*

ANSWERS

A1. RT-PCR can detect the invariant chimeric mRNA species.

A2. t(9;22)(p34;q11.21).

A3. The gene product of the *BCR–ABL* fusion gene is a protein that is typically 210 kDa. This is the case in patients who have established CML then enter blast crisis. Patients with de novo ALL usually have a 190 kDa version of the protein.

A4. Recall that many oncogenes and oncoproteins derive from normal genes and proteins. The *ABL* gene at 9p34.1 codes for a tyrosine kinase.

A5. Chromosomes 5 and 7 are characteristically involved.

A6. t(12;21) has a favorable prognosis.

A7. No. Nonquantitative PCR is not sensitive enough in assessing for MRD in the t(1;19) cases and other ALL rearrangements. Quantitative PCR (Q-PCR) is a better choice

A8. Here, RT-PCR is useful. Detection correlates with relapse.

A9. No, not necessarily. The translocation has been shown to persist in the cells of long-term survivors of AML M2.

A10. Chromosome 14q32.

A11. True.

A12. Lane E1 shows the 190 kDa fusion product of most cases of Ph+ ALL. Lane B2 shows the 210 kDa fusion product of CML. Lane M is the molecular size marker, or ladder, and lane N is the negative control, which is performed on all PCRs.

A13. PCR advantages – easy, rapid (few days), little DNA required, paraffin-fixed tissue OK.

PCR disadvantages – labile to micromolecular alterations (a small change in a gene may result in nonhybridization and a subsequent false-negative), mutations in patient sample may prevent primer from binding leading to failure (this occurs in some B-cell lymphomas).

SBH advantages – gold standard, binds to large regions of DNA and is thus not as sensitive as PCR to micromolecular alterations.

SBH disadvantages – laborious, costly, time-consuming (2–3 weeks), requires fresh or frozen tissue (not paraffin).

A14. PCR. If cases are difficult to interpret, then go to SBH.

A15. The BCL2 protein plays an antiapoptotic role in cells.

A16. Chromosome 18q21.

A17. Mantle cell lymphoma. It is occasionally seen in prolymphocytic leukemia, splenic lymphoma with villous lymphocytes, and CLL.

A18. The large size of the breakpoints and the high number of different breakpoints found in mantle cell lymphoma make SBH and PCR less sensitive for this translocation. FISH picks up this fusion gene more effectively.

A19. The BCL6 protein is critical to normal germinal center development and to T-cell-dependent antibody responses.

A20. *BCL6* translocations are described as promiscuous. There are so many that no clear translocation characteristic of *BCL6*-positive lymphomas has emerged. Occasionally, we will see the classic translocation with the *IgH* gene; this is t(3;14)(q27;q32).

A21. t(8;14)(q24;q32) – Ig heavy chain.
t(2;8)(p12;q24) – κ light chain.
t(8;22)(q24;q11) – λ light chain.

A22. c-Myc forms a DNA-binding complex with another protein, Max. This initiates transcription of genes that are necessary for cells to enter the cell cycle and to proliferate. One can easily see how unregulated activity by c-Myc/Max can lead to neoplasia.

A23. PCR assays in general are sensitive. PCR is specific in this translocation because the fusion mRNA is constant. You are always looking for the same mRNA transcript. Keep in mind that this translocation is associated with a favorable prognosis.

A24. Anaplastic large cell lymphoma and classic Hodgkin lymphoma.

A25. These are both proprietary platforms that employ quantitative PCR, a technology that is particularly useful in evaluation of minimal residual disease.

CHAPTER 72

Molecular diagnosis of genetic diseases

QUESTIONS

• Q 1

What molecular technique is particularly applicable to detecting known point mutations in genes? *(p. 1324)*

• Q 2

Applications of molecular techniques in medical genetics fall into five categories: carrier screening, newborn screening, diagnostic gene testing, presymptomatic DNA testing, and prenatal testing. Which of the five categories is suggested by the following descriptions? *(p. 1325)*

a. Obviates need for fetal tissue biopsy in phenylketonuria if mother has the disease:

_____

b. Used chiefly as a backup to simpler biochemical tests in a large patient population:

_____

c. Performed on a symptomatic individual: _____

d. Use for aid in family planning: _____

e. Used in such diseases as Huntington's and in familial cancer syndromes:

_____

• Q 3

A mother has Marfan's syndrome and has four children, two of whom have been found to have the gene. One of her children is tall with long limbs and has lens ectopia. The other is normally proportioned with no apparent manifestations. This is an example of: *(p. 1326)*

Q 4

Two boys in a family are both affected with cystic fibrosis due to the F508 mutation in chromosome 7. One of them has severe pulmonary infections and struggles to maintain his weight. His brother has a significantly less severe course, with fewer, milder infections. This can be explained by the concept of: *(p. 1326)*

Q 5

Anticipation is typically associated with what type of genetic disorders? *(p. 1326)*

Q 6

X-chromosome inactivation is achieved in females by epigenetic changes occurring after fertilization of the ovum. What chemical modification takes place to silence the genes on the X chromosome? *(p. 1326)*

Q 7

What are the two main difficulties that have been encountered in DNA testing for cystic fibrosis? *(p. 1327)*

Q 8

Duchenne muscular dystrophy (DMD) is caused by one of many possible deletions in this large gene in two-thirds of cases, but because the gene is so large (2.5 million bp) and has so many (79) exons, it is laborious to screen for them all. What molecular method has allowed for screening of multiple different deletions at once? *(Fig. 72–4, p. 1328)*

Q 9

Can one use the restriction endonuclease *Ms*II or *Dde*I to diagnose the hemoglobin C mutation? *(Fig. 72–1, pp. 1324, 1328–1329)*

Q 10

What is the amino acid substitution in coagulation factor V that results in factor V being resistant to activated protein C? *(p. 1329)*

_____ replaces _____ at position _____

on factor V.

Q 11

In 1991, the trinucleotide repeat expansion disorders were discovered. Several diseases are now known to fit into this category, and some are characterized by anticipation, or by transmission sex bias, in which the sex of the parent passing on the gene influences the severity of the disorder. Does fragile XA syndrome exhibit either of these characteristics? *(Table 72–2, p. 1330)*

Q 12

A mother with normal intelligence has three sons. They are ages 2, 3, and 5. As there is some suggestion of developmental delay in two of them, all three undergo testing for fragile X. Given the number of CGG triplet repeats, classify each son as normal, premutation, or full mutation. *(Table 72–2, p. 1330)*

2-year-old – 325 repeats: _____

3-year-old – 180 repeats: _____

5-year-old – 75 repeats: _____

Q 13

Several trinucleotide diseases are associated with a CAG expansion. All are autosomal dominant except _____ which is X-linked.

(Table 72–2, p. 1330)

Q 14

Friedreich ataxia is unique among the majority of trinucleotide repeat disorders for several reasons. List three. *(Table 72–2, pp. 1330, 1332)*

Q 15

A 2-year-old girl demonstrates progressive myotonia and has cataracts. She is tested for myotonic dystrophy (DM) and is found to have 1375 repeats. Which parent transmitted the disease? *(p. 1331)*

Q 16

What are the two main methods of diagnosing trinucleotide repeats? *(p. 1332)*

Q 17

Prader–Willi syndrome (PWS) and Angelman syndrome (AS) are classic examples of the phenomenon of imprinting. In PWS, a deletion of 15q11–13 on the (circle correct choices)

maternal   paternal

chromosome is pathologic. In AS, it is the

maternal   paternal

chromosome that suffers a deletion. *(p. 1332)*

Q 18

True/False. Tumorigenesis in multiple endocrine neoplasia (MEN) 2A and 2B follow the patten of the two-hit hypothesis. One allele is mutated in the germline. When the other allele is mutated as a random event, malignancies such as medullary thyroid carcinoma develop. *(p. 1334)*

Q 19

What genetic defect does hereditary nonpolyposis colon cancer have in common with Fanconi anemia? *(Table 72–3, pp. 1333–1334)*

Q 20

Clinical Consultation: A clinician calls you about a 34-year-old male with a serum transferrin saturation of 95% and diabetes mellitus. She wants to evaluate him for hereditary hemochromatosis (HH). *(pp. 1336–1337)*

Is the race of the patient relevant? _____

_____

What molecular technique will you use as a first-line test? _____

_____

What sort of abnormality are you looking for in the protein HFE?

_____

ANSWERS

A1. PCR. Variations on PCR include digesting PCR products with certain restriction enzymes if the mutant PCR product creates a new, unique restriction site; and multiplex PCR, where many different probes are used in a solid support medium to screen for several mutations in a single test.

A2. a. Prenatal screening.
b. Neonatal screening.
c. Diagnostic genetic testing.
d. Carrier screening.
e. Presymptomatic testing.

A3. Penetrance. Penetrance is an all-or-nothing phenomenon. If you inherit the gene, either you have some expression or you don't have any. Marfan's disease and neurofibromatosis exhibit variable penetrance. Remember that, even if you do not manifest the disease, if you inherit the gene you can pass it on to your offspring.

A4. Expressivity. Expressivity, in contrast to penetrance, is a spectrum phenomenon. Some people have mild disease, while others suffer severe manifestations. Cystic fibrosis is characterized by variable expressivity.

A5. Trinucleotide repeat disorders, such as Huntington's, myotonic dystrophy, and fragile X syndrome.

A6. Methylation of cytosines at cytosine–purine–guanine (CpG) dinucleotides silences genes.

A7. The length of the gene; it is over 250 000 base pairs long.
    The great number of mutations; over 1700 have been discovered.
    While the F508 three-base pair deletion accounts for some 70% of cases, it does not account for the other 30%. With such a large gene, there are many other sites for deletions and mutations to occur. We cannot test for them all.

A8. Multiplex PCR can pick up 98% of the cases due to a deletion. Now, only two thirds of the cases are due to a deletion and the remaining one third are due to mutations or microdeletions/insertions.

A9. No. Hb C mutation is an A replacing a G at position 6 on the β-globin gene. This point mutation does not destroy the restriction site for either of the two endonucleases because it is at a flexible position for the endonucleases. The digest for Hb C looks just like that for Hb A, so it is not useful for diagnosis of Hb C.

A10. Glutamine (Q) replaces arginine (R) at position 506. This is abbreviated R506Q.

A11. Fragile XA exhibits both, with maternal sex bias.

A12. Greater than 200 repeats is considered a full mutation, so the 2-year-old has fragile X syndrome. The other two sons are in the range of 50–200 repeats, which is considered a premutation. These boys do not have fragile X but they can pass on chromosomal instability to their daughters and, in their daughter's meiosis, the full mutation can occur. These daughters may then pass on the disease to their sons.

A13. Kennedy disease is X-linked. Like the other CAG repeat disorders, it is characterized by expanded polyglutamine sequences in proteins, with subsequent neuronal toxicity.

A14. Friedreich ataxia is autosomal recessive, does not demonstrate anticipation, and manifests the repeats in introns rather than coding regions (exons).

A15. In cases of over 1000 repeats, transmission is always maternal.

A16. PCR and Southern blot. In cases where there are greatly expanded trinucleotide repeats, Southern blot is preferable. Otherwise, PCR is favored due to its speed and simplicity.

A17. PWS – paternal deletion.
AS – maternal deletion.

A18. False. Just one allele with a mutation is enough in the *RET* oncogene associated with medullary thyroid carcinoma.

A19. Both are examples of DNA repair defects, as are ataxia telangiectasia, Bloom syndrome, and xeroderma pigmentosum. These defects occur all in different genes, however.

A20. HH is a disease of Caucasians. PCR amplification works well for single nucleotide substitutions, as is the case in HH, where tyrosine replaces cysteine at amino acid 282, written C282Y, in 80–90% of cases. Thus, you are looking for single missense mutation.

CHAPTER 73

Identity analysis:
use of DNA polymorphisms in parentage and forensic testing

QUESTIONS

Q 1

Define obligatory paternal genes. *(p. 1344)*

Q 2

A child in a parentage dispute has an HLA genotype of HLA B7 and B3. The mother has B7 and B10. The alleged father is homozygous for B12. The alleged father is ruled (circle correct choices)

in   out   by   direct   indirect   exclusion. *(p. 1345)*

Q 3

From the 1930s through the 1970s, what genetic markers were used in cases of disputed parentage? *(p. 1340)*

• Q 4

DNA testing by polymerase chain reaction (PCR) has replaced traditional serologic markers for the identification of individuals. Briefly outline the advantages of DNA testing over the older methods. *(p. 1341)*

• Q 5

What is the anticoagulant of choice for DNA testing, particularly for blood samples collected in a Vacutainer? *(p. 1341)*

• Q 6

What are the two most common methodologies forming the basis of DNA analysis in parentage testing? *(p. 1342)*

• Q 7

Study Figure 73.1 below and review case 2 in this RFLP analysis. Here, two probes, A and B, are employed to analyze two loci called D12S11 and D17S79. When we use restriction endonucleases to cut DNA, we come up with DNA fragments of varying but characteristic lengths, which we can compare among individuals in a manner very similar to what we used to do with HLA antigens. Instead of HLA A3 and B27, we now have D12S11 and D17S79. Probe A = D12S11, probe B = D17S79. In case two, we test the mother (M), child (C), alleged father (AF), and a mixture of C's and AF's DNA (m). A DNA ladder is at the far right. *(pp. 1344–1345)* (circle correct choices)

Probe A is a: match   indirect exclusion   direct exclusion

Probe B is a   match   direct exclusion   indirect exclusion

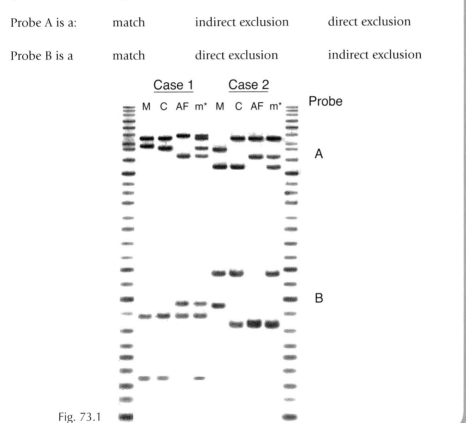

Fig. 73.1

● Q 8

Study Figure 73.2 *(Fig. 73–6, p. 1347)*, in which a parentage study was performed when the alleged father was deceased. Both of the AF's parents were analyzed to reconstruct his possible genotype. Does this study support the paternity of the deceased man in this case?

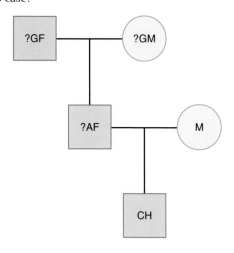

System	Child	Mother	OG	?GF*	?GM*	Possible phenotypes of ?AF	Formula to calculate system index
CSF1PO	10, 12	9, 12	*10*	10, 13	10, 11	10; 10,11; 10, 13; 11,13	0.5/p
D3S1358	14, 15	14, 17	*15*	15, 16	16, 17	15, 16; 15, 17; 16, 17; 16	0.25/p
D7S820	10, 11	10, 11	*10 or 11*	8, 9	11	8, 11; 9, 11	0.5/p + q
D16S539	9, 12	9, 13	*12*	10, 12	12	10, 12; 12	0.75/p
TPOX	8	8, 11	*8*	8	8	8	1/p
vVWA31/A	18	18	*18*	18	18	18	1/p

• Q 9

Study Figure 73.3 *(Fig. 73–7, p. 1348)*, and review this parentage study. Here, the mother is deceased, leaving behind four children and two alleged fathers. The probable maternal marker for each system is underlined and in bold type. AF 1 is possibly the father of child(ren) ———————————————— and is excluded from parentage of child(ren) ————————————————. In the case of AF 2 and child 3, the markers D3S1358 and THO1 are both examples of what type of exclusion?

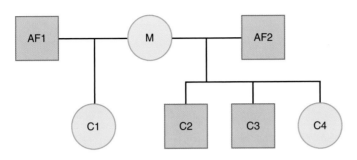

System	AF1	AF2	Child 1	Child 2	Child 3	Child 4
CSF1PO	10, 11	11, 12	10, **14**	12, **14**	**9**, 12	11, **14**
D3S1358	15, 17	15, 17	**14**, 17	17	**14**, 16	**14**, 15
D5S818	13, 14	11, 12	**10**, 14	**10**, **12**	12	12
D7S820	8, 9	10, 13	8, **11**	10, **11**	10, **14**	13, **14**
D13S317	11, 12	8, 10	12, **14**	8, **10**	10, **14**	**10**
D16S539	12, 15	9, 11	**8**, 15	**8**, 11	11, **13**	9, **13**
vWA31/A	14, 20	16, 17	**15**, 20	**15**, 17	16, **18**	17, **18**
TH01	8, 9	6, 9	8, **9.3**	6, **9.3**	8, **9.3**	9, **9.3**
TPOX	8, 22	8, 10	**8**	**8**, 12	**8**, 12	**8**
Amelogenin	Male	Male	Female	Male	Male	Female
DYS390	23	23		23	23	
DYS391	10	11		11	11	

• Q 10

The mainstay of DNA testing in the forensic DNA testing community uses ———— ———————————————— genetic loci identified by the FBI, which have been standardized for use in obtaining genetic profiles. How many nucleotides long is each short tandem repeat (STR) locus? *(p. 1342)*

• Q 11

True/False. The majority of cases in which DNA evidence is tested are resolved through plea-bargaining and do not go to trial. *(p. 1344)*

• Q 12

What type of DNA sequencing may be performed on shed hairs, which lack nuclear DNA? *(p. 1342)*

• Q 13

What region of DNA is used more often in testing – coding or noncoding (junk DNA)? *(p. 1341)*

• Q 14

True/False. The cumulative probability of exclusion is a mathematical estimate of probability that demonstrates diminishing returns as more and more systems are used. *(p. 1345)*

• Q 15

Review *Table 73–6 (p. 1347)* to answer the following question. Of the 10 STR loci evaluated, which represent obligatory paternal genes, meaning that they are present in the fetal tissue but are absent in the mother?

STR Locus	Obligatory Gene
CSF1PO	
D3S1358	
D5S818	
D7S820	
D8S1179	
D13S317	
D16S539	
D18S51	
D21S11	
vWA31/A	

• Q 16

The paternity index (PI) of tested man 1 (TM 1) is 2.19×10^6. Is this adequate, based on the AABB Standards required to determine parentage? *(p. 1346)*

• Q 17

Study Figure 73.4 and analyze the Amplitype DNA probe. *(pp. 1344–1345)* Does the blood match the reference sample of the victim, suspect 1 or suspect 2? _____

_____ .

The hair found on the victim matches with _____

_____ .

Can suspect 1 be excluded as the donor of both the hair and the blood?_____

_____

• Q 18

Review Figure 73.5 *(Fig. 73–2, p. 1343)*

This is a PCR amplification of an alleged father (AF). The child has the D21S11 alleles 20, 21. What type of exclusion is shown, if any? _____

At D2S1338, the child has alleles 12 and 19. Is this an exclusion for the AF?

_____

At allele VWA, the child inherited allele 18 from the mother, who is homozygous at this locus, and has alleles 17, 18. Is this an exclusion? _____

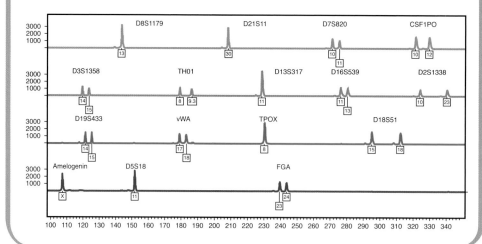

• Q 19

What is Amelogenin? *(p. 1342)*

• Q 20

What is the 'Chelex' method? *(p. 1342)*

ANSWERS

A1. Often abbreviated OG, the obligatory paternal gene refers to an allele present in the child but not present in the mother. It is thus obligatory in the father.

A2. The alleged father is ruled out by indirect exclusion. Keep in mind that one indirect exclusion does not fully exclude the alleged fathers. However, two indirect exclusions are usually sufficient.
Let's take a moment to clarify two common terms in paternity cases.
Direct exclusion – when a child has a marker that the alleged father lacks.
Indirect exclusion – when a child lacks a marker for which the alleged father is apparently homozygous.

A3. The blood group systems, first ABO and Rh, and then MNSs, Kell, Duffy, and Kidd were used in paternity cases. Polymorphic serum proteins and red cell enzymes were sometimes employed as well.

A4. Sensitivity is far greater with DNA, as PCR can amplify minute amounts of the molecule. DNA is robust, resisting acids, alkalis, detergents, and environmental factors. Even denatured DNA will often (not always) retain its nucleotide sequence, allowing meaningful analysis.

A5. Ethylenediaminetetraacetic acid (EDTA) is the anticoagulant of choice. Heparin is not recommended.

A6. DNA testing relies on PCR and restriction length fragment polymorphisms (RFLP). The only sample needed is nucleated cells, any kind.

A7. Both probes are matches.

A8. Yes. Every OG was found in one of the child's presumed grandparents.

A9. AF 1 is possibly the father of child 1. He is excluded as the father of children 2, 3, and 4. AF 2 has been directly excluded from paternity of child 3. In both these markers, the child has a marker that the alleged father lacks.

A10. The forensic community uses 13 STRs. Each is 3–7 nucleotides long.

A11. True.

A12. Mitochondrial DNA sequencing, although performed at few laboratories, is useful when nuclear DNA is extremely degraded or absent.

A13. Noncoding regions contain variable number tandem repeats, which show polymorphism among individuals.

A14. True. The curve flattens out as more systems are used, so you get less bang for your buck.

A15.

STR Locus	OG
CSF1PO	None
D3S1358	16
D5S818	11
D7S820	None
D8S1179	None
D13S317	10
D16S539	9
D18S51	17
D21S11	None
vWA31/A	17

A16. Yes. AABB requires a PI of at least 100, and TM1 is far beyond that.

A17. Blood, found in apartment of suspect, matches that of victim. Hair, found on victim, matches suspect 2. Suspect 1 is excluded as donor of both blood and hair.

A18. The AF is homozygous for D21S11 (allele 30), so this is an indirect exclusion. The AF shows D2S1338 (alleles 10, 23), so this is a direct exclusion. AT VWA, the AF is a match, as he could have given allele 17 to the child.

A19. Amelogenin is a sex-determination system utilizing the different sizes of alleles on the X compared to the Y chromosome.

A20. The 'Chelex' method is a DNA extraction technique that involves boiling the sample to release cellular contents, then adding Chelex-100 to bind metal ions, thus inactivating nucleases and polymerases. This method replaced the classical chloroform/phenol and ethanol extraction, which was cumbersome, although reliable.

Part IX

Clinical pathology of cancer

CHAPTER 74

Diagnosis and management of cancer using serologic tumor markers

QUESTIONS

• Q 1

Are tumor markers generally more useful as screening tools or to monitor patients with established malignancies? *(p. 1354)*

• Q 2

State the reasons why carcinoembryonic proteins are not suitable for screening for cancer. *(p. 1360)*

• Q 3

How has hybridoma technology improved sensitivity and specificity in the detection of tumor markers? *(p. 1355)*

• Q 4

Despite some improvements in sensitivity and specificity in tumor marker assays, they are generally not recommended for screening. How is it that prostate-specific antigen (PSA) is an effective screening tool? *(p. 1362)*

• Q 5

Clinical Consultation: A 64-year old man with hemochromatosis, inadequately treated, is status post-resection of his left colon for colon cancer 2 years ago. On a routine recheck, his CEA is elevated. A computed tomography (CT) scan of his liver shows no mass lesions. What is the likely cause of his elevated CEA, and what explains his CT scan? *(p. 1357)*

• Q 6

What modification to serum α-fetoprotein (AFP) measurement can help distinguish between primary hepatoma and benign liver diseases? *(p. 1357)*

• Q 7

What group of malignancies may be monitored with β_2-microglobulin? *(p. 1360)*

• Q 8

Sialylated lacto-*N*-fucopentaose II is the epitope for what tumor marker? *(p. 1360)*

_____

What sort of patient would be negative for this marker even in the presence of the appropriate malignancy? _____

In what racial group would this test be less useful? _____

• Q 9

In what benign condition of the female genital tract is CA 125 elevated? *(p. 1360)*

• Q 10

What malignancy is likely to be monitored with CA 15-3? Is CA 15-3 used to screen patients, per FDA regulations? *(p. 1360)*

• Q 11

What is the chief drawback of CA 72-4? *(p. 1361)*

• Q 12

Would the utility of CEA as a marker of recurrence of a gastrointestinal cancer be limited in a patient with cirrhosis? Explain why or why not? *(p. 1360)*

• Q 13

The protein encoded by *c-erb*B-2 shows structural and functional homology with what normal protein? *(p. 1361)*

• Q 14

True/False. The *HER2* ELISA test can still be used to monitor breast cancer patients on the monoclonal antibody Herceptin because different antigen epitopes are targeted by the ELISA platform than are targeted by the drug. *(p. 1361)*

• Q 15

What percentage of patients with seminomas have elevated beta-human chorionic gonadotropin (β-hCG)? *(p. 1361)*

• Q 16

What domain of the p53 protein is the site of mutation in human cancers? *(p. 1361)*

• Q 17

What percentage of free PSA to total PSA is usually associated with benign prostatic hypertrophy? *(p. 1362)* _____
What percentage supports a diagnosis of prostatic cancer? _____
_____

• Q 18

Define PSA velocity as a mathematical formula. What PSA velocity is a strong, specific predictor of prostate cancer? *(p. 1363)*

ANSWERS

A1. Assays for tumor markers are typically neither sensitive nor specific enough for screening; measurements of particular markers such as carcinoembryonic antigen (CEA) over time in a patient with colon cancer is reasonable and useful.

A2. Although CEA is a marker of malignancy, it is seen in several cancers, including those of lung, liver and breast. Crossreactivity of the antibodies directed against the proteins yields false positives; this, coupled with the incidence of colon cancer, makes the positive predictive value low. Also, these proteins do not appear early enough in the disease course to be of use for asymptomatic persons.

A3. Production of several monoclonal antibodies in mice and subsequent selection of the antibody that binds a particular epitope on the tumor cell has improved specificity and sensitivity.

A4. PSA is specific for the prostate gland, as suggested by its name. Also, the prevalence of prostate carcinoma is high enough for a useful positive predictive value to be generated by a positive test. Recall from your study of statistics that positive predictive value depends strongly on the prevalence of the disease in question.

A5. This person could well have a recurrence of his colon cancer with liver metastases. Untreated hemochromatosis can lead to cirrhosis. With impaired hepatic clearance of the CEA, it is possible that lesions undetectable by CT scan would produce CEA that was not cleared by the liver and was detectable by serum sample.

A6. Some tumors alter the structure of tumor markers with the addition of carbohydrate moieties. In primary hepatoma, an additional fucose is added to AFP, which causes AFP from hepatoma to react to lentil lectin. Thus, identifying lentil lectin activity in AFP suggests hepatoma over a benign process.

A7. B-cell lymphoid malignancies can be monitored with this marker.

A8. CA 19–9.

Someone who is Le a–b–, as this marker is related to the Lewis blood group antigens.

22% of African Americans are Le a–b–, so it would be helpful to know an African American patient's Lewis antigen status before using this test on him/her.

A9. Endometriosis.

A10. CA 15-3 can be used to monitor and predict the outcome of patients with breast cancer. It is found in adenocarcinomas of other organs, but has FDA approval only for monitoring breast cancer patients.

A11. CA 72–4 has poor sensitivity. It is only moderately elevated in most carcinomas.

A12. Yes. CEA is metabolized in the liver, and liver disease results in decreased clearance of CEA with subsequently higher serum levels.

A13. Epidermal growth factor receptor (EGFR).

A14. True. This is advantageous, because many women with *HER2*-positive tumors are treated with Herceptin.

A15. 10–30% of seminomas are β-hCG positive.

A16. p53 is usually mutated in the DNA-binding domain.

A17. More than 23% free PSA usually indicates a benign process, such as benign prostatic hypertrophy. <6% is associated with cancer of the prostate.

A18. PSA velocity = (current PSA – previous PSA)/ years between measurements. A velocity of 0.75 ng/year has a specificity of 95% to predict cancer.

CHAPTER 75

Oncoproteins and early tumor detection

QUESTIONS

Q 1

The signal transduction pathway that regulates the cell cycle is a complex cascade of events that is normally regulated at many steps to prevent continuous mitogenic signaling, which leads to neoplasia. Two nuclear transcription factors, which form a heterodimer to induce transcription of cyclin, a mitogenic protein, are at the end of this pathway. These two factors are: *(Fig. 75-1, p. 1368)*

Q 2

The signal transduction pathway is divided into four elements. Proteins are known in each of these pathway elements which are mutated or overexpressed in certain cancers. To familiarize yourself with the players in oncogenesis, list the examples of these oncoproteins which are described in this chapter. *(pp. 1369–1372)*

Growth factors: _____

Growth factor receptors: _____

Cytosolic proteins: G proteins: _____

Nuclear oncoproteins: _____

Q 3

What malignancy would best be followed with serum measurements of TGF-β? *(p. 1369)*

Q 4

Platelet-derived growth factor is elevated in a small percentage of patients with many different types of cancer, so it lacks both sensitivity and specificity as a diagnostic tool. However, it does correlate well with the stage of which type of cancer? *(p. 1370)*

Q 5

True/False. Increased levels of hepatocyte growth factor are found in hepatocellular carcinoma (HCC) but not in cirrhosis. *(p. 1370)*

Q 6

What is the primary utility of HER-2/*neu* in breast cancer? It is a valid predictor of (circle correct choice): *(p. 1370)*

histologic type   early detection   prognosis   response to radiation

Q 7

The p21^{ras} G protein undergoes conformational changes to become permanently activated in several different types of cancer. The two cancers that correlate most strongly to *ras* activation, with a high percentage of tumors demonstrating *ras* mutations, are: *(p. 1372)*

Q 8

True/False. Because G proteins are intracellular, attempting serum measurements of the G protein p21 to screen for or monitor cancer is fruitless. *(p. 1372)*

Q 9

Describe the action of normal p53. *(p. 1372)*

Q 10

Qualitatively, how sensitive (how many false negatives) is serum p53 in diagnosing hepatocellular carcinoma, breast, lung, and colon cancers? *(p. 1373)*

Q 11

The Myc protein is probably a transcription factor, which has what effect on cell replication in the normal cell? *(p. 1373)*

Q 12

Describe the enzyme-linked immunosorbent assay (ELISA) test for transitional cell carcinoma (TCC) that has been approved by the US Food and Drug Administration (FDA) for follow-up for TCC patients already treated for this disease. *(p. 1374)*

Q 13

What technology evaluates complex patterns of serum proteins and protein ion fragments by mass spectroscopy to assist in the diagnosis of malignancy? *(p. 1374)*

· ·

ANSWERS

A1. These are *fos* and *jun*. These are considered oncogenes, but bear in mind that most oncogenes are normal elements of the cell cycle which have undergone mutation or are being overexpressed.

A2. The growth factors are TGF-α and TGF-β, FGF, PDGF, and EGF.
The growth factor receptors are EGFR, and a key player in oncogenesis – HER-2/*neu*.
The main G-protein is p21^{ras}.
Two key nuclear oncoproteins are p53 and Myc; others are NMP22 and BTA.

A3. Hepatocellular carcinoma.

A4. Serum levels of PDGF correlate well with the stage of breast cancer.

A5. False. HGF is elevated in nonmalignant liver diseases, so it is not as useful as a tumor marker.

A6. HER-2/*neu* is an indicator of prognosis. It is also useful in selecting patients who may benefit from Herceptin, the monoclonal antibody therapy used in treating these breast cancers.

A7. Pancreatic and colon cancer. Over 90% of pancreatic cancers and 75% of colon cancers show *ras* mutations.

A8. False. Through an unknown mechanism, p21 proteins gain access to the extracellular environment and are found in serum as well as in the tumors themselves.

A9. Normal p53 binds to certain regions of DNA to repress mitosis. When p53 is mutated, then it fails to repress mitosis, and cell replication proceeds unchecked. Again, keep clear in your mind that these oncoproteins have a function in the normal cycling of the cell. Also bear in mind that some of these, such as p53, normally function to inhibit the cell cycle.

A10. Sensitivity is poor, with 8–34% of patients with these cancers having elevated serum levels of p53.

A11. Myc normally derepresses replication, to allow replication to go forward.

A12. This ELISA provides antibodies to the nuclear matrix protein NMP22 as its reagent. NMP22 is a protein involved in the formation of the mitotic spindle, which is specific for TCC, as it is present in tumor cells at levels above 10 U/mL compared with levels of below 10 U/mL in normal bladder cells. NMP22 is shed in the urine of many patients with invasive or in situ TCC. A patient urine sample is applied to the ELISA well. If NMP22 is present, it binds to the kit antibody and produces a visible result.

A13. This is proteomics.

CHAPTER 76

Diagnostic and prognostic impact of high-throughput genomic and proteomic technologies in the post-genomic era

QUESTIONS

• Q 1

True/False. Despite the fact that the Human Genome Project (HGP) and previous studies have identified thousands of single-gene disorders, many common diseases and almost all cancers arise from multigenic and multifactorial causes. *(p. 1381)*

• Q 2

The HGP discovered widespread genetic variation among individuals, in the form of single nucleotide polymorphisms (SNPs). Here, two individuals have the same DNA sequence for a number of base pairs, then just one base pair is different, then they are the same again, then another single nucleotide is different, and so on. How frequently do these SNPs occur? *(p. 1383)*

• Q 3

The HGP also discovered that we humans do not have quite so many protein-coding genes as we expected to. How many protein-coding genes were estimated by the draft sequence? *(p. 1383)*

Q 4

What is the goal/achievement of genomic high-throughput technologies? *(p. 1383)*

Q 5–7

Several genomic high-throughput technologies have been developed to increase our knowledge base of the expression of genes. For each description provided, name the technology. *(pp. 1384–1385)*

Q 5

This method makes cDNA from mRNA and then uses anchoring and tagging enzymes to isolate and sequence several thousand short (10–14 bp) tags from the cDNA. *(pp. 1384–1385)*

Q 6

This method requires previous knowledge of the gene sequence and employs an 80–100 bp sequence that is identical to the gene of interest except for a single point mutation. Amplification reactions on the reagent and 'real' gene are run in parallel to quantify gene expression. *(pp. 1384–1385)*

Q 7

This method uses cDNA immobilized onto a solid support media, which will bind complementary RNA in a hybridization reaction. *(pp. 1384–1385)*

Q 8

A recent study employed a technique called 'neighborhood analysis' to aid in discriminating between AML and ALL. What is the principle underlying this technique? *(p. 1388)*

Q 9

Define proteomics. *(p. 1389)*

Q 10

Briefly discuss the limitations of the new field of proteomics. *(pp. 1392–1393)*

ANSWERS

A1. True.

A2. SNPs occur at about 1 per 1250 base pairs.

A3. Only about 30 000 were estimated. The sequence revision, which filled in the gaps of the draft, estimates even fewer, about 20 000–25 000.

A4. This technology quantifies the level of mRNA to measure gene expression. Every cell nucleus contains the DNA to code for every gene product, but a particular cell only expresses certain genes and produces certain proteins according to its specific function. By learning which genes are expressed and to what degree they are expressed, we can gain a better understanding of that cell's function.

A5. This is serial analysis of gene expression (SAGE).

A6. This is real competitive polymerase chain reaction (PCR).

A7. This is DNA microarrays.

A8. 'Neighborhood analysis' uses the principle of differential ranking of gene expression to aid in classification of leukemias. In this study, 50 genes were selected that were highly expressed in one of the leukemias, but poorly expressed in the other. So, if you saw high expression of one gene, this was a 'vote' for AML, not ALL, and so on.

A9. Proteomics is the analysis of differences in patterns of protein expression in various cancers. In a similar fashion to the above-described 'neighborhood analysis' of gene expression, proteomics looks at protein expression to aid in the discrimination of certain types of cancers. This technology uses mass spectroscopy to analyze proteins and protein-ions by mass-charge ratios.

A10. The key limitations are tissue heterogeneity (various numbers of tumor cells in different areas of the tumor), overfitting of predictive models (sometimes algorithms work for groups of patients but break down when applied to an individual patient), and the failure to identify causative disease proteins (some proteins have been determined to be just inflammatory markers, or bystanders).

Appendix A

Image simulation examination

QUESTIONS

The following 50 questions utilize some of the photomicrographs in several sections of Henry. These questions are to simulate the computer-based image section of the clinical pathology board examination. When photomicrographs from the text are used, the figure reference is provided to aid in your study.

Put ✗ in the box next to the correct word or phrase.

Q 1

This urine sediment demonstrates:

○ A. Acute tubular necrosis.
○ B. Transitional cell carcinoma.
○ C. Likely urinary tract infection.
○ D. Benign renal tubular epithelial cells.
○ E. Renal cell carcinoma.
(Fig. A.1 *(Fig, 27–6, p. 411)*

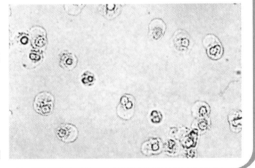

Fig. A.1

Q 2

In a 25-year-old female with fever, right flank pain, and a recent urinary tract infection, this urine sediment supports a diagnosis of:

- ○ A. Lower urinary tract infection, recurrent.
- ○ B. Acute pyelonephritis.
- ○ C. Renal tubular acidosis.
- ○ D. Hemolytic uremic syndrome.
- ○ E. Nephrotic syndrome.

(Fig. A.2 *(Fig. 27–19, p. 413)*;
Fig. A.3 *(Fig. 27–22, p. 414)*)

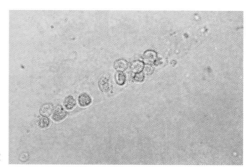

Fig. A.2

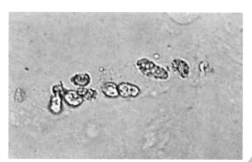

Fig. A.3

Q 3

These crystals are associated with all of the following except:

- ○ A. Neutral urine.
- ○ B. Acidic urine.
- ○ C. Ingestion of large amounts of vitamin C.
- ○ D. Ingestion of ethylene glycol.
- ○ E. Solubility in acetic acid.

(Fig. A.4 *(Fig. 27–32, p. 415)*;
Fig. A.5 *(Fig. 27–33, p. 415)*)

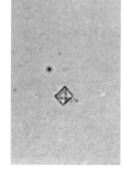 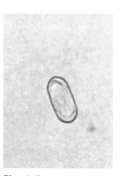

Fig. A.4   Fig. A.5

Q 4

This urine sediment demonstrates:

○ A. A clinically insignificant finding.
○ B. A large protozoan parasite.
○ C. A malignant cell.
○ D. A reactive renal epithelial cell.
○ E. A cestode ovum.

(Fig. A.6 *(Fig. 27–49, p. 419)*)

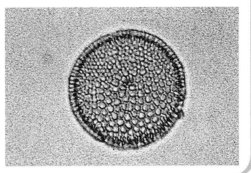

Fig. A.6

Q 5

These cells from cerebrospinal fluid (CSF) support a diagnosis of:

○ A. Bacterial meningitis.
○ B. Tubercular meningitis.
○ C. Subarachnoid hemorrhage.
○ D. Cryptococcosis.
○ E. Metastatic carcinoma.

(Fig. A.7 *(cf. Fig. 28–5, p. 430)*)

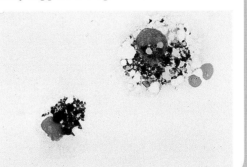

Fig. A.7

Q 6

In an elderly patient, the most likely agent to be cultured from this CSF is:

○ A. *Neisseria meningitidis.*
○ B. Group B streptococcus.
○ C. *Mycobacterium tuberculosis.*
○ D. *Streptococcus pneumoniae.*
○ E. *Escherichia coli.*

(Fig. A.8 *(not shown in text)*)

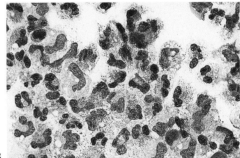

Fig. A.8

Q 7

This pleural fluid demonstrates:

- ○ A. Mesothelial cells.
- ○ B. Metastatic adenocarcinoma.
- ○ C. Metastatic breast carcinoma (ductal type).
- ○ D. Anaplastic large cell lymphoma.
- ○ E. Burkitt lymphoma.

(Fig. A.9)

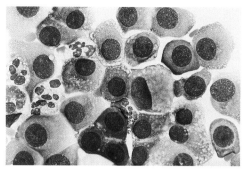

Fig. A.9
(From Kjeldsberg CR, Knight JA: Body fluids: laboratory examination of amniotic, cerebrospinal, seminal, serous and synovial fluids, 3rd edn American Society of Clinical Pathologists, Chicago, 1993, with permission.)

Q 8

In a 65-year-old male with a WBC of 70 000/μL and ascites, these cells support a diagnosis of:

- ○ A. Metastatic adenocarcinoma (colon).
- ○ B. Chronic lymphocytic leukemia.
- ○ C. Chronic myelogenous leukemia.
- ○ D. Metastatic carcinoma (prostate).
- ○ E. Leukemoid reaction.

(Fig. A.10 (*cf. Fig. 32–42, p. 574*))

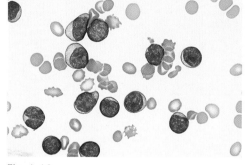

Fig. A.10

Q 9

This peripheral blood smear represents:

- ○ A. Normal lymphocyte and neutrophil morphology.
- ○ B. Toxic granulation consistent with sepsis.
- ○ C. A normal neutrophil and a large granular lymphocyte.
- ○ D. A mature neutrophil and a band neutrophil.
- ○ E. Pelger–Huët anomaly.

(Fig. A.11 (*not shown in text*))

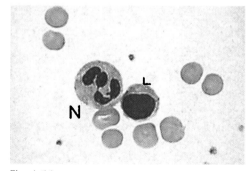

Fig. A.11

Q 10

These intact two cells may be seen in what two conditions?

- A. Acute myeloid leukemia with minimal differentiation (AML M0) and AML without maturation (AML M1).
- B. AML M0 and leukemoid reaction.
- C. Acute lymphoblastic leukemia (ALL) and AML M1.
- D. Chronic lymphocytic leukemia (CLL) and ALL.
- E. Chronic myelogenous leukemia (CML) and leukemoid reaction.

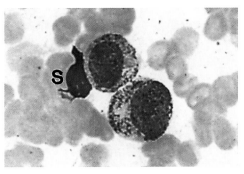

Fig. A.12

(Fig. A.12 *(cf. Fig. 32–12, p. 558)*)

Q 11

In this bone marrow aspirate, the cells labeled PN (polychromatophilic normoblast):

- A. Are normal erythroid precursors.
- B. Are more mature than the cell labeled BN (basophilic normoblast).
- C. May be seen in peripheral blood in severe hemolytic anemia.
- D. A and B are true.
- E. A, B, and C are true.

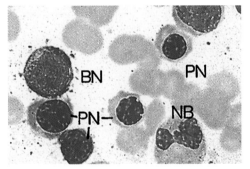

Fig. A.13

(Fig. A.13 *(cf. Figs. 30–3, 30–4, pp. 487–488)*)

Q 12

If this photomicrograph were taken from the peripheral blood of a 48-year-old female, it would prompt a chromosomal study for what translocation?

- A. t(8;14).
- B. t(1;19).
- C. t(9;22).
- D. t(4;11).
- E. t(11;14).

(Fig. A.14 *(cf. Fig. 32–12, p. 558)*)

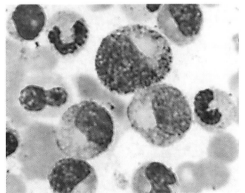

Fig. A.14

Q 13

This multinucleated cell from a bone marrow aspirate is:

- ○ A. Normal megakaryocyte.
- ○ B. Normal osteoclast.
- ○ C. Normal osteoblast.
- ○ D. Megakaryocyte demonstrating endoreduplication.
- ○ E. Micromegakaryocyte.

(Fig. A.15 *(not shown in text)*)

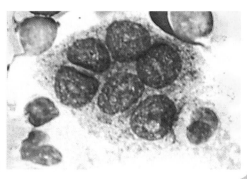

Fig. A.15

Q 14

This touch preparation from an enlarged epitrochlear lymph node in a 15-year-old boy suggests a diagnosis of:

- ○ A. Nodular sclerosing Hodgkin lymphoma.
- ○ B. Diffuse large B cell lymphoma.
- ○ C. Small lymphocytic lymphoma.
- ○ D. Reactive lymphadenopathy.
- ○ E. Burkitt lymphoma.

(Fig. A.16 *(not shown in text)*)

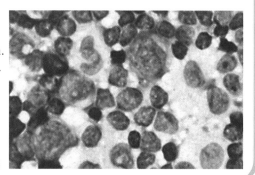

Fig. A.16

Q 15

This Prussian blue stain of bone marrow demonstrates a disease characterized by all of the following statements except:

- ○ A. Elevated serum iron with a greatly elevated percent iron saturation.
- ○ B. Hereditary forms are more common than acquired forms.
- ○ C. Hereditary forms may be X-linked, autosomal dominant, or recessive.
- ○ D. Some patients with the acquired form respond to pyridoxine.
- ○ E. Electron microscopy shows characteristic changes in mitochondria.

(Fig. A.17 *(Fig. 31–5, p. 506)*)

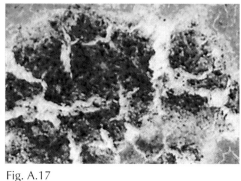

Fig. A.17

Q 16

The patient, a 71-year-old female suffering from fatigue and dark stools, with this peripheral blood smear would have all of the following serum findings except:

- ○ A. Low serum iron.
- ○ B. Low serum ferritin.
- ○ C. Low iron saturation.
- ○ D. Low total iron-binding capacity.
- ○ E. Low mean corpuscular volume.

(Fig. A.18 *(cf. Fig. 29–10, p. 470)*)

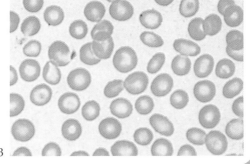

Fig. A.18

Q 17

The patient with this peripheral smear may have all of the following laboratory findings except:

- ○ A. Low serum folate.
- ○ B. Elevated RBC folate.
- ○ C. Low B$_{12}$.
- ○ D. Abnormal Schilling test, part one.
- ○ E. Normal Schilling test, part two.

(Fig. A.19 *(cf. Fig. 31–6, p. 507)*)

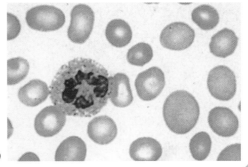

Fig. A.19

Q 18

The patient with this peripheral blood smear:

- ○ A. Has a single amino acid substitution on the beta chain of hemoglobin.
- ○ B. Will have a positive sickle solubility test.
- ○ C. Will typically require transfusions to maintain adequate oxygenation.
- ○ D. Will pass on an abnormal gene to half of his offspring.
- ○ E. Requires acid pH electrophoresis to distinguish his Hb from D and G.

(Fig. A.20 *(Fig. 31–23, p. 527)*)

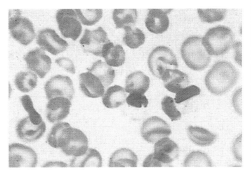

Fig. A.20

Q 19

The patient with this peripheral smear:

- A. Will pass on an abnormal gene to half of his offspring.
- B. Will demonstrate splenomegaly in adulthood.
- C. Will likely require treatment with desferroxamine.
- D. Requires acid electrophoresis to distinguish his Hb from E and O.
- E. Has a mutation on chromosome 16.

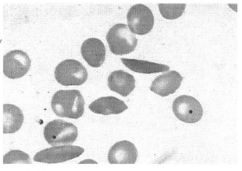

Fig. A.21

(Fig. A.21 *(cf. Fig. 31–22, p. 526)*)

Q 20

The patient with this peripheral blood smear has a platelet count of 50 000/μL with several giant platelets. All of the following statement are true about this disease except:

- A. The pale blue inclusions in the neutrophils are characteristic of this disorder.
- B. The patient will likely have a benign course.
- C. This patient has an autosomal dominant condition.
- D. The inclusions resemble Döhle bodies, but are structurally different on EM.
- E. This is a common condition, often found incidentally.

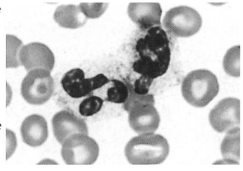

Fig. A.22

(Fig. A.22 *(cf. Fig. 32–3, p. 550)*)

Q 21

These two images represent the same condition. All of the following are features of this condition except:

○ A. Autosomal recessive inheritance.

○ B. Frequent fungal infections, especially with *Candida* spp.

○ C. Partial albinism.

○ D. Fusion of abnormal lysosomes in leukocytes.

○ E. Markedly shortened lifespan.

(Fig. A.23; Fig. A.24 *(cf. Figs. 32–5, 32–7, pp. 550, 551)*)

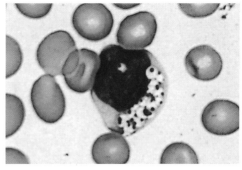

Fig. A.23

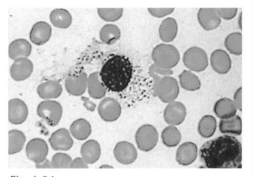

Fig. A.24

Q 22

This bone marrow aspirate of a 30-year-old female with acute leukemia demonstrates increased eosinophils. Which finding is characteristic?

○ A. Poor prognosis compared to other acute myeloid leukemias.

○ B. Staining with chloroacetate esterase, but not with α-naphthyl esterase.

○ C. Negative staining with Sudan Black B.

○ D. t(8;21).

○ E. inv16(p13q22).

(Fig. A.25 *(cf. Fig. 32–25, p. 567)*)

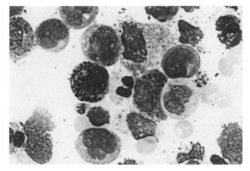

Fig. A.25

Q 23

This is a peripheral smear from a 73-year-old female with an elevated WBC. Which of the following is true about her condition?

○ A. Her diagnosis rests on finding >20% prolymphocytes among the leukemic cells.

○ B. This disease is more common in women than in men.

○ C. She likely has massive splenomegaly.

○ D. This is probably a clonal disorder of T cells.

○ E. Her WBC is probably less than 40 000/μL.

(Fig. A.26 (*cf. Fig. 32–43, p. 574*))

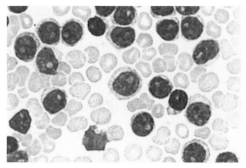

Fig. A.26

Q 24

This marrow aspirate from a 10-year-old male typically shows all of the findings except:

○ A. Monoclonal surface immunoglobulin.

○ B. CD19.

○ C. CD20.

○ D. TdT.

○ E. t(8;14).

(Fig. A.27 (*cf. Fig. 32–64, p. 581*))

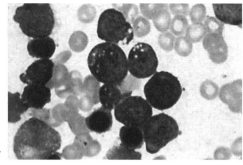

Fig. A.27

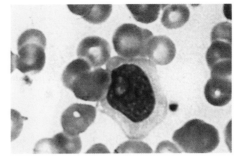

Q 25

All three of these peripheral blood smears demonstrate the same cell type. Which of the following is true about this cell?

- A. It is a T lymphocyte.
- B. It is CD4 positive.
- C. It bears a receptor for a complement protein.
- D. It is characteristic of pertussis.
- E. Both A and C are true.

(Fig. A.28; Fig. A.29; Fig. A.30
(cf. Fig. 32–10, p. 555))

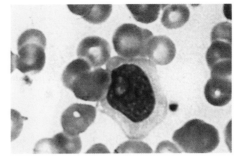

Fig. A.28

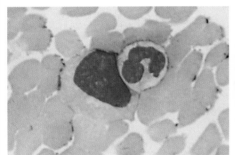

Fig. A.29

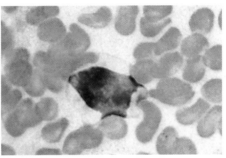

Fig. A.30

Q 26

Differentiation of the species of the bacteria shown here can be made from various common biochemical tests. Which statement is true regarding Gram-negative cocci?

- A. *Moraxella catarrhalis* ferments maltose only.
- B. *Neisseria meningitidis* ferments glucose and maltose.
- C. *Neisseria gonorrhoeae* ferments glucose and sucrose.
- D. Thayer–Martin medium differentiates between *N. gonorrhoeae* and *N. meningitidis*.
- E. Oxidase reaction differentiates between *Neisseria* spp. and *Moraxella*.

(Fig. A.31 *(Fig. 56–12, p. 1028)*)

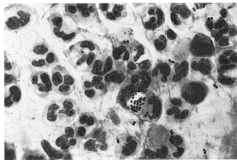

Fig. A.31

Q 27

This photograph compares growth of a fungal organism in Sabouraud dextrose agar with and without added peanut oil. All of the following are true regarding this organism except:

- ○ A. It is a common skin commensal in humans.
- ○ B. Systemic infection is associated with intravenous hyperalimentation.
- ○ C. Systemic infection is fatal in up to 25% of cases.
- ○ D. It is the agent of tinea versicolor.
- ○ E. KOH preparation of skin scrapings resembles spaghetti and meatballs.

(Fig. A.32 *(Fig. 60–20, p. 1100)*)

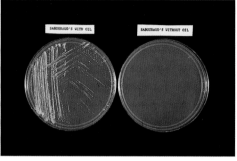

Fig. A.32

Q 28

Here is a composite of 24 drawings of a blood parasite, outlining its maturation. All of the following statements regarding this parasite are true except:

○ A. The characteristic dots are also seen in *Plasmodium ovale*.

○ B. Immunity may be conferred by absence of Duffy blood group antigens.

○ C. All stages may be seen in peripheral blood.

○ D. Fever with this parasite typically follows a quartan periodicity.

○ E. Recurrences are common if not fully treated.

(Fig. A.33
(Fig. 61–2, p. 1129))

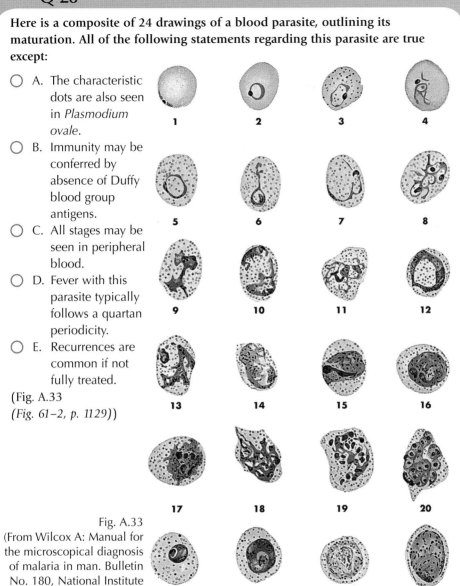

Fig. A.33
(From Wilcox A: Manual for the microscopical diagnosis of malaria in man. Bulletin No. 180, National Institute of Health, 1942.)

Q 29

Here is another composite of 28 drawings of a malarial species. Which statement accurately describes the typical peripheral blood findings for this parasite?

A. Drawings 21–24 demonstrate the most common form in infected patients.

B. Drawing 8, with a parasitemia rate of 15%, is characteristic of this species of malaria.

C. Drawing 26 is commonly seen in mild–moderate ill patients.

D. Drawings 9 and 12 demonstrate Schuffner's dots.

E. The double chromatin dots in drawings 3 and 4 are also seen in *Plasmodium malariae*.

(Fig. A.34
(*Fig. 61–4, p. 1131*))

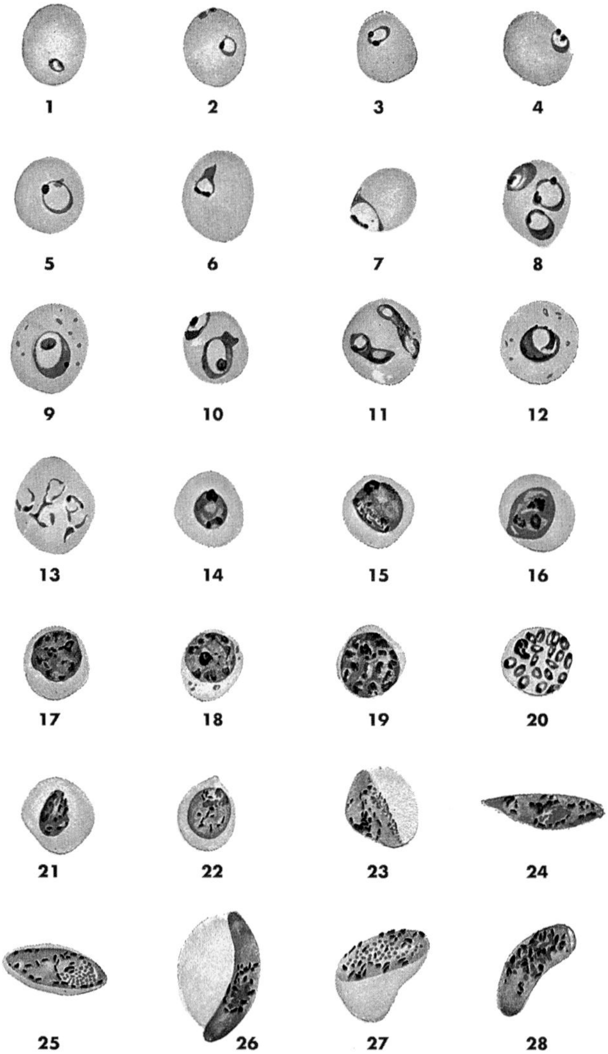

1   2   3   4

5   6   7   8

9   10   11   12

13   14   15   16

17   18   19   20

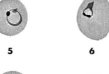
21   22   23   24

25   26   27   28

Fig. A.34
(Courtesy of National Institute of Health, USPHS.)

Q 30

This peripheral blood smear is from a febrile 30-year-old male from Connecticut. He has no history of travel outside the USA. Which statement is true regarding his illness?

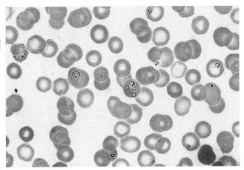

Fig. A.35

- ○ A. The vector is a mosquito of the *Anopheles* genus.
- ○ B. Splenectomy may be indicated to control hemolysis.
- ○ C. This parasite must be distinguished from hemoflagellates by serology.
- ○ D. A characteristic skin rash usually precedes clinical symptoms.
- ○ E. Multiple rings inside erythrocytes forming a Maltese cross is a helpful clue.

(Fig. A.35 *(Fig. 61–6A, p. 1134)*)

Q 31

This peripheral blood smear demonstrates an extracellular parasite. All of the following are true regarding the genus except:

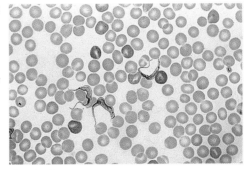

Fig. A.36

- ○ A. This photomicrograph is of an amastigote.
- ○ B. Two species cause sleeping sickness in Africa.
- ○ C. In Central and South America, it is transmitted by the reduviid bug.
- ○ D. Persons infected in equatorial Africa have a worse outcome than persons infected in western Africa.
- ○ E. The vector in Africa is a fly of the *Glossina* species.

(Fig. A.36 *(not shown in text)*)

Q 32

This photomicrograph is from the autopsy of a 22-year-old male who died of a rapid-onset meningoencephalitis. One week ago, he and his friends had been diving at a local reservoir. This etiologic agent of his illness is:

- A. *Acanthamoeba* spp.
- B. *Naegleria fowleri.*
- C. *Trypanosoma cruzi.*
- D. *Toxoplasma gondii.*
- E. *Leishmania mexicana.*

(Fig. A.37 *(Fig. 61–8A, p. 1137)*)

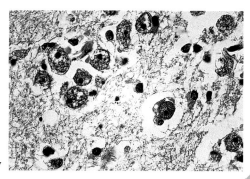

Fig. A.37

Q 33

This hematoxylin and eosin stained photomicrograph taken at oil immersion came from a 35-year-old female with abdominal pain and diarrhea. All of the following are true regarding this organism except:

- A. It is an ameba.
- B. It is morphologically identical to a nonpathogenic member of the same genus.
- C. Cyst forms may have eight nuclei.
- D. Serologic tests are helpful in diagnosing extraintestinal cases.
- E. It is spread through contaminated food and water.

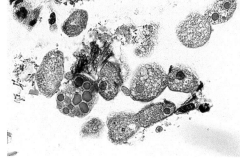

Fig. A.38

(Fig. A.38 *(Fig. 61–11C, p. 1140)*)

Q 34

This duodenal biopsy is from a 50-year-old male living in rural North Carolina. He presented with diarrhea and steatorrhea over a 2-week period. Which statement regarding this organism is true?

○ A. A diagnosis of *Chilomastix mesnili* is considered, but less likely because *C. mesnili* is a nonpathogen, and this patient is symptomatic.

○ B. The patient should be questioned about his water supply.

○ C. Diarrheic stools typically show cyst forms, while formed stools show trophozoites.

○ D. A and B are correct.

○ E. A, B, and C are correct.

(Fig. A.39 *(Fig. 61–14E, p. 1144)*)

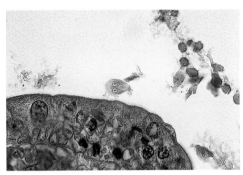

Fig. A.39

Q 35

This small bowel biopsy came from a 3-year-old girl who is believed to have contracted diarrhea at her daycare center. The microorganisms present measured 5 μm on average. What is the diagnosis?

○ A. *Cyclospora cayetanensis*.

○ B. Microsporidia.

○ C. *Isospora belli*.

○ D. *Cryptosporidium parvum*.

○ E. *Balantidium coli*.

(Fig. A.40 *(Fig. 61–15C, p. 1146)*)

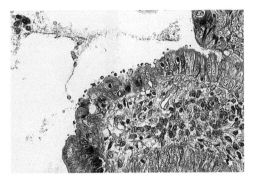

Fig. A.40

Q 36

Shown here are adult forms as well as an ovum of an intestinal parasite. Which statement regarding this parasite is true?

- ○ A. It is a nematode.
- ○ B. Autoinfection may occur in the immunocompromised host.
- ○ C. Adults live in the ileum of the human host.
- ○ D. Infective larva penetrating the skin is the mode of transmission.
- ○ E. A and C are true.

(Fig. A.41 *(Fig. 61–17F, p. 1148)*; Fig. A.42 *(Fig. 61–17G, p. 1148)*)

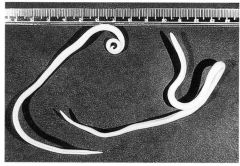

Fig. A.41
(From A Pictorial Presentation of Parasites: A cooperative collection prepared and/or edited by H Zaiman.)

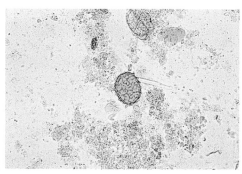

Fig. A.42

Q 37

This stool specimen is viewed at 400× magnification. It came from an anemic 13-year-old girl living in Mississippi. The diagnosis is:

- ○ A. *Necator americanus.*
- ○ B. *Ancylostoma duodenale.*
- ○ C. *Strongyloides stercoralis.*
- ○ D. *Ascaris lumbricoides.*
- ○ E. *Trichuris trichiura.*

(Fig. A.43 *(Fig. 61–18A, p. 1149)*)

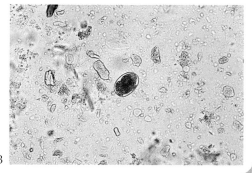

Fig. A.43

Q 38

This stool specimen is viewed at 400 × magnification. The diagnosis is:

- A. *Hymenolepis nana.*
- B. *Fasciolopsis buski.*
- C. *Clonorchis sinensis.*
- D. *Paragonimus westermani.*
- E. *Diphyllobothrium latum.*

(Fig. A.44 (*cf. Fig. 61–20F, p. 1151*))

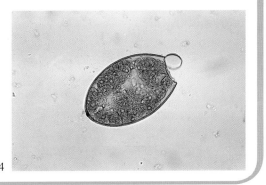

Fig. A.44

Q 39

Displayed here are a lymph node biopsy and peripheral blood smear from a 42-year-old male with lymphadenopathy and massive lymphedema. Which statement regarding this parasite is true?

- A. It is the leading cause of blindness in endemic areas.
- B. Microfilariae circulate with nocturnal periodicity.
- C. The vector is a *Chrysops* species.
- D. This filarial form lacks a sheath.
- E. It is geographically restricted to Southeast Asia.

(Fig. A.45 (*Fig. 61–24A, p. 1155*); Fig. A.46 (*Fig. 61–24B, p. 1155*))

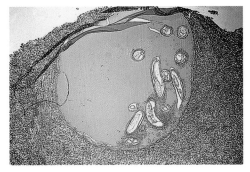

Fig. A.45

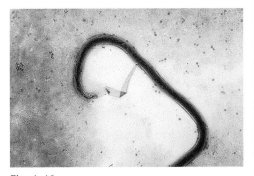

Fig. A.46

Q 40

This autopsy specimen was taken from a 35-year-old female from Mexico with a history of headaches and seizures over 2 weeks prior to her death. How did she acquire this infection?

- A. She was bitten by a reduviid bug.
- B. She ingested *Taenia solium* ova.
- C. She was bitten by an *Aedes* spp. mosquito.
- D. She ate undercooked pork.
- E. She ate undercooked beef.

(Fig. A.47 *(Fig. 61–26A, p. 1158)*)

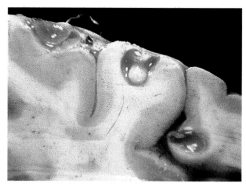

Fig. A.47
(From A Pictorial Presentation of Parasites: A cooperative collection prepared and/or edited by H Zaiman.)

Q 41

A 73-year-old male in septic shock has a blood pH of 7.2 and $P_{a}O_2$ of 40 mmHg. Which statement is true?

- A. He is in metabolic alkalosis with an oxygen saturation of 90%.
- B. He is in metabolic acidosis with an oxygen saturation of 90%.
- C. He is in metabolic acidosis with an oxygen saturation of 65%.
- D. He is in metabolic acidosis with an oxygen saturation of 73%.
- E. He is in respiratory acidosis with an oxygen saturation of 73%.

(Fig. A.48 *(Fig. 8–3, p. 85)*)

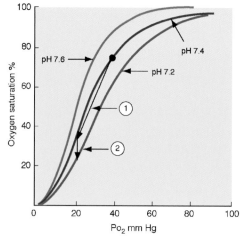

Fig. A.48

Q 42

Review the laboratory budget below. Which statement is true?

○ A. Salaries for the next year will increase by 4%.
○ B. Salaries for the next year will account for approximately an equal percentage of the expenses as they do for the current year.
○ C. The cost per test will increase by 4% to achieve a 4% increase in revenue.
○ D. The cost per test will decrease by 4% to achieve a 4% increase in revenue.
○ E. The cost per test will not change in the coming year.

(Table A.1 *(Table. 12–7, p. 128)*)

Table A.1   Pro Forma Laboratory Budget

Category	Current year	Assumptions	Change	Projection for new year
Revenue	$ 3 000 000	4% growth	$ 120 000	$ 3 120 000
Total tests	$ 370 000	4% growth	$ 14 800	$ 384 800
Revenue/test	$ 8.11			$ 8.11
Expenses				
Salaries	$ 950 000	3% cost of living increase	$ 28 500	$ 978 500
Laboratory supplies	$ 421 000	4% growth (no price increase)	$ 16 840	$ 437 840
Reference lab fees	$ 250 000	4% growth	$ 10 000	$ 262 600
		1% price increase (on projected $260 000)	$ 2600	
Phlebotomy supplies	$ 35 500	4% growth	$ 1420	$ 36 920
Maintenance contracts	$ 40 000	No change		$ 40 000
Total expense	$ 1 696 500		$ 59 360	$ 1 755 860
Cost per test	$ 4.59			$ 4.56

Q 43

Review the spreadsheet for the analysis of a payback period for the purchase of a new analyzer for your laboratory. As it is initially determined, the payback period is 4 years. You would like to decrease that period to 3.5 years. What would you need to charge per test to achieve this goal if you perform 100 000 tests/year?

- ○ A. $5.71
- ○ B. $5.50
- ○ C. $9.38
- ○ D. $6.14
- ○ E. $5.07

(Table A.2 *(Table. 12–10, p. 130)*)

Table A.2   Financial Evaluation of a New Automated Analyzer

Given		
Investment (cost of analyzer)		$200 000
Discount rate (rate of inflation or interest rate of borrowed money)		10.00%
Useful life of analyzer		5 years
Annual depreciation expense	$200 000/5 years	$40 000
Annual revenue	100 000 tests at $5.00/test	$500 000
Annual labor expense	100 000 tests at $2.50/test	$250 000
Annual supply expense	100 000 tests at $2.00/test	$200 000
Annual net revenue (Annual revenue − annual Expense)	$500 000 − ($250 000 + $200 000)	$50 000
Net revenue per test (Test revenue − Test expense)	$5.00 − ($2.50 + $2.00)	$0.50

Calculations		
PAYBACK PERIOD = Investment/ Annual net revenue	$200 000/$50 000	4 years
BREAKEVEN Per year = Depreciation/Net revenue per test	$40 000/$0.50	80 000 tests
Life of analyzer = Investment/ (Net revenue per test)	$200 000/$0.50	400 000 tests
RETURN ON INVESTMENT (ROI) = Annual net revenue/Investment	$50 000/$200 000	25% per year
NET PRESENT VALUE (NPV) = Present value of the sum of future net revenue (cash flows) minus investment. Note: Present value interest factor (PVIF) for each year based on 10% discount rate is multiplied by net revenue to determine present value. PVIF is available from any financial data resource. NPV can also be calculated with financial calculator		

Today's investment	($200 000)	
Year 1 Net revenue × PVIF	$50 000 × 0.9091 = $45 455	
Year 2 Net revenue × PVIF	$50 000 × 0.8264 = $41 320	
Year 3 Net revenue × PVIF	$50 000 × 0.7513 = $37 565	
Year 4 Net revenue × PVIF	$50 000 × 0.6830 = $34 150	
Year 5 Net revenue × PVIF	$50 000 × 0.6209 = $31 045	
Present value of sum of future net revenue	$189 535	
NPV		$(10 465)

INTERNAL RATE OF RETURN (IRR) = Discounted interest rate at which NPV = 0. Note: financial calculator is used to determine IRR by entering cash flow and discount rate

Today's investment	($200 000)	
Year 1 Net revenue × PVIF	$50 000 × 0.9265 = $46 326	
Year 2 Net revenue × PVIF	$50 000 × 0.8585 = $42 923	
Year 3 Net revenue × PVIF	$50 000 × 0.7954 = $39 769	
Year 4 Net revenue × PVIF	$50 000 × 0.7369 = $36 847	
Year 5 Net revenue × PVIF	$50 000 × 0.6828 = $34 140	
Present value of sum of future net revenue	$200 000	
NPV	$0	
IRR		8%

Q 44

This radiograph is from the hand of a 52-year-old woman with solitary benign neck mass. She likely manifests all of the following biochemical changes except:

- ○ A. Decreased parathyroid hormone due to negative feedback.
- ○ B. Increased serum calcium due to increased bone resorption.
- ○ C. Increased serum calcium due to increased renal calcium absorption.
- ○ D. Increased serum calcium due to increased renal $1,25(OH)_2D_3$ biosynthesis.
- ○ E. Decreased serum phosphate due to phosphate diuresis.

(Fig. A.49 *(Fig. 15–4A, p. 177)*)

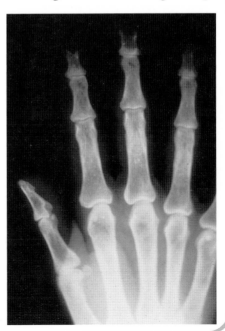

Fig. A.49

Q 45

What is the location of the metabolic defect which results in Dubin–Johnson syndrome?

○ A. Step A.
○ B. Step B.
○ C. Step C.
○ D. Step D.
○ E. Step E.

(Fig. A.50
(Fig. 21–2, p. 264))

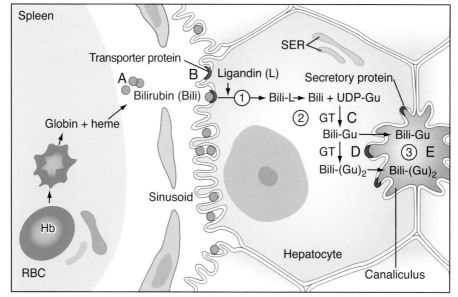

Fig. A.50

Q 46

Which statement regarding this molecule is true?

- A. It increases blood pressure and heart rate.
- B. It is the most common hormone produced by pituitary adenomas.
- C. It is the precursor of the hormone which lowers blood glucose.
- D. It is the active hormone which lowers blood glucose.
- E. It is the active form of vitamin D.

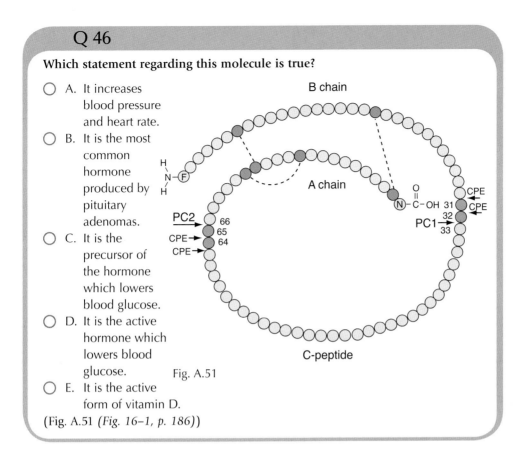

Fig. A.51

(Fig. A.51 *(Fig. 16–1, p. 186)*)

Q 47

This technology would most likely be used to measure:

○ A. Plasma glucose.
○ B. Blood cocaine metabolites.
○ C. Serum total protein.
○ D. Plasma HIV (quantitative).
○ E. Serum potassium.
(Fig. A.52 *(Fig. 4–21, p. 48)*)

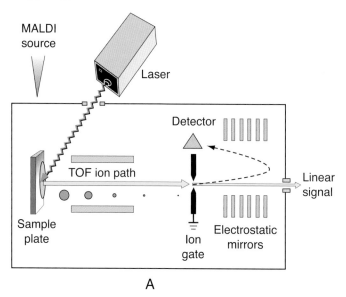

A

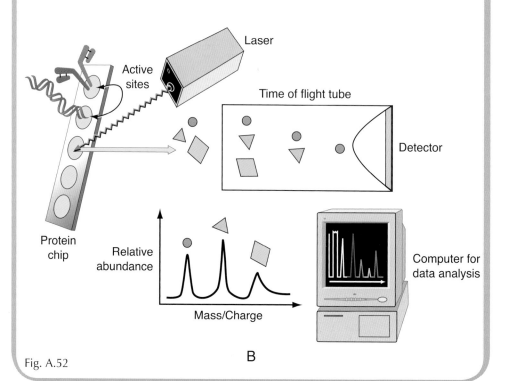

B

Fig. A.52

QUESTIONS

Q 48

These three chemical compounds are all:

- A. Opiates.
- B. Barbiturates.
- C. Tricyclic antidepressants.
- D. Cocaine metabolites.
- E. Sedative-hypnotics.

(Fig. A.53 *(Fig. 23–7, p. 304)*)

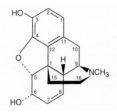
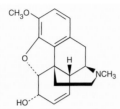
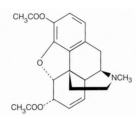

Fig. A.53

Q 49

All of the following statements are true regarding the *FRAXA* locus in the family analyzed below except:

- A. Family member 5 has mental retardation.
- B. Methylation of the X chromosome represented by the 5.2-kb band explains why family member 8 is not a carrier.
- C. Expansion of the repeats occurred in utero in family member 5.
- D. Expansion of the repeats occurred in family members 3 and 4
- E. Family member 3 is at risk for having an affected son.

(Fig. A.54 *(Fig. 72–6A and B, p. 1331)*)

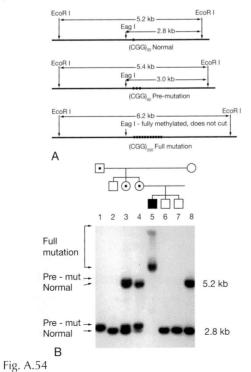

Fig. A.54

Q 50

All of the following statements are true regarding the disorders demonstrated in this PCR analysis except:

○ A. PWS is due to either maternal deletion at 15q12 or uniparental disomy.

○ B. AS manifests are mental retardation and inappropriate laughter.

○ C. AS is due to a deletion of a gene at 15q12 which is normally only expressed in the female.

○ D. Uniparental disomy for maternal chromosome 15 can cause PWS.

○ E. The basis for both PWS and AS is normal methylation of a gene on one allele, followed by abnormal deletion of the corresponding locus on the alternative allele.

(Fig. A.55 *(Fig. 72–7, p. 1332)*)

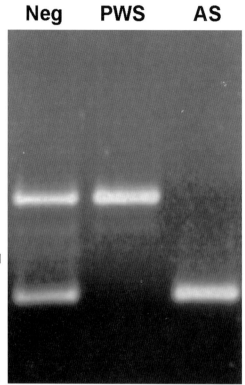

Fig. A.55

A1. C

A2. B

A3. E

A4. A

A5. C

A6. D

A7. A

A8. B

A9. A

A10. E

A11. E

A12. C

A13. B

A14. D

A15. B

A16. D

A17. B

A18. A

A19. C

A20. E

A21. B

A22. E

A23. C

A24. D

A25. A

A26. B

A27. C

A28. D

A29. B

A30. E

A31. A

A32. B

A33. C

A34. D

A35. D

A36. A

A37. A

A38. E

A39. B

A40. B

A41. C

A42. B

A43. E

A44. A

A45. D

A46. C

A47. B

A48. A

A49. C

A50. A

Appendix B
Math examination

....

QUESTIONS

The following 30 questions are written to simulate problems on the boards where calculations and analysis of graphs and diagrams are required. As a calculator is allowed on the boards, you may use one here. Although the real boards will be in a multiple choice format, write in the correct response format here.

Q 1

Answer the following questions using the Levey–Jennings plot in Figure B.1.

○ A. What is the target mean? _____

○ B. If the control limits are set at ±2 SD, what is the value of the SD? _____

○ C. What is the Westgard notation for week 3 (days 15–21)? _____

○ D. What sort of bias is demonstrated in this plot? _____

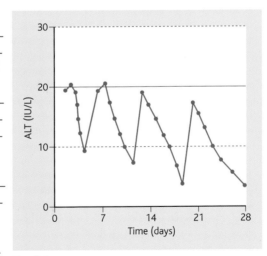

Fig. B.1

Q 2–4

For questions 2–4, use the following data. In a small town with 350 adults, a screening program for disease X was undertaken using a new test methodology, polymerase chain reaction (PCR). All 350 blood samples were then evaluated by a confirmatory method (gold standard). 20 townspeople were found to have disease X by the gold standard method. 17 of these had positive PCR tests, and had 3 negative PCR. 25 persons had a positive PCR, but were negative by the gold standard.

Q 2

What is the sensitivity of PCR to detect disease X? _____

Q 3

What is the specificity of PCR to detect disease X? _____

Q 4

What is the positive predictive value of PCR in this town for disease X? _____

Q 5

Answer the following questions using the receiver operator curve in Figure B.2.

○ A. What point on the curve maximizes diagnostic efficiency? _____
_____

○ B. At a sensitivity of 95%, what is the false-positive percentage of this diagnostic test? _____
_____
_____

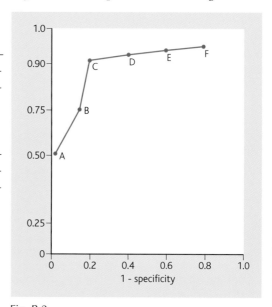

Fig. B.2

Q 6

Using the receiver operator curve in Figure B.3, answer the following questions. Tests X and Y are being evaluated as screening tests for prostate cancer.

○ A. At a specificity of 90%, what is the sensitivity of test X? _____
_____

○ B. At a sensitivity of 90%, what is the false-positive percentage of test Y? _____
_____
_____

○ C. What point marks the maximum diagnostic efficiency of test X? _____
_____
_____

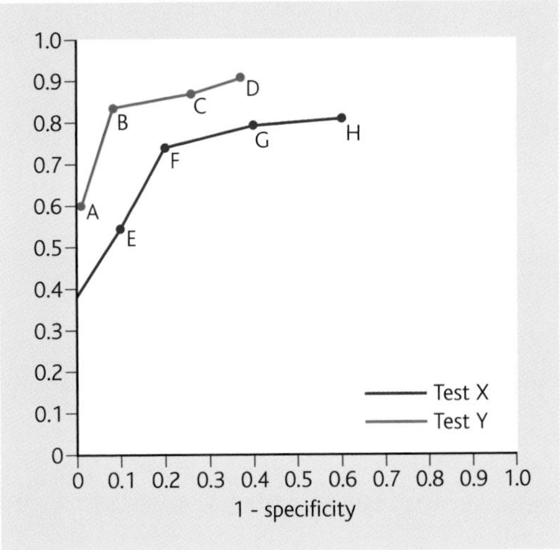

○ D. The maximum diagnostic efficiency of test Y combines a sensitivity of _____% and a specificity of _____%.

○ E. Overall, the superior test in terms of sensitivity and specificity is _____.

Fig. B.3

Q 7

A 26-year-old female with autoimmune hemolytic anemia has an RBC of $2.8 \times 10^{-6}/\mu L$, an Hct of 25% (nl = 40%) and a reticulocyte percentage of 11% (nl = 1%). The maturation time for reticulocytes at an Hct of 25% is 2.0 days.

Calculate the absolute reticulocyte count: _____
Calculate the reticulocyte production index (RPI): _____

Q 8

An 8-year-old boy with beta-thalassemia major has a Hb = 8.1 g/dL, Hct = 24.0%, RBC = $4.14 \times 10^{-6}/\mu L$.

Calculate the MCV: _____
Calculate the MCH: _____
Calculate the MCHC: _____

Q 9

A 20-year-old male with a brisk hemolytic anemia has 8 nucleated red cells per 100 WBCs and an uncorrected WBC = 8300/μL.

Calculate the corrected WBC: _____

Q 10

A 40-year-old female with AML has been getting less of an increment from her platelet transfusions over the past week. Analyze her most recent transfusion. Her pretransfusion platelet count = 6000/μL and the 30-minute post-transfusion count = 18000/μL. She received 1 unit of apheresis platelets labeled as 6.8 equivalent, where 6.0 is equivalent to 6 standard random-donor units. Her BSA is 1.5 m².

What is her corrected count increment (CCI)? _____

_____

Is this adequate? _____

Q 11

A 61-year-old male is to undergo plasmapheresis for CIDP. He will have 1.5 plasma volumes (PV) exchanged and receive 5% albumin as 65% of his replacement fluid and normal saline as the other 35%. Estimate his blood volume as 5.0 L. His Hct = 43% today.

What is his PV? _____
What is his exchange volume (EV)? _____
What volumes of 5% albumin and normal saline will you reinfuse? Albumin: _____
_____; saline _____

Q 12

A 28-year-old male with chronic relapsing TTP has a blood volume of 4.8 L, an Hct = 29%, and requires daily plasmapheresis of 1.7 PV over the next 3 days. What amount of what replacement fluid will you need to support him for the next 3 days of treatment?

_____

Q 13

A 40-year-old female with the exact minimum acceptable Hb concentration for donation gives a unit of blood. She weighs 41 kg and gives an exact amount commensurate with her weight.

How much blood may she donate? _____

Q 14

An 83-year-old male with an Hct = 25% receives 2 units of PRBCs. What is his expected post-transfusion Hct?

_____

Q 15

A 50-year-old female in DIC has a fibrinogen of 50 mg/dL. How many bags of cryoprecipitate would be required to raise her fibrinogen to 150 mg/dL. Assume a BV of 5.0 L, an Hct = 28%, and 250 mg fibrinogen per unit of cryo.

_____

Q 16

A 26-year-old male with hemophilia A presents to the ER with a large hemarthrosis in his right knee. His weight is 70 kg and his Hct = 27%. You have no factor VIII concentrate, and must use cryoprecipitate. Assume a factor VIII level of essentially zero to start and calculate the number of bags of cryoprecipitate to raise his factor VIII level to 50% (50 units/dL).

_____

Q 17

Calculate the FE_{Na} in the following patient, who weighs 70 kg: plasma Cr = 4.7 mg/dL; plasma Na = 140 mmol/L; plasma K^+ = 3.9 mmol/L; urine Cr = 5 mg/kg/day; urine Na = 200 mEq/day.

_____

Q 18

Calculate the anion gap (AG) in the following patient: Na = 141; Cl = 93; HCO_3 = 16.

_____

Q 19

A patient admitted to the ICU has a measured osmolality of 327 mOsm/kg. His other admission results are: Na = 148; glu = 52; BUN = 18. Normal osmolality = 282 mOsm/kg.

What is his calculated osmolality? _____

What is his osmolal gap? _____

Q 20

Estimate the GFR in a 73-year-old male who weighs 65 kg and has a Cr = 6.1 mg/dL.

_____

Q 21

Calculate the Hct in a person with an MCV = 84 fL and an RBC = 4.8×10^{-6}/μL.

_____

Q 22

Calculate the reticulocyte production index in a patient with an Hct = 21% (nl = 45), a reticulocyte percentage of 10% (nl = 1). The maturation time in days is given for several Hcts below.

Hct	Maturation	RPI _____
45	1.0	
35	1.5	
25	2.0	
15	2.5	

Q 23–27

In a population of 800 adults aboard a cruise ship, a gastroenteritis outbreak has a prevalence of 38%, based on the gold standard of active diarrhea. A new test to diagnose Norwalk virus, the suspected etiologic agent, has a sensitivity of 92% and a specificity of 81% based on the manufacturer's trials. It is used to test all the passengers, sick or healthy.

Q 23

What will be the number of true positives? _____

Q 24

What will be the number of true negatives? _____

Q 25

What will be the number of false positives? _____

Q 26

What will be the number of false negatives? _____

Q 27

What is the positive predictive value of a positive result on this cruise ship? ___
_____

Q 28–30

The cumulative probability of exclusion (CPE) is determined by the formula:

$$CPE = 1 - (1 - P1)(1 - P2)(1 - P3) \dots (1 - Pn)$$

Here, P is the average power of exclusion for each system used in exclusion testing, and is also abbreviated A. Using *Table B–1 (Table 73–4, p. 1345)*, calculate the cumulative exclusion in the following three examples.

Table B-1 Power of Exclusion (*A*): Selected Test System

System	*A*
Classical	
ABO	0.166
RH	0.283
ACP	0.239
Restriction fragment length polymorphism	
D2S44	0.95
D10S28	0.96
Short tandem repeats	
D7S820	0.523
D13S317	0.417
vWA31/A	0.65
Values vary in different populations	

QUESTIONS

Q 28

Systems used: ABO, RH, ACP. CPE = _____

Q 29

Systems used: D7S820, D13S317, WA31/A. CPE = _____

Q 30

Systems used: D2S44, D10S528. CPE = _____

ANSWERS FOR MATH EXAMINATION

Refer to key formulae on the following pages as a guide to the solutions for selected questions.

A1. A. 20 IU/L   B. 5 IU/L   C. 3 2s   D. Negative bias

A2. 17/20 = 85%

A3. 305/330 = 92%

A4. 17/(17 + 25) = 40%

A5. A. Point C   B. 80% (Point F)

A6. A. 55%   B. 38%   C. Point F
    D. 85% sensitivity and 92% specificity   E. Test Y

A7. Absolute reticulocyte count = $0.308 \times 10^{-6}/\mu L$. RPI = 3.44

A8. MCV = 58 fL. MCH = 19.6 pg. MCHC = 34 g/dL

A9. 7685/μL

A10. CCI = 5294. Above 7500 is considered adequate.

A11. PV = 2.85 L. EV = 4.28 L. Reinfuse with 2.78 L albumin and 1.5 L saline

A12. 17.38 L of FFP

A13. She donates 430 mL whole blood (10.5 mL/kg)

A14. 31%

A15. 14.4 bags

A16. 22.36 bags

A17. 1.95%

A18. 32

A19. Calculated osmolality = 304.6; the osmolal gap = 22.6

A20. 9.92 mL/min

A21. 40.3%

A22. RPI = 2.12. This problem requires interpolation of the values for maturation. Use 2.2 days as maturation time

A23. TP = 280

A24. TN = 402

A25. FP = 94

A26. FN = 24

A27. PPV = 75%

A28. 0.545

A29. 0.903

A30. 0.998

A2–4. Disease

	+	−
Test +	A	B
−	C	D

Sensitivity = A/(A + C)

Specificity = D/(B + D)

PPV = A(A + B)

A7. Abs retic count = Retic% × RBC

$$RPI = \frac{Pt\ retic\ \%}{Nl\ retic\ \%} \times \frac{Pt\ Hct}{Nl\ Hct} \times \frac{1}{Mat\ time}$$

Nl retic % = 1%, Nl Hct = 45%

A8. $MCV = \dfrac{Hct\ (\%) \times 10}{RBC\ (millions/\mu L)}$

$MCH = \dfrac{Hb\ (g/dL) \times 10}{RBC\ (millions/\mu L)}$

$MCHC = \dfrac{Hb\ (g/dL)}{Hct\ (decimal)}$

A9. $Corr\ WBC = Uncorr\ WBC \times \dfrac{100}{100 + NRBCs}$

A10. $CCI = \dfrac{(Plt\ count\ post\text{-}trans - Plt\ count\ pre\text{-}trans) \times BSA\ (m^2)}{Platelets\ transfused \times (10^{11})}$

For this question, the patient received a greater number of platelets than in a standard apheresis unit. Multiply 3 (the standard number of platelets) by 6.8/6.0 to determine the denominator.

A11. PV = (1 − Hct) × BV.

A12. PV = (1 − Hct) × BV.   EV = 3 days × 1.7 × PV in this case.

A13. For lightweight donors, maximum amount of blood = Donor weight (Kg) × 10.5 mL/kg.

A14. Expected increment = number of units PRBCs × 3%/unit.

A15. PV = (1 − Hct) × BV. In this case, it is 72% × 5.0 L = 3.6 L = 36 dL.
Necessary increment in fibrinogen = (Post − Pre) = (150 − 50 mg/dL) = 100 mg/dL.
Required fibrinogen = Increment (mg/dL) × PV (dL) = 100 mg/dL × 36 dL = 3600 mg.
Number of bags of cryo = Req fibrinogen/Fibrinogen per bag = 3600 mg/ 250 mg/bag = 14.4 bags.

A16. BV = Weight (kg) × 70 mL/kg. In this case, it is 70 kg × 70 mL/kg = 4900 mL.

PV = (1 − Hct) × BV. Here, it is 73% × 4900 mL = 3577 mL = 35.8 dL.

1 unit factor VIII raises the factor VIII level 1% per dL PV.

Required factor VIII = PV (dL) × 1 unit/dL × % increment. Here, this is 35.8 dL × 1 unit/dL × 50 = 1790 units.

Number of bags of cryo = Required factor VIII (units)/Units per bag.

There are 80 units of factor VIII per bag, so 1790/80 = 22.36 bags.

A17. $FE_{Na} = \dfrac{U_{Na} \times P_{Cr}}{U_{Cr} \times P_{Na}} \times 100$

A18. Anion gap = Na − (Cl + HCO$_3$).

A19. $Osm = 2Na + \dfrac{BUN}{3} + \dfrac{Glu}{20}$

Osmolal gap = Measured osm − Calculated osm.

A20. $GFR = \dfrac{(140 - Age) \times Wt\ (kg)}{Cr \times 72}$

A21. $MCV = \dfrac{Hct\ (\%) \times 10}{RBC\ (million)}$

A22. $RPI = \dfrac{Pt\ retic\ \%}{Nl\ retic\ \%} \times \dfrac{Pt\ Hct}{Nl\ Hct} \times \dfrac{1}{Mat\ time}$

A23–27. Use same 2 × 2 table as for Q 2–4.

A28–30. Formula is provided in the question.

Appendix C

Comprehensive examination

QUESTIONS

This is a 100-question examination. All questions are in a single best answer format. There are no photomicrographs or calculations beyond simple arithmetic. If you would like to time yourself, give yourself 90 minutes to complete the exam.

Put ✗ in the box next to the correct word or phrase.

Q 1

What is the mechanism of action of the preservative and anticoagulant in a green top blood collection tube?

- ○ A. Inhibition of thrombin formation.
- ○ B. Chelation of calcium.
- ○ C. Inhibition of glycolysis.
- ○ D. Clot activation.
- ○ E. RBC preservation.

Q 2

What organization regulates hazardous substances in hospital and laboratories?

- ○ A. CDC.
- ○ B. MSDS.
- ○ C. CLIA.
- ○ D. OSHA.
- ○ E. ADA.

Q 3

Physician-performed microscopy includes all of the following procedures except:

- ○ A. Potassium hydroxide preparations.
- ○ B. Urine sediment examinations.
- ○ C. WBC differential counts.
- ○ D. Pinworm examinations.
- ○ E. Cervical wet mounts.

Q 4

The Beckman Array 360 Protein/Drug System measures the rate of insoluble immunoprecipitation products resulting from specific antibody–antigen interaction, at an angle of 90% from the light source. This is an example of:

- ○ A. Nephelometry.
- ○ B. Refractometry.
- ○ C. Turbidimetry.
- ○ D. Electrophoresis.
- ○ E. Osmometry.

Q 5

Chronic renal failure may be characterized by all of the following laboratory findings except:

- ○ A. Burr cells.
- ○ B. Normochromic, normocytic anemia.
- ○ C. Elevated serum phosphate.
- ○ D. Hypocalcemia.
- ○ E. Increased $1,25(OH)_2$ vitamin D.

Q 6

What laboratory test is useful in discriminating between SIADH and other common causes of hyponatremia?

- ○ A. Serum sodium.
- ○ B. Serum potassium.
- ○ C. 24-Hour urine sodium.
- ○ D. Random urine sodium.
- ○ E. Urine osmolality.

Q 7

In statistics, a Type II error is:

○ A. Stating that two groups are not statistically different when they really are.
○ B. Stating that two groups are statistically different when they really are not.
○ C. Mathematically related to statistical power.
○ D. The likelihood of a positive test when the patient has the disease of interest.
○ E. Both A and C are correct.

Q 8

The Westgard rule indicated by 2_{2s} is translated as:

○ A. The last two control results were within 2% of each other.
○ B. The next two control results must be within 2% of each other, or the instrument must be shut down for analysis.
○ C. The last two patient samples were greater than 2 SD from the reference mean.
○ D. The last two control results were more than 2 SD from the target mean.
○ E. The last two control results were greater than 2% away from the target mean.

Q 9

A patient presents to an emergency department obtunded with the following laboratory values: Na = 140 mmol/L, glu = 60 mg/dL, BUN = 21 mg/dL, Cl = 98 mmol/L, HCO_3 = 22 mmol/L. His plasma osmolality is measured at 385 mOsm/kg. What is the most likely explanation?

○ A. Diabetic ketoacidosis.
○ B. Severe vomiting.
○ C. Ethanol toxicity.
○ D. Addisonian crisis.
○ E. Barbiturate coma.

Q 10

What acid–base disorder is suggested by the following laboratory values: P_{CO_2} = 53 mmHg, HCO_3 = 33 mmol/L, Cl = 97 mmol/L, Na = 141 mmol/L?

○ A. Metabolic acidosis, anion gap.
○ B. Respiratory acidosis.
○ C. Respiratory alkalosis.
○ D. Metabolic acidosis, nonanion gap.
○ E. Metabolic alkalosis.

Q 11

A 40-year-old female presents with acute-onset abdominal pain with vomiting, fever to 100.3°F, and bizarre behavior. She has had similar episodes several times before, most recently when she took oral contraceptives. Skin lesions are not present. Urine aminolevulinic acid and porphobilinogen are markedly elevated, and urine uroporphyrins are mildly elevated. Which statement is true regarding her illness?

- A. It is inherited in an autosomal recessive manner.
- B. Liver functions tests will consistently be within the reference range.
- C. It is prevalent in South African white people.
- D. More than 90 different mutations in the PBG deaminase gene make screening difficult.
- E. The enzyme defect is in uroporphyrinogen decarboxylase.

Q 12

All of the following are true regarding Wilson's disease except:

- A. Serum ceruloplasmin levels correlate with disease severity.
- B. The gene defect is on chromosome 13.
- C. The gene codes for a copper-transporting ATPase.
- D. Many patients are compound heterozygotes rather than true recessives.
- E. Serum copper levels are of little diagnostic value.

Q 13

Which one of the following sets of glycogenoses and clinical or biochemical features is incorrect?

- A. McArdle's – myasthenia after exercise.
- B. Andersen's – amylopectinosis.
- C. Pompe's – glucose-6-phosphatase deficiency.
- D. Von Gierke's – hepatomegaly.
- E. Cori's – amylo-1,6-glucosidase deficiency.

Q 14

All of the following are true regarding familial hypercholesterolemia except:

- A. There is an increased band in the beta fraction on SPEP.
- B. It is type IIa in the Frederickson classification.
- C. Levels of LDL are markedly increased in homozygotes.
- D. Tendon xanthomas are a characteristic feature.
- E. Plasma is cloudy.

Q 15

All of the following are causes of low HDL except:

- ○ A. Dysbetalipoproteinemia.
- ○ B. Anabolic steroid use.
- ○ C. Tangier disease.
- ○ D. ApoA-I deficiency.
- ○ E. Lecithin:cholesterol acyltransferase deficiency.

Q 16

Alpha-1-antitrypsin deficiency is characterized by all of the following except:

- ○ A. Heterozygotes for M will have a normal trypsin inhibitory capacity.
- ○ B. The ZZ phenotype is seen in 1 in 4000 individuals.
- ○ C. Liver disease is not seen in all homozygotes for ZZ.
- ○ D. 10% of white people are heterozygotes for the Z allele.
- ○ E. AAT is able to neutralize elastase.

Q 17

Electrophoresis is characterized by all of the following except:

- ○ A. A low ionic strength will cause the faster protein separation at a given current.
- ○ B. Prealbumin may be seen as a faint band cathodal to albumin.
- ○ C. Endosmotic flow may carry globulins toward the cathode.
- ○ D. Acetic acid can act as a fixative as it precipitates proteins at their positions.
- ○ E. Polyacrylamide gel electrophoresis may be used to increase resolution of bands.

Q 18

Which set of autoimmune liver disease – autoantibodies is incorrect?

- ○ A. Primary sclerosing cholangitis – perinuclear antineutrophil cytoplasmic antibody.
- ○ B. Autoimmune hepatitis type 1 – antinuclear antibody.
- ○ C. Autoimmune hepatitis type 2 – anti-liver–kidney microsomal antigens.
- ○ D. Primary biliary cirrhosis – antimitochondrial antibody type M1.
- ○ E. Isoniazid-induced hepatitis – antimitochondrial antibody type M6.

Q 19

What is the most likely etiology of liver disease in a 23-year-old male with an ALT of 4100 IU/L, AST of 4900 IU/L, a prothrombin time of 19.2 seconds, and a total bilirubin of 1.2 mg/dL?

- ○ A. Acute alcohol intoxication.
- ○ B. Chronic alcohol abuse.
- ○ C. Acute hepatitis C infection.
- ○ D. Acute toxin ingestion, 12 hours ago.
- ○ E. Acute toxin ingestion, 48 hours ago.

Q 20

In a patient with chronic biliary obstruction who undergoes a surgical correction, the chief reason for a slow return to normal of bilirubin is:

- ○ A. Alkaline phosphatase interferes with conjugation of insoluble portion.
- ○ B. Delta bilirubin is elevated and bound to albumin.
- ○ C. Conjugated bilirubin is poorly excreted in urine.
- ○ D. Conjugated bilirubin is poorly excreted in feces.
- ○ E. Unconjugated bilirubin remains high due to ongoing hemolysis.

Q 21

Which of the following is true regarding a competitive inhibitor?

- ○ A. The x-intercept is closer to the origin than the line for no inhibitor on a Lineweaver–Burke plot.
- ○ B. The inhibitor binds to a site apart from the enzyme catalytic site.
- ○ C. The inhibitor decreases V_{max}.
- ○ D. K_M is decreased.
- ○ E. Citrate's inhibition of alkaline phosphatase is an example.

Q 22

All of the following are true regarding myoglobin except:

- ○ A. It is the earliest marker to become abnormal in cardiac injury.
- ○ B. Sensitivity as a marker of cardiac injury is high, 95–100%.
- ○ C. Its half-life in plasma is about 4 hours if renal function is normal.
- ○ D. Plasma levels are related to muscle mass in healthy individuals.
- ○ E. It is a highly specific marker of cardiac injury.

Q 23

All of the following drugs increase thyroid-binding globulin except:

- ○ A. Glucocorticoids.
- ○ B. Methadone.
- ○ C. Estrogen.
- ○ D. Clofibrate.
- ○ E. 5-Fluorouracil.

Q 24

All of the following are true regarding hyperaldosteronism except:

○ A. Patients with primary hyperaldosteronism are hypertensive.
○ B. Patients with secondary hyperaldosteronism are typically not hypertensive.
○ C. Renin is decreased in secondary causes of hyperaldosteronism.
○ D. Patients with primary hyperaldosteronism are hypokalemic.
○ E. Cirrhosis, nephrosis and congestive heart failure are common causes of secondary hyperaldosteronism.

Q 25

All of the following drugs have a similar four fused ring structure except:

○ A. Codeine.
○ B. Heroin.
○ C. Methadone.
○ D. Naloxone.
○ E. Morphine.

Q 26

Which of the following accurately describes the alcohols?

○ A. Isopropyl alcohol intoxication is associated with blindness.
○ B. Methanol is metabolized to acetone.
○ C. Methanol is a cause of increased anion and osmolal gaps.
○ D. The production of NAD is measured at 340 nm in ethanol assays.
○ E. Peak plasma levels of ethanol occur 3–4 hours after ingestion.

Q 27

All of the following are associated with an increased risk of Down syndrome except:

○ A. Decreased inhibin A.
○ B. Increased HCG.
○ C. Decreased MSAFP.
○ D. Decreased unconjugated estriol.
○ E. Advanced maternal age.

Q 28

All of the following proteins are commonly seen in urine in glomerular disease except:

○ A. Albumin.
○ B. Transferrin.
○ C. Alpha-1-glycoprotein.
○ D. Beta-lipoprotein.
○ E. Alpha-1-antitrypsin.

Q 29

Which of the following accurately describes the sodium nitroferrocyanide reagent strip method of testing for urine ketones?

- ○ A. It correlates well with total blood ketones.
- ○ B. Phenylketones may produce false-negatives.
- ○ C. All manufacturers' strips measure 3-hydroxybutyrate.
- ○ D. None of the manufacturers' strips measure acetone.
- ○ E. Most manufacturers' strips measure acetoacetic acid.

Q 30

What is the most common cause of WBC casts in urine sediment?

- ○ A. Glomerulonephritis.
- ○ B. Chronic renal failure.
- ○ C. Pyelonephritis.
- ○ D. Lupus nephritis.
- ○ E. Acute tubular necrosis.

Q 31

What is the predominant cell type in the CSF of neonates?

- ○ A. Neutrophil.
- ○ B. Lymphocyte.
- ○ C. Monocyte.
- ○ D. Eosinophil.
- ○ E. Ependymal cell.

Q 32

All of the following are causes of xanthochromia except:

- ○ A. Subarachnoid hemorrhage.
- ○ B. Viral meningitis.
- ○ C. Bilirubinemia.
- ○ D. Polyneuritis.
- ○ E. Rifampin therapy.

Q 33

All of the following are associated with group II (inflammatory) effusions of joint spaces except:

- ○ A. Rheumatoid arthritis.
- ○ B. Osteoarthritis.
- ○ C. Systemic lupus erythematosus.
- ○ D. Reiter's syndrome.
- ○ E. Psoriatic arthritis.

Q 34

Which of the following is true regarding celiac disease?

- A. It is associated with type 1 DM, IgA deficiency, and Down syndrome.
- B. The gold standard for diagnosis is positive antigliadin antibodies.
- C. Antiendomysial antibodies lack sufficient sensitivity for routine testing.
- D. It is most common in Caucasians of Mediterranean descent.
- E. It carries an increased risk for GI carcinoid tumors.

Q 35

What is the characteristic red cell morphology seen in extravascular hemolysis?

- A. Schistocytes.
- B. Macro-ovalocytes.
- C. Hypochromic.
- D. Spherocytes.
- E. Burr cells.

Q 36

The translocation t(11;14) involving the Bcl-1 protein is best described as:

- A. Stimulating entry into the cell cycle and occurring in marginal zone lymphoma.
- B. Stimulating entry into the cell cycle and occurring in small lymphocytic lymphoma.
- C. Binding DNA and occurring in Burkitt lymphoma.
- D. Overexpressing cyclin D1 and occurring in mantle cell lymphoma.
- E. Inhibiting apoptosis and occurring in follicular lymphoma.

Q 37

Increased levels of RBC protoporphyrin may be seen in:

- A. Lead poisoning.
- B. Iron deficiency.
- C. Thalassemia minor.
- D. Both A and B.
- E. A, B, and C.

Q 38

An infant is found to have a severe megaloblastic anemia with an MCV of 125 fL and an Hct of 23%. Serum cobalamin is within the reference range, as are serum and red cell folate. What is the likely explanation?

- A. Deficiency of intrinsic factor.
- B. Malabsorption syndrome, such as cystic fibrosis.
- C. Deficiency of transcobalamin II.
- D. Deficiency of a haptocorrin.
- E. Inadequate intake of animal products.

Q 39

What embryonic hemoglobin chain is the analog of the alpha chain?

- A. Zeta.
- B. Epsilon.
- C. Gamma.
- D. Delta.
- E. Beta.

Q 40

What is the translocation seen in follicular lymphoma?

- A. t(11;14)
- B. t(14;18)
- C. t(9;22)
- D. t(8;14)
- E. t(11;22).

Q 41

Which of the following laboratory findings is least consistent with iron deficiency anemia?

- A. Elevated TIBC.
- B. Low free erythrocyte protoporphyrin.
- C. Elevated red cell distribution width.
- D. Low transferrin saturation.
- E. Low mean corpuscular volume.

Q 42

Fanconi's anemia shares a common pathophysiology with all of the following disorders except:

- A. Diamond–Blackfan anemia.
- B. Bloom syndrome.
- C. Ataxia-telangiectasia.
- D. Xeroderma pigmentosum.
- E. Cockayne syndrome.

Q 43

All of the following laboratory findings are seen in isolated vitamin B_{12} deficiency except:

- A. Low serum cobalamin.
- B. Increased methylmalonic acid in urine.
- C. Increased serum homocysteine.
- D. Normal serum folate.
- E. Normal red cell folate.

Q 44

Which of the following cell surface markers is not typically seen in hairy cell leukemia?

- A. HLA-DR.
- B. CD11c.
- C. CD22.
- D. CD23.
- E. CD25.

Q 45

A patient with a bleeding disorder and grayish platelets on a peripheral blood smear would have decreased levels of which platelet biomolecule?

- A. Serotonin.
- B. P-selectin.
- C. ADP.
- D. ATP.
- E. Both C and D are correct.

Q 46

All of the following statements are true regarding Glanzmann's thrombasthenia except:

- A. Platelets may suggest May–Hegglin anomaly on peripheral smear.
- B. Glycoprotein IIb and/or IIIa are defective.
- C. Inheritance is autosomal recessive.
- D. Platelet count is usually within the reference range.
- E. Platelet aggregation study with epinephrine is abnormal.

Q 47

All of the following statements regarding low-molecular-weight heparin (LMWH) are true except:

- A. The incidence of heparin-induced thrombocytopenia is reduced compared to traditional heparin.
- B. Clearance is impaired in patients with renal failure.
- C. The half-life is about 4 hours.
- D. It binds to platelet factor 4 to a lesser degree than heparin does.
- E. It is a direct inhibitor of factor IIa.

Q 48

Which statement accurately describes the ristocetin cofactor assay?

○ A. It measures ristocetin-mediated binding of reagent vWF to patient platelets.
○ B. It measures ristocetin-mediated binding of patient vWF to reagent platelets.
○ C. It is reported as positive or negative.
○ D. It is paradoxically normal in type 3 vWD.
○ E. It is synonymous with the ristocetin-induced platelet aggregation test.

Q 49

All of the following statements are true regarding emergency issue of red cells except:

○ A. Type-specific blood is given if time permits.
○ B. Group O-negative blood is given if time does not allow for type and crossmatch.
○ C. Physician signs release for accepting uncrossmatched blood.
○ D. Crossmatch is performed after release of uncrossmatched blood.
○ E. Antibody screen is not performed after release of uncrossmatched blood.

Q 50

A leukocyte-reduced unit of RBCs contains less than _____ WBCs.

○ A. 5.5×10^{-10}.
○ B. 5×10^{-6}.
○ C. 3×10^{-11}.
○ D. 1.0×10^{-10}.
○ E. 3×10^{-9}.

Q 51

All of the following are true regarding pheresis platelets except:

○ A. Contain at least 3×10^{-11} platelets (based on QC counts).
○ B. Have a shelf life of 5 days.
○ C. Volume is approximately 150 mL.
○ D. Stored at 20–24°C.
○ E. Minimize HLA exposure for chronic transfusion patients.

Q 52

All of the following fetal red cell antigens may stimulate HDN except:

○ A. ABO.
○ B. Duffy.
○ C. P.
○ D. Kell.
○ E. Kidd.

Q 53

RhIg (Rh immunoglobulin) therapy is indicated in all of the following conditions except:

- ○ A. Within 72 hours of delivery of an Rh-positive infant to an Rh-negative mother.
- ○ B. At 36 weeks' gestation to an Rh-negative mother with an Rh titer of $1:128$.
- ○ C. At 28 weeks' gestation to an Rh-negative woman.
- ○ D. After spontaneous abortion in an Rh-negative woman.
- ○ E. After percutaneous umbilical cord sampling in an Rh-negative woman.

Q 54

What are the goals of a red cell exchange transfusion in sickle cell anemia?

- ○ A. Hct = 30%, Hb S <30%.
- ○ B. Hct = 30%, Hb S <10%.
- ○ C. Hct = 30%, Hb S <5%.
- ○ D. Hct = 40%, Hb S <30%.
- ○ E. Hct = 40%, Hb S <15%.

Q 55

Which statement accurately describes the mechanisms of hypersensitivity?

- ○ A. Delayed-type involves the formation of immune complexes.
- ○ B. NK cell type II is antibody independent.
- ○ C. Immediate hypersensitivity involves IgE binding to basophils.
- ○ D. Type III typically involves activation of complement.
- ○ E. Type I is the basis for the purified protein derivative skin test.

Q 56

All of the following are true regarding radioimmunoassay except:

- ○ A. In competitive assays, the amount of bound radioactive label varies inversely with the amount of patient analyte.
- ○ B. The Scatchard plot evaluates antibody performance with a plot of bound/free antibody vs. analyte concentration.
- ○ C. The second antibody technique provides more precise data.
- ○ D. The short shelf life of ^{125}I is a disadvantage.
- ○ E. It has been replaced largely because of poor sensitivity.

Q 57

All of the following are true regarding homogeneous immunoassays except:

- ○ A. They eliminate the washing steps.
- ○ B. They are more sensitive than heterogeneous or radioimmunoassay methods.
- ○ C. The enzyme-multiplied immunoassay (EMIT) conjugates inactive haptens to reagent enzymes to mimic the analyte of interest.
- ○ D. They may be competitive or noncompetitive.
- ○ E. They are readily adapted to automated systems.

Q 58

All of the following cytokines are part of the type I T-cell response except:

- ○ A. IL-10.
- ○ B. IL-2.
- ○ C. IFN-γ.
- ○ D. IL-12.
- ○ E. All of the above are part of the type I response.

Q 59

Which of the following accurately characterizes IgE?

- ○ A. It fixes complement by the classical pathway.
- ○ B. Synthesis is promoted by IL-4 secreted by Th-2 cells.
- ○ C. Crosslinking of IgE molecules on the surface of mast cells stimulates bradykinin release.
- ○ D. It crosses the placenta.
- ○ E. Synthesis in the human fetus begins in the third trimester.

Q 60

Which of the following sets of disease states and hyperimmunoglobulinemias is incorrect?

- ○ A. AIDS – polyclonal, all classes.
- ○ B. Congenital syphilis – polyclonal IgG.
- ○ C. Waldenström's – monoclonal IgM.
- ○ D. Visceral larva migrans – polyclonal IgE.
- ○ E. AA amyloidosis – polyclonal, all classes.

Q 61

All of the following complement or complement receptor protein deficiencies are associated with recurrent pyogenic infections except:

- ○ A. Factor H.
- ○ B. Factor D.
- ○ C. C3.
- ○ D. C4.
- ○ E. CR3.

Q 62

A deficiency of early classical pathway complement components such as C1, C4, or C2 is associated with:

- ○ A. Systemic lupus erythematosus.
- ○ B. Recurrent pyogenic infections.
- ○ C. Disseminated neisserial infections.
- ○ D. Hereditary angioedema.
- ○ E. Paroxysmal nocturnal hemoglobinuria.

Q 63

A T cell deficiency is suggested by all of the following except:

- ○ A. Giant cell pneumonia after a rubeola vaccine.
- ○ B. Neonatal tetany due to deficient calcium homeostasis.
- ○ C. Recurrent infection with *Haemophilus* or *Streptococcus* species.
- ○ D. Graft-versus-host disease after a blood product infusion.
- ○ E. Overwhelming pneumonia after varicella infection.

Q 64

All of the following may be seen in chronic mucocutaneous candidiasis except:

- ○ A. Elevated levels of IgM.
- ○ B. Granulomatous skin lesions.
- ○ C. Hypoadrenalism.
- ○ D. Hypoparathyroidism.
- ○ E. Other endocrinopathies.

Q 65

A nucleolar pattern of autoantibodies in immunofluorescence suggests what disease?

- ○ A. Systemic lupus erythematosus.
- ○ B. Rheumatoid arthritis.
- ○ C. Scleroderma.
- ○ D. Sjögren's syndrome.
- ○ E. Polymyositis.

Q 66

Which statement is true regarding autoantibodies in systemic lupus erythematosus?

- ○ A. Most patients have a single autoantibody.
- ○ B. Anti-Sm is seen in the majority of patients.
- ○ C. Antiphospholipid antibodies are seen in 10–15% of patients.
- ○ D. Anti-native DNA and anti-Sm are specific for lupus.
- ○ E. Patients with drug-induced lupus usually have SS-A or SS-B antibodies.

Q 67

All of the following are true regarding Takayasu's arteritis except:

- ○ A. Most cases occur in young women.
- ○ B. It is a granulomatous vasculitis.
- ○ C. The aortic arch and pulmonary arteries are the main sites of inflammation.
- ○ D. Rheumatoid factor and antinuclear antibodies are usually positive.
- ○ E. ESR is elevated in most patients with active disease.

Q 68

What is the predominant direct immunofluorescence pattern in bullous pemphigoid?

- ○ A. Linear IgA in basement membrane zone.
- ○ B. Linear C3 and IgG, or C3 alone in basement membrane zone.
- ○ C. Granular IgM In basement membrane zone.
- ○ D. Coarse granular IgG and C3 in basement membrane zone.
- ○ E. Linear intercellular IgG and C3 without basement membrane staining.

Q 69

IgA is the predominant immunoglobulin in which glomerular disease?

- ○ A. Acute poststreptococcal glomerulonephritis.
- ○ B. Membranoproliferative glomerulonephritis type I.
- ○ C. Membranous lupus nephritis.
- ○ D. Dense deposit disease.
- ○ E. Henoch–Schönlein purpura.

Q 70

Despite its low sensitivity, this marker is used to manage patients with gastric carcinoma.

- ○ A. c-erb-2.
- ○ B. CA 15-3.
- ○ C. CA 125.
- ○ D. CEA.
- ○ E. CA 72-4.

Q 71

Some protection against certain strains of malaria is provided by all of the following except:

- ○ A. Primaquine prophylaxis.
- ○ B. G6PD deficiency.
- ○ C. Lewis a–b– RBCs.
- ○ D. Sickle cell trait.
- ○ E. Duffy a–b– RBCs.

Q 72

All of the following regarding parvovirus B19 are true except:

- ○ A. Culturing on BAP is diagnostic but takes over 1 week in most cases.
- ○ B. Infects erythroid precursors in marrow.
- ○ C. Is one cause of hydrops fetalis.
- ○ D. Is the agent of erythema infectiosum.
- ○ E. Ground glass nuclear inclusions are characteristic.

Q 73

All of the following are true regarding the agent of scarlet fever except:

○ A. Is PYR hydrolysis negative.
○ B. Is sensitive to bacitracin.
○ C. Is beta-hemolytic.
○ D. Belongs to a Lancefield group.
○ E. Is catalase negative.

Q 74

Which of the following accurately describes the genus *Pseudomonas*?

○ A. Oxidase-negative aerobes causing infections in burn victims.
○ B. Nonmotile Gram-negative bacilli causing pneumonia.
○ C. Motile, strictly aerobic, oxidase-positive rods causing pneumonia in CF patients.
○ D. Nonmotile, oxidase-negative bacilli producing a slime polysaccharide.
○ E. Gram-negative rods with growth and tumbling motility at 4°C.

Q 75

What is the etiologic agent of undulant fever?

○ A. *Francisella tularensis*.
○ B. *Bordatella pertussis*.
○ C. *Borrelia recurrentis*.
○ D. *Brucella abortus*.
○ E. *Streptobacillus moniliformis*.

Q 76

Which statement accurately describes the VDRL test?

○ A. It is a specific test for treponemal antigens.
○ B. It may be falsely positive in connective tissue diseases.
○ C. It is a specific test for treponemal antibodies.
○ D. It is persistently positive after treatment of early cases.
○ E. It has the greatest sensitivity when performed in the primary stage of syphilis.

Q 77

Which statement accurately describes *Mycobacterium tuberculosis*?

○ A. It is a rapid grower, with colonies evident in less than 1 week.
○ B. It is a photochromagen.
○ C. It is niacin negative.
○ D. It has the same biochemical properties as *M. avium-intracellulare*.
○ E. It may be provisionally distinguished from *M. kansasii* by pigmentation.

Q 78

All of the following support a diagnosis of *Cryptococcus neoformans* except:

- ○ A. A positive phenol oxidase test.
- ○ B. Growth in cyclohexamide.
- ○ C. A positive latex agglutination test for capsular polysaccharide antigen.
- ○ D. A positive India ink preparation.
- ○ E. Demonstration of melanin pigment with Fontana–Masson stain.

Q 79

All of the following support a diagnosis of *Candida albicans* except:

- ○ A. A positive germ tube test in 3 hours.
- ○ B. Characteristic chlamydospores from culture, stained with lactophenol.
- ○ C. Presence of pseudohyphae.
- ○ D. Root-like structures at the base of hyphae.
- ○ E. Growth in cyclohexamide.

Q 80

Which person is least likely to develop disseminated coccidioidomycosis?

- ○ A. Black male.
- ○ B. HIV-positive female.
- ○ C. Ashkenazi Jewish male.
- ○ D. Filipino female.
- ○ E. Native American female.

Q 81

Which statement regarding *Apergillus* spp. is true?

- ○ A. They are hyphomycetes.
- ○ B. Disseminated disease is usually due to *A. fumigatus* and *A. flavus*.
- ○ C. Colonies of *A. fumigatus* are blue-green in color.
- ○ D. The black fruiting heads of *A. niger* give colonies a salt and pepper look.
- ○ E. All of the above are true.

Q 82

All of the following are true regarding *Plasmodium vivax* except:

- ○ A. It preferentially infects senescent RBCs.
- ○ B. All stages of the life cycle may be seen in a single film.
- ○ C. True relapse may occur if treatment is incomplete.
- ○ D. Shuffner's dots are characteristic.
- ○ E. Periodicity is tertian.

Q 83

Which hemoflagellate does not cause clinical illness?

- ○ A. *Trypanosoma brucei*.
- ○ B. *Trypanosoma cruzi*.
- ○ C. *Trypanosoma rangeli*.
- ○ D. *Leishmania donovani*.
- ○ E. *Leishmania infantum*.

Q 84

Which statement accurately describes *Toxoplasma gondii*?

- ○ A. Mature oocysts are passed by felines.
- ○ B. Serology is the primary approach to diagnosis.
- ○ C. Humans are the only described accidental host.
- ○ D. Primary infection in the third trimester accounts for most congenital cases.
- ○ E. Felines act as an intermediate host.

Q 85

What is the most reliable method of diagnosing *Entamoeba histolytica* in a patient with a liver abscess on CT scan and a history, now resolved, of diarrhea?

- ○ A. Formed stool demonstrating trophozoites.
- ○ B. Serologic titer for *E. histolytica*.
- ○ C. Diarrhea demonstrating cysts.
- ○ D. String test.
- ○ E. Stool culture.

Q 86

Which of the following intestinal flagellates is a considered a pathogen?

- ○ A. *Trichomonas hominis*.
- ○ B. *Chilomastix mesnili*.
- ○ C. *Enteromonas hominis*.
- ○ D. *Dientamoeba fragilis*.
- ○ E. *Retortamonas intestinalis*.

Q 87

All of the following regarding *Cryptosporidium parvum* are true except:

- ○ A. Incubation period is 3–5 days.
- ○ B. Acid-fast staining helps demonstrate organisms.
- ○ C. Oocysts are refractory to usual water chlorination procedures.
- ○ D. Outbreaks may occur in day-care centers.
- ○ E. Oocysts measure 4–6 µm in diameter.

Q 88

All of the following regarding *Strongyloides stercoralis* are true except:

- A. A free-living variant life cycle may occur in areas with high humidity.
- B. Autoinfection occurs chiefly in immunocompromised hosts.
- C. Short buccal cavity is a key morphologic feature.
- D. Adults mature and live in the cecum and colon.
- E. Reproduction is parthenogenetic.

Q 89

All of the following are morphologic features of *Diphyllobothrium latum* except:

- A. Adults may reach a length of 10 meters.
- B. Eggs are oval and operculate.
- C. Eggs may be confused with those of *Taenia* spp.
- D. Gravid proglottids are wider than they are long.
- E. Bothria in the scolex replace usual suckers.

Q 90

Which statement accurately characterizes *Wuchereria bancrofti* and *Brugia malayi*?

- A. *W. bancrofti* usually causes more severe disease than *B. malayi*.
- B. *W. bancrofti* exhibits diurnal periodicity, while *B. malayi* is nocturnal.
- C. *B. malayi* is seen chiefly in the islands of Timor and Flores.
- D. *B. malayi* may be distinguished morphologically by its lack of sheath.
- E. *W. bancrofti* may be distinguished by the presence of nuclei in its tail.

Q 91

Which of the following conditions would ensure only the most perfectly matched duplexes in a nucleic acid hybridization?

- A. High temperature, high salt, high formamide.
- B. High temperature, high salt, no formamide.
- C. High temperature, low salt, high formamide.
- D. Low temperature, high salt, no formamide.
- E. Low temperature, low salt, no formamide.

Q 92

All of the following are elements of strand-displacement amplification except:

- A. Thermal cycling method used.
- B. Used to detect *M. tuberculosis*.
- C. Used to detect *C. trachomatis*.
- D. Used to detect *N. gonorrhoeae*.
- E. High sensitivity when thermostable polymerases used.

Q 93

What is the most common mutation in cystic fibrosis?

○ A. F508, chromosome 3.
○ B. F508, chromosome 13.
○ C. F508, chromosome 7.
○ D. C282Y, chromosome 7.
○ E. C282Y, chromosome 6.

Q 94

In uniparental heterodisomy, a child inherits:

○ A. One chromosome from each parent.
○ B. Two copies of the chromosome from one parent and a single copy from the other parent.
○ C. Two copies of the same chromosome from one parent.
○ D. Two heterozygous chromosomes from the same parent.
○ E. Three copies of the chromosome from the same parent.

Q 95

T cell chronic lymphocytic leukemia may involve an abnormality of chromosome:

○ A. 5.
○ B. 8.
○ C. 9.
○ D. 12.
○ E. 14.

Q 96

All of the following are true regarding Kallman syndrome except:

○ A. Patients have hypogonadism.
○ B. The gene *KAL1* is localized to chromosome 22p.
○ C. It represents a microdeletion syndrome.
○ D. Inability to smell is a feature.
○ E. The gene is close to the STS gene for ichthyosis.

Q 97

All of the following are true regarding Gorlin syndrome except:

○ A. It is a familial cancer syndrome.
○ B. Inheritance is autosomal recessive.
○ C. The gene is located at 9q22.
○ D. Affected persons have increased incidence of basal cell carcinomas.
○ E. Affected persons have increased incidence of medulloblastoma.

Q 98

Which of the following is true regarding Cowden syndrome?

- ○ A. It is associated with an increased incidence of both breast and thyroid cancer.
- ○ B. The gene is located at 17q21.
- ○ C. Inheritance is autosomal recessive.
- ○ D. The gene product is the p53 protein.
- ○ E. It is primarily a DNA repair defect.

Q 99

Compound heterozygotes for these two mutations may be affected with hemochromatosis.

- ○ A. C282P and F508.
- ○ B. F508 and H63D.
- ○ C. C282Y and H65D.
- ○ D. C282Y and H63D.
- ○ E. C63D and H282Y.

Q 100

What is the standard method today to determine parentage?

- ○ A. Red blood cell antigens.
- ○ B. Restriction length fragment polymorphisms.
- ○ C. Human leukocyte antigens.
- ○ D. Polymerase chain reaction-based assay of DNA segments.
- ○ E. Red blood cell enzymes systems.

ANSWERS FOR COMPREHENSIVE EXAMINATION

A1. A

A2. D

A3. C

A4. A

A5. E

A6. E

A7. E

A8. D

A9. C

A10. B

A11. D

A12. A

A13. C

A14. E

A15. A

A16. A

A17. B

A18. D

A19. D

A20. B

A21. A

A22. E

A23. A

A24. C

A25. C

A26. C

A27. A

A28. D

A29. E

A30. C

A31. C

A32. B

A33. B

A34. A

A35. D

A36. D

A37. D

A38. C

A39. A

A40. B

A41. B

A42. A

A43. E

A44. D

A45. B

A46. A

A47. E

A48. B

A49. E

A50. B

A51. C

A52. C

A53. B

A54. A

A55. C

A56. E

A57. B

A58. A

A59. B

A60. B

A61. D

A62. A

A63. C

A64. A

A65. C

A66. D

A67. D

A68. B

A69. E

A70. E

A71. C

A72. A

A73. A

A74. C

A75. D

A76. B

A77. E

A78. B

A79. D

A80. C

A81. E

A82. A

A83. C

A84. B

A85. B

A86. D

A87. A

A88. D

A89. C

A90. A

A91. C

A92. A

A93. C

A94. D

A95. E

A96. B

A97. B

A98. A

A99. D

A100. D

ANSWERS